SOCIAL DETERMINANTS, HEALTH DISPARITIES AND LINKAGES TO HEALTH AND HEALTH CARE

RESEARCH IN THE SOCIOLOGY OF HEALTH CARE

Series Editor: Jennie Jacobs Kronenfeld

RESEARCH IN THE SOCIOLOGY OF HEALTH CARE
VOLUME 31

SOCIAL DETERMINANTS, HEALTH DISPARITIES AND LINKAGES TO HEALTH AND HEALTH CARE

EDITED BY

JENNIE JACOBS KRONENFELD

Department of Sociology, Arizona State University, USA

United Kingdom – North America – Japan
India – Malaysia – China

Emerald Group Publishing Limited
Howard House, Wagon Lane, Bingley BD16 1WA, UK

First edition 2013

British Library Cataloguing in Publication Data
A catalogue record for this book is available from the British Library

ISBN: 978-1-78190-587-6
ISSN: 0275-4959 (Series)

ISOQAR certified
Management System,
awarded to Emerald
for adherence to
Environmental
standard
ISO 14001:2004.

ISOQAR
REGISTERED
Certificate Number 1985
ISO 14001

INVESTOR IN PEOPLE

CONTENTS

PART 4: CHRONIC CARE AND SERIOUS HEALTH PROBLEMS

PART 5: COMPARATIVE AND POLITICAL ISSUES

LIST OF CONTRIBUTORS

Martha I. Arrieta	Center for Healthy Communities, University of South Alabama, Mobile, AL, USA
Stephanie Ayers	Southwest Interdisciplinary Research Center, Arizona State University, Phoenix, AZ, USA
Elyas Bakhtiari	Department of Sociology, Boston University, Boston, MA, USA
Jason Beckfield	Department of Sociology, Harvard University, Cambridge, MA, USA
Neale R. Chumbler	Department of Health Policy and Management, College of Public Health, University of Georgia, Athens, GA, USA
Kathryn Connors	Department of Obstetrics and Gynecology, Maricopa Integrated Health System/District Medical Group, Phoenix, AZ, USA
Dean V. Coonrod	Department of Obstetrics and Gynecology, Maricopa Integrated Health System/District Medical Group, Phoenix, AZ, USA; University of Arizona College of Medicine-Phoenix, Phoenix, AZ, USA
Cindy Dinh	John F. Kennedy School of Government, Harvard University, Cambridge, MA, USA
Christopher R. Freed	Department of Sociology, Anthropology and Social Work, University of South Alabama, Mobile, AL, USA
Bridget K. Gorman	Department of Sociology, Rice University, Houston, TX, USA

James W. Grimm	Department of Sociology, Western Kentucky University, Bowling Green, KY, USA
Patricia Habak	Department of Obstetrics and Gynecology, University of Arizona, Phoenix, AZ, USA
Shantisha T. Hansberry	Center for Healthy Communities, University of South Alabama, Mobile, AL, USA
Anne M. Hewitt	Seton Hall University, South Orange, NJ, USA
Hanna Jokinen-Gordon	Florida State University, Tallahassee, FL, USA
Jennie Jacobs Kronenfeld	Sanford School of Social and Family Dynamics, Arizona State University, Tempe AZ, USA
Nancy G. Kutner	School of Medicine, Emory University, Atlanta GA, USA
Tamara Leech	Indiana University School of Liberal Arts, Indiana University-Purdue University Indianapolis, Indianapolis, IN, USA
A. E. Luloff	Department of Agricultural Economics, Sociology, and Education, The Pennsylvania State University, University Park, PA, USA
Flavio Marsiglia	School of Social Work, Arizona State University Phoenix, AZ, USA
Sigrun Olafsdottir	Department of Sociology, Boston University, Boston, MA, USA
Harry Perlstadt	Department of Sociology, Michigan State University, East Lansing, MI, USA
Jill Quadagno	Florida State University, Tallahassee, FL, USA

Teresa L. Scheid	Department of Sociology, University of North Carolina at Charlotte, Charlotte, NC, USA
D. Clayton Smith	Department of Sociology, Western Kentucky University, Bowling Green, KY, USA
Galen H. Smith, III	Department of Political Science and Public Administration, University of North Carolina at Charlotte, Charlotte, NC, USA
Mark Tausig	Department of Sociology, The University of Akron, Akron, OH, USA
Gene L. Theodori	Department of Sociology, Sam Houston State University, Huntsville, TX, USA
Ann Marie Wood	Department of Sociology, University of Missouri at Kansas City, Kansas City, MO, USA
Rebecca Zhang	Rollins School of Public Health, Emory University, Atlanta GA, USA

PART 1
INTRODUCTION TO VOLUME

SOCIAL DETERMINANTS AND HEALTH DISPARITIES

Jennie Jacobs Kronenfeld

ABSTRACT

Purpose – *This chapter provides both an introduction to the volume and a review of literature on health disparities and social determinants.*

Methodology/approach – *Literature Review.*

Findings – *The chapter argues for the importance of greater considera-tion of social determinants of health disparities. This includes a consideration of race/ethnicity and socioeconomic status factors, geographic and place factors, and disparities especially linked to particular diseases.*

Originality/value of paper – *Reviews the topic of health disparities and social determinants and previews this book.*

Keywords: Health disparities; health care disparities; social determinants; race/ethnicity; socioeconomic status; geography

This chapter is an introduction to Volume 31 in the Research in the Sociology of Health Care series. The beginning of this chapter reviews some of the more important material about health disparities, and some of

Social Determinants, Health Disparities and Linkages to Health and Health Care
Research in the Sociology of Health Care, Volume 31, 3–19
ISSN: 0275-4959/doi:10.1108/S0275-4959(2013)0000031003

the social factors that link to health disparities. The last part of this chapter reviews the overall contents of the volume and the structure of the volume.

HEALTH DISPARITIES

Fields have different areas of research that both grow and decline in popularity and scholarly interest over the years. In medical sociology for the past decade, one of the more robust areas of research has been an interest in health disparities and this interest is not limited only to medical sociology, but is also an area of high interest in epidemiology, public health, and health services research. Beyond researchers, it has also become an area of high interest to providers of care and policymakers, especially within the United States. What do we mean by disparities or differences in health and health care? There are a number of different answers to this question both from within medical sociology and from related fields. The Institute of Medicine (IOM) defines health care disparities as differences in treatment or access between population groups that cannot be justified by different preferences for services or differences in health (McGuire, Alegria, Cook, Wells, & Zaslavsky, 2006). Within the United States, much of the focus on health care disparities has turned to differences in access and quality across racial and ethnic groups, although these are not the only social characteristics that are of interest either sociologically or from a policy perspective. Very importantly, differences based on socioeconomic status (SES) and some of its components such as education and income are of research and policy interest as are factors such as geographic location, gender, sexuality, and even types of health problems. Beyond research and thinking about policy implications, health care disparities matter even more if they result in health disparities, defined as differences in health outcomes across population groups (Schnittker & McLeod, 2005).

Within sociology, some of the focus on health disparities has looked particularly at issues of race/ethnicity and SES. In an address given at the 2008 annual meeting of the American Sociological Association and later published in *Journal of Health and Social Behavior*, Aneshensel (2009) argued that mental health disparities refer to the disproportionate amount of psychopathology among persons of low social status. Following this definition, we can think of disparities in health status as the dispropor-tionate amount of pathology among people, disparities that are often linked to SES, to race/ethnicity, to gender, or to other social factors. In that same address, Aneshensel argued that health disparities have complex causes and are due to both biological differences and social inequalities, as Adler and Rehkopf (2008) have also pointed out. Sociologists and other social scientists particularly tend to focus more on social inequalities because they may be avoidable and are unjust. In this volume, it is the social inequalities and social determinants that are the focus. While the Aneshensel article entitled "Toward Explaining Mental Health Disparities" focuses on mental rather than physical health, this volume will consider all aspects of health. This chapter is in agreement with one of her conclusions in her article that research that examines differences and disparities in health is somewhat different from research that might focus on improving the mental health (or in this case also physical health) of the population overall. Disparities research has a goal ultimately of helping to connect to interventions that might alleviate health disparities. This is something that is less likely to occur directly from the kinds of research discussed in papers in this volume, but papers focusing on how social inequities become health disparities can eventually also connect to more policy-oriented research.

The large interest in research about social differences in health and health disparities was summarized well by the Adler and Rehkopf (2008) review of US disparities in health by examining literature for the term "health disparities" and finding that while this was a key word in only one article in 1980, and fewer than 30 in the 1990s, it went up to over 400 articles from 2000 to 2004. If the term "health inequalities" was used instead, the pattern of increase was similar.

The interest in this topic is broader than just in the United States and the importance of this in British studies is especially strong. In 1980, the Black Report in Great Britain was one of the first in that country to apply the term inequality to an examination of health differences. Some studies from the late 1970s and early 1980s in Great Britain found significant differences in cardiovascular disease and mortality by occupational level within a population of office-based workers (Marmot, Rose, Shipley, & Hamilton, 1978; Marmot, Shipley, & Rose, 1984), another indication of interest in that country in health differences. In the United States in this same time period, studies did link together death and health information with information on SES from sources such as the Current Population Study, the US Census, and Social Security Administration records (Kitagawa & Hauser, 1978; Kliss & Scheuren, 1978). These studies reported higher age-adjusted mortality rates for nonwhites, for individuals with less education and lower income, and for certain occupational categories.

Within the United States, some of these earlier studies and traditions in various fields including sociology of research into variation in health, health

care utilization, and health services issues by SES and race/ethnicity led to
the now well-known efforts in the United States to examine and try to
eliminate health disparities due to race/ethnicity and SES in the *Healthy
People* series. From the federal government level, one of the pushes for more
research on health care inequalities came from the passage of Public Law
106-129, the Healthcare Research and Quality Act of 1999. That law directed
the Agency for Healthcare Research and Quality (AHRQ) to develop two
annual reports, one focused on quality and one focused on disparities.
AHRQ's responsibility was to track prevailing disparities in health care
delivery as they relate to racial and socioeconomic factors among priority
populations such as low-income groups, racial and ethnic minorities, women,
children, the elderly, individuals with special health care needs, the disabled,
people in need of long-term care, people requiring end-of-life care, and places
of residence (rural communities). The first National Healthcare Disparities
Report (2004) was built on previous efforts by the federal government,
especially Healthy People 2010 (U.S. Department of Health and Human
Services, 2000) and the IOM Report, Unequal Treatment: Confronting
Racial and Economic Disparities in Healthcare (Smedley, Stith, & Nelson,
2003). Elimination of disparities in health was a goal of Healthy People,
2010. Unequal Treatment extensively documented health care disparities in
the United States and focused on those related to race and ethnicity, but not
on SES, a weakness of the report. The IOM report on Unequal Treatment
also looked at factors related to providers of care and argued that providers'
perceptions and, from that, their attitudes toward patients can be influenced
by patient race or ethnicity (Smedley et al., 2003).

The National Healthcare Disparities Report (2004) did focus on the
ability of Americans to access health care and variation in quality of care.
Disparities related to SES were included, along with racial/ethnic disparities.
As part of this, the report began an exploration of the relationship between
race/ethnicity and socioeconomic position. Some key findings from the
report are important to review. First, inequality in quality of care continues
to exist. These disparities often are particularly true for some more serious
health care problems, such as minorities being diagnosed with cancer at later
stages, less often receiving optimal care when hospitalized for cardiac
problems, and higher rates of avoidable hospital admissions among blacks
and poorer patients. Differential access to health care may lead to disparities
in quality of care actually received. In addition, opportunities to provide
preventive care may be missed.

In 2005, the third National Healthcare Disparities Report (2005)
was released. One advantage of continuing reports is a comparison to

previous years. The 2005 report focused on findings from a set of core report measures. The two measures of access covered were facilitators and barriers to care and health care utilization. The overall summary indicated that disparities still exist, but some disparities are diminishing, an encouraging result, but one that clearly leaves opportunities for further improvement. Disparities remain in areas of access, quality, and across many levels and types of care including preventive care, treatment of acute conditions, and management of chronic disease. This applies to a variety of specific clinical conditions including cancer, diabetes, end stage renal disease, heart disease, HIV disease, mental health and substance abuse, and respiratory diseases.

Looking at access more specifically, major issues of disparity occur for poor people and Hispanics, with lesser but important issues for Blacks, American Indians, and Asians. Poor people have worse access to care than high-income people for all eight core report measures. Hispanics have worse access for 88 percent of the core report measures, while Blacks and American Indians have worse access on half of the measures. Asian Americans have worse access on 43 percent of the measures. The 2005 report also tracks changes in the core measures over time. For each core report measure, racial, ethnic, and socioeconomic groups were compared with a designated comparison group at various points in time. For racial minorities, more disparities in quality of care were becoming smaller rather than larger, while for Hispanics, 59 percent were becoming larger and 41 percent smaller. For poor people, half of disparities were becoming smaller and half were becoming larger (National Healthcare Disparities Report, 2005)

Federal government's focus on these efforts has continued, with the Healthy People 2020 publication, much of which is now easily obtainable through US government websites (U.S. Department of Health and Human Services, 2013). For the 2020 effort, the report points out that in Healthy People 2000, the goal was to reduce health disparities among Americans, and in Healthy People 2010 the goal was to eliminate, not just reduce, health disparities. By Healthy People 2020, that goal was expanded even further: to achieve health equity, eliminate disparities, and improve the health of all groups. Healthy People 2020 defines health equity as attaining the highest level of health for all people. It points out that both efforts to eliminate disparities and achieve health equity have focused primarily on diseases or illnesses and on health care services.

The Centers for Disease Control and Prevention (CDC) is another US federal agency that works on issues linked to health differences and health disparities. In a special report they issued in 2011, the agency consolidated the most recent national data available on disparities in mortality, morbidity, behavioral risk factors, health care access, preventive health services, and social determinants of critical health problems in the United States by using selected indicators (Truman et al., 2011). Persistent gaps between the healthiest persons as well as states as units were shown on outcomes such as income, morbidity, mortality, and self-reported healthy days. The report includes data on the gaps but also has analytic essays that recommend some applied interventions, some of which have high rates of success such as close to elimination of disparities in certain vaccination rates among children.

In the United States, in addition to federal government efforts, some important private foundations such as the Commonwealth Foundation now have programs that focus on health differences and health disparities (Commonwealth Fund, 2013). The goals of the Commonwealth Fund's Program on Health Care Disparities are to improve the overall quality of health care delivered to low-income and minority Americans, and to eliminate racial and ethnic health disparities. This program builds on efforts to improve quality of care in the United States. A particular focus is to improve the performance of minority serving safety-net hospitals and ambulatory care providers in order to reduce disparities in access to high-quality care.

RACE/ETHNICITY AND SES FACTORS AND DISPARITIES

In the early years of sociology within the United States, there was a major focus on social class differences, to the extent that data were available. In addition, there was also early consideration of both racial and ethnic issues within the United States as well. As differences in recent years have become redefined as disparities with the growth of federal government efforts in health, there has been more focus on race/ethnicity than on SES. Partially, this was due to greater data availability and partially a belief, especially in the United States, that a policy focus necessitated more attention to race/ethnicity than to class. In the past few years, there is now a growing consensus whether in the United States or in Great Britain that looking only at data on race/ethnicity without a consideration of social class differences is problematic (Adler & Rehkopf, 2008; Davey Smith, 2000;

Kawachi, Daniels, & Robinson, 2005). I have already discussed some of this material in greater depth in an earlier volume within this series (Kronenfeld, 2012). If studies focus on race/ethnicity and ignore social class issues, it is too easy to conclude that differences are linked either specifically to race/ethnicity or even to biological differences that may be linked to race and ethnicity (Issacs & Schroeder, 2004).

In a recent review type article, Takeuchi, Walton, and Leung (2010) argue that there is an important role played by segregation as a social process. It contributes to differential exposure to many particular environments and contexts and these different opportunity structures and community structures may influence health by shaping social processes. Similarly, a recent review article about the Hispanic paradox by Dubowitz, Bates, and Acevado-Garcia (2010) points out how the sociopolitical context and patterns of migration contribute to health and to the paradox that Hispanics/Latinas have higher life expectancies than would be expected based on their higher representation among the poor. The more factors researchers consider in trying to understand the complexity between health differences, immigration, race/ethnicity, and SES, the more confusing and conflicting results researchers sometimes find. Perhaps some of the studies in this volume will add to better understanding as well as the growing complexity of this confusing literature.

Some of the same concerns about how information is gathered and disparate results depending on the exact ways data are gathered apply to the issue of SES and health disparities. Three traditional ways of measuring SES are occupation, income, and education. Each of these factors have somewhat different associations with health outcomes (Adler & Rehkopf, 2008; Kitagawa & Hauser, 1978; Kliss & Scheuren, 1978). In addition, another newer way to consider SES is social capital (Kawachi, 2010). In the United States, most studies now use income and education more often than occupation, because those questions are much simpler to ask and to code. In addition, in the United States, weaker associations have been found with measures of occupation as compared with income and education, perhaps because of the difficulty of having more standardized measures across studies (Adler & Rehkopf, 2008; Braveman et al., 2005). Some authors argue that education is the key to socioeconomic differentials in health (Ross & Mirowsky, 2010). A slightly different way to look at SES and its relationship to health disparities is the fundamental cause argument (Link & Phelan, 2010). Again, I have discussed some of these issues in greater depth in an earlier article (Kronenfeld, 2012).

GEOGRAPHICAL AND PLACE FACTORS AND DISPARITIES

In some ways, it is difficult to discuss the issue of geographical and place factors, since they become so intertwined with SES and race/ethnicity as discussed in the previous part. Thus this part will provide a few additional thoughts on the role of place and geography within the development of health disparities, recognizing the importance and interaction with SES and race/ethnicity. Thoughts about the relevance of place are not all new, and one could go far back in sociology and health and find some studies on rural–urban differences, or look at the more recent literatures (the past thirty years and its greater focus on health disparities) to find how some theoretical approaches such as Bandura (1986, 2001) and his social cognitive theory have discussed different factors that construct an environment that not only interacts with the individual, but can also be influenced by the individual's behavior. His approach recognizes the dynamic interaction between individual, environment, and behavior, and has become one way to integrate social ecology approaches into population health improvement efforts. These can then be tied into more recent discussions about health disparities. More narrowly within health education, there has been a concern to include the environment as part of the social ecological approach (Parcel & Baranowski, 1981, 2002). Social ecological theory emphasizes a holistic approach to environmental factors, although some newer social determinant approaches recognize that these elements are part of a system that also includes medical care and that the community or place is extremely important.

Moving away from these more theoretical approaches and looking at more applied articles, there has also been growth in recent years in articles that look at geographic factors as one component of disparity in use of health care services and health outcomes. Some articles focus on more serious and less common health problems, adding in geographic factors such as a recent examination of both geographic and socioeconomic disparities in PET (positron emission tomography) use by Medicare beneficiaries with cancer (Onega et al., 2012). PET is a nuclear medical imaging technique that produces a three-dimensional image or picture of functional processes. The use of this approach among Medicare beneficiaries with cancer increased from 2004 to 2008, with higher rates observed among white, higher SES groups, and in higher Medicare spending areas. Another cancer-related article with a geographic focus on health disparities looked at utilization of sentinel lymph node biopsy for certain types of melanoma and found that patients from the South were less likely to receive this approach (Martinez, Shah, Maverakis, & Yang, 2012). Another article has focused on place and geography for chronic kidney disease (McClellan, Plantinga, & McClellan, 2012). This article was a review article that included geographic attributes such as diversity in the physical environment as well as socioeconomic and medical care characteristics of the environment. Outside of the United States, examining differences between rural and urban areas in terms of health variations has been particularly important in Canada, and a recent article points out that not only are there rural urban differences, but that heterogeneity in health is also found within rural areas and that the variation may be even larger than the simpler rural urban differences (Lavergne & Kephart, 2012). Using US data from the 2006–2007 Current Population Survey, Chahine, Subramanian, and Levy (2011) look at sociodemographic and geographic variability in smoking at the US state, core-based statistical areas (CBSA) during a time period when smoking prevalence in the United States had decreased substantially yet disparities remained. Sociodemographic covaries were significant predictors of smoking, but explained more variance at the CBSA level than at the state level while contextual factors such as indoor smoking legislation and cigarette taxes at the state level explained a large proportion of variance at the state level but individually had modest statistical significance, illustrating the complex associations when trying to consider both sociodemographic and contextual factors.

Especially within research in the United States, an important set of studies examining geographic disparities in health care use have been those linked with the Dartmouth Atlas Project (Fisher & Wennberg, 2003; Wennberg, 1984; Wennberg & Gittelsohn, 1973). This project, beginning with early work in the 1970s and continuing into the present, has demonstrated the importance of what were initially called small area variations (focusing on geographic differences) in the types and amounts of health care used within the United States. As the work of this group has expanded, they have looked at cost and quality variations as well, and documented major variations in how medical resources are distributed and used in the United States. Today, the research group maintains a website that provides much greater detail on their current research, much of which uses Medicare data to provide information and analysis about national, regional, and local markets, as well as hospitals and their affiliated physicians (Dartmouth Atlas of Health Care, 2013). In a recent article examining some of these studies as well as others looking at the differences between high-spending and low-spending regions for health care in the United States and the future impact of the Affordable Care Act, as its major provisions become law in 2014, Cooper argues that meaningful health care reform will need to accept the reality that poverty and its cultural extensions are the major causes of geographic variation in health care utilization and also a major source of escalating health care spending (Cooper, 2011).

HEALTH PROBLEMS AND DISPARITIES

In many ways, looking at health problems is not always one of the ways we think about health disparities, because disparities in health outcomes are often seen as resulting from disparities in health care and utilization outcomes, the very thing being studied in health disparities research. So, as compared with the previous parts on race/ethnicity and SES as well as geography and place as social determinants of health disparities, this part is briefly reviewing some of the recent work on health problems and disparities and trends within that, rather than looking at these as one of the social determinants of disparities. The chapter has already referenced some studies that look at specific disease-type outcomes, especially in the part on geography and place. This part will review a few interesting studies on heart disease-related mortality trends, specialty care use with chronic diseases, and also one study that examines functional limitations across states and helps researchers as well as policy makers better understand how to track health disparities across communities and places. Looking at the latter issue first, in a recent article in the *Milbank Quarterly*, Asada, Yoshida, and Whipp (2013) point out that among the challenges of reporting on health disparities, one often overlooked is how best to report health disparities associated with multiple attributes. The focus of this article was to propose a new approach that measures health disparities associated with multiple attributes at the same time and summarizes them as the overall health disparity in the population. This is an important issue in research in health disparities, and especially as relates both to health outcomes and to social determinants, the theme of this volume. Asada et al. (2013) conclude that it is difficult to draw conclusions across different factors, using functional limitations in states as the outcome of interest. In their data, they report a general lack of consistency in the rankings of overall and attribute-specific disparities in functional limitation across states. Wyoming has the smallest overall disparity and West Virginia the largest. But, picking out states as the best and worst is an enormous oversimplification because they found in each of the four attribute-specific health disparity rankings that most of the best- and worst-performing states in regard to overall health disparity are not consistently good or bad and the factors underlying the differences also vary. In their analysis, they found three different disparity profiles across states: (1) the largest contribution from race/ethnicity (thirty-four states), (2) roughly equal contributions of race/ethnicity and socioeconomic factor(s) (ten states), and (3) the largest contribution from socioeconomic factor(s) (seven states).

The two heart disease-related studies both use major US databases to examine coronary artery disease mortality trends and stroke mortality trends. The article on coronary heart disease (CHD) mortality trends uses the US mortality files for 1977–2007, as obtained from the Centers for Disease Control and Prevention in the United States (Gillum, Mehari, Curry, & Obisesan, 2012). They found higher death rates for African American men and women as compared to European American men and women. While rates declined in all groups over the time period studied, in women, rates declined more in later years of life. For men, rates declined less for African Americans. Rates were higher in the Ohio and Mississippi River areas. In the study looking at stroke mortality over the same time period, rates declined in all groups, but declined less for African American males (Gillum, Kwagyan, & Obisesan, 2011). Among those males, rates declined less in east and south central divisions of the United States.

In the last article mentioned here, specialty care use in US patients with chronic diseases is examined, paying some attention to differences by racial, and ethnic groups as the social determinants of importance (Bellinger et al., 2010). Using data from the Commonwealth Fund 2006 Health Care Quality Survey, they examined variation in specialty care utilization by chronic disease status. Poor perceived health, minority status, and lack of health insurance were all associated with both reduced specialty care use and chronic disease diagnosis.

These articles all report complicated and at time contrasting patterns of health outcomes depending on the outcome being studied as well as upon the social determinants being considered. This brief review helps to point out some of these complexities, as do several of the chapters in this volume, both the ones more focused on chronic disease outcomes and some of the other chapters. The last part of this chapter will briefly review the other chapters in this volume.

REVIEW OF CONTENTS OF THE VOLUME

Part 1 of this volume contains one chapter, the introduction to the volume. Part 2 of this volume is entitled Geographical and Place Factors and Disparities and includes four chapters related to this theme. The first chapter by Ann M. Hewitt deals with understanding place in the role of social determinant interventions. This chapter presents a conceptual explanation of social determinants approaches and describes the potential impact for traditional health promotion activities that target the at-risk populations. The chapter uses two major resources, the Health Impact Assessment Toolkit and the HHS Disparities Action Plan, to help review this material. The second chapter by Neale Chumbler and Tamara Leach also looks at issues linked to place and geography, but they examine the impact of neighborhood cohesion on the self-rated health status (SRHS) of individuals. Using aspects of collective efficacy theory, this chapter hypothesized that older individuals who perceived that their neighborhood has high levels of social cohesion around elderly issues will have better SRHS. The chapter uses data from a telephone survey of Indianapolis, Indiana residents, along with some court data, and census information. They find that both social cohesion and low income are statistically significant predictors of poor self-rated health status. The third chapter in this part uses data gathered from 13 semistructured focus groups, plus three semistructured interviews. Freed and colleagues report about both structural and hidden barriers to the local primary health care infra-structure. Structural barriers include transportation, clinic, and appoint-ment wait time, and co-payments and health insurance. Hidden barriers consist of knowledge about local health care services, nonphysician gatekeepers, and fear of medical care. The fourth chapter by Grimm et al. focuses on rural settings for care as part of their consideration of geography and space. The chapter looks at the effects of two rural community residential advantages – economic growth and availability of health services – upon residents' health and emotional well-being using household survey data they collected. Both residential advantages were necessary for improved health while the most important negative net effect on health was aging.

Part 3 of the volume looks at race/ethnicity and SES factors as social determinants of health and health care disparities. This part includes four chapters on these topics. The first chapter by Gorman and Dinh examines ethnic group differences in the utilization of preventive medical services among foreign-born Asians and Latinos, using the Andersen Behavioral

Model of health services use. Among Latinos, a much lower proportion of Mexican immigrants reported a preventive medical care visit during the last year than either Cuban or Puerto Rican immigrants. Asian immigrants showed less variation in use, but significant differences still existed with Filipino immigrants reporting the highest level of use, followed by Vietnamese and the then Chinese immigrants. This study demonstrates the importance of not just examining Asians and Latinos as homogeneous groups. The second chapter focuses on one ethnic group, low-income Latina mothers, and looks at the impact of an educational intervention designed to reduce health disadvantages of these women by providing social support during and after pregnancy. Using a randomized control-group design, and recruiting 440 pregnant Latina women, 88 percent of whom were first generation, the study does not find an improvement in birth outcomes for those in the social support intervention group. Jokinen-Gordon and Quadagno in the third chapter discuss the variations in parents' perceptions of children's medical treatment and tests whether greater dissatisfaction is associated with less preventive care and unmet medical need. Parents' dissatisfaction scores are significantly higher for racial/ethnic minorities, non-English speakers, lower SES respondents, and the uninsured. Parent dissatisfaction has a significant and strong association with lack of preventive care and reports of unmet medical need. The last chapter in this part by Smith and Scheid examines the race concordance hypothesis which suggests that matching patients and health providers on the basis of race improves communication and patients' perceptions of health care, and therefore also encourages patients to seek and utilize health care, which may reduce health disparities. While blacks (compared to whites) used less primary care and had more emergency care visits, race concordance was not a statistically significant predictor of either primary care or emergency room use. Patients' satisfaction with primary care providers was associated with significantly fewer primary care and emergency care visits while trust in one's provider was associated with more primary care visits.

Part 4 includes three chapters that deal with serious and chronic health care problems. The first chapter in this part by Wood deals with issues connected with AIDS and HIV, looking particularly at disparities by age in attention paid to these health issues. As Wood points out, older adults are often omitted from HIV/AIDS prevention programs. Through qualitative research with state policymakers and AIDS service organizations, she points out how there is often too little attention paid to these issues for people 50 and above, a group in the United States in which there is currently an increase in new infections and diagnoses. The second chapter by Tausig explores issues of self care management for chronic illness. This chapter is a review and synthesis of research literature, and has a goal of development of an explanation for how chronic illnesses are managed at home as a way to improve the sociological perspective on health care for persons with chronic illness. Two important insights from the chapter are that first, chronic illness care occurs in the context of the household, neighborhood, and community and, therefore, there is great importance in understanding the caregiving social network around the patient and second, that the risk of chronic illness and the resources available to deal with it are socially (and unequally) distributed, so that "health care" interventions need to take account of disparities in risks and resources that impact the patient's ability to successfully comply with self-care regimens. The last chapter in this part is by Kutner and Zhang and focuses on social capital, gatekeeping, and access to kidney transplantation. The authors hypothesized that early opportunities for discussion of kidney transplantation potentially generate social capital that serves as a resource for patients as they navigate the transplantation pathway. Using a national sample of first-year dialysis patients, they examined whether kidney transplantation had been discussed with them before and after starting dialysis treatment. Time to placement on the kidney transplant waiting list was significantly shorter for patients who reported that transplantation had been discussed with them before, as well as after, starting dialysis. Likelihood of reported discussion varied by patient's age, employment and insurance status, cardiovascular comorbidity burden, and perceived health status.

Part 5 of the volume includes two chapters which have a focus on comparative and political issues. The first chapter focuses on the need for comparative research on social inequalities in health care. It points out that much of the research on disparities in the United States has been US-centric and too rarely takes a cross-national comparative approach to answering its questions. The chapter argues that the central methodological challenges to comparative research include issues of comparable measurement, the identification of causal mechanisms and lag structures, the nonindependence of cases selected for macro-level comparisons, and case selection and unmeasured heterogeneity. It also links the US-centric focus to the emphasis on race in the United States. The second chapter in this part by Perlstadt looks at political ideology, party identification, and perceptions of health disparities. The chapterapplies theories of cognitive dissonance to the topic and uses data from a statewide telephone survey in Michigan. Political ideology was important as was political party identity to a lesser extent. Liberals were most likely to believe that minorities were unable to get routine care when needed and Democrats that ability to speak English meant differential treatment. Respondents with low education were most likely to believe people were treated unfairly based on insurance, while those with lower incomes were more likely to believe that minorities received higher quality of care than whites.

REFERENCES

Adler, N. E., & Rehkopf, D. H. (2008). U.S. disparities in health: Descriptions, causes and mechanisms. *Annual Review of Public Health, 29*, 235–252.

Aneshensel, C. S. (2009). Toward explaining mental health disparities. *Journal of Health and Social Behavior, 50*(December), 377–394.

Asada, Y., Yoshida, Y., & Whipp, A. M. (2013). Summarizing social disparities in health. *Milbank Quarterly, 91*(1), 5–36.

Bandura, A. (1986). *Social foundations of thought and action.* Englewood Cliffs, NJ: Prentice Hall.

Bandura, A. (2001). Social cognitive theory: An agent perspective. *Annual Review of Psychology, 52*, 1–26.

Bellinger, J. D., Hassan, R. M., Rivera, P. A., Cheng, Q., Williams, E., & Glover, S. H. (2010). Specialty care use in US patients with chronic diseases. *International Journal of Environmental Research and Public Health, 7*(3), 975–990.

Braveman, P. A., Cubbin, C., Egerter, S., Chideya, S., Marchi, K. S., Metzler, M., & Posner, S. (2005). Socioeconomic status in health research – one size does not fit all. *Journal of the American Medical Association, 294*, 2879–2888.

Chahine, T., Subramanian, S. V., & Levy, J. I. (2011). Sociodemographic and geographic variability in smoking in the U.S.: A multilevel analysis of the 2006-2007 current population survey, tobacco use supplement. *Social Science and Medicine, 73*(5), 752–758.

Commonwealth Fund (2013, March). Retrieved from http://www.commonwealthfund.org/ Program-Areas/Archived-Programs/Health-Care-Disparities.aspx

Cooper, R. A. (2011). Geographic variation in health care and the affluence poverty nexus. *Advances in Surgery, 45*, 63–82.

Dartmouth Atlas of Health Care. (2013). Retrieved from http://www.dartmouthatlas.org/. Accessed on April 4, 2013.

Davey Smith, G. (2000). Learning to live with complexity: Ethnicity, socioeconomic position and health in britain and the united states. *American Journal of Public Health, 90*, 1694–1698.

Dubowitz, T., Bates, L. M., & Acevado-Garcia, D. (2010). The latino health paradox: Looking at the intersectionality of sociology and health. In C. E. Bird, P. Conrad, A. M. Fremont & S. Timmermans (Eds.), *Handbook of medical sociology* (5th ed.). Nashville, TN: Vanderbilt University Press.

Fisher, E. S., & Wennberg, J. E. (2003). Health care quality, geographic variations, and the challenge of supply-sensitive care. *Perspectives in Biology and Medicine, 46*(1), 69–79.

Gillum, R. F., Kwagyan, J., & Obisesan, T. O. (2011). Ethnic and geographic variation in stroke mortality trends. *Stroke, 42*(11), 3294–3296.

Gillum, R. F., Mehari, A., Curry, B., & Obisesan, T. O. (2012). Racial and geographic varia-
    tion in coronary heart disease mortality trends. *BMC Public Health, 12*(June 6), 410.
    doi:10.1186/1471-2458-12-410
Issacs, S. L., & Schroeder, S. A. (2004). Class-the ignored determinant of the nation's health.
    New England Journal of Medicine, 351(11), 1137–1142.
Kawachi, I. (2010). Social capital and health. In C. E. Bird, P. Conrad, A. M. Fremont &
    S. Timmermans (Eds.), *Handbook of medical sociology* (5th ed.). Nashville, TN:
    Vanderbilt University Press.
Kawachi, I., Daniels, N., & Robinson, D. E. (2005). Health disparities by race and class:Why
    both matter. *Health Affairs, 24*, 343–352.
Kitigawa, E., & Hauser, P. (1978). *Differential mortality in the united states.* Cambridge, MA:
    Harvard University Press.
Kliss, B., & Scheuren, F. J. (1978). The 1973 CPS-IRS-SSA exact match study. *Social Security
    Bulletin, 42*, 14–22.
Kronenfeld, J. J. (2012). Health care system issues and race/ethnicity, immigration, SES
    and gender as sociological issues linking to health and health care. In J. J. Kronenfeld
    (Ed.), *Issues in health and health care related to race/ethnicity, immigration, SES and
    gender* (Vol. 30). Research in the Sociology of Health Care. London, England: Emerald
    Press.
Lavergne, M. R., & Kephart, G. (2012). Examining variations in health within rural canada.
    Rural Remote Health, 12, 1848. Epub Feb 29.
Link, B. G., & Phelan, J. C. (2010). Social conditions as fundamental causes of health
    inequalities. In C. E. Bird, P. Conrad, A. M. Fremont & S. Timmermans (Eds.),
    Handbook of medical sociology (5th ed.). Nashville, TN: Vanderbilt University Press.
Marmot, M. G., Rose, G., Shipley, M. J., & Hamilton, P. J. S. (1978). Employment grade and
    coronary heat disease in British civil servants. *Journal of Epidemiology and Community
    Health, 32*, 244–249.
Marmot, M. G., Shipley, M. J., & Rose, G. (1984). Inequalities in death-specific explanations of
    a general pattern. *Lancet, 323*, 1003–1006.
Martinez, S. R., Shah, D. R., Maverakis, E., & Yang, A. D. (2012). Geographic variation in
    utilization of sentinel lymph node biopsy for intermediate thickness cutaneous
    melanoma. *Journal of Surgical Oncology, 106*(7), 807–810.
McClellan, A. C., Plantinga, L., & McClellan, W. M. (2012). Epidemiology, geography
    and chronic kidney disease. *Current Opinion in Nephrology and Hypertension, 21*(3),
    323–328.
McGuire, T., Alegria, M., Cook, B. L., Wells, K. B., & Zaslavsky, A. M. (2006). Implementing
    the Institute of Medicine definition of disparities: An application to mental health care.
    Health Services Research, 41, 1979–2005.
National Healthcare Disparities Report. (2005, December). *Agency for Healthcare Research and
    Quality*, Rockville, MD. AHRQ Publication No. 06-0017. Retrieved from www.ahrq.
    gov/qual/nhdr05/nhdr05.pdf
National Healthcare Disparities Report: Summary. (2004, February). *Agency for Healthcare
    Research and Quality*, Rockville, MD. Retrieved from http://www.ahrq.gov/qual/
    nhdr03/nhdrsum03.htm
Onega, T., Tosteson, T. D., Wang, Q., Hillner, B. E., Song, Y., Siegel, B., & Tosteson, A. N. A.
    (2012). Geographic and sociodemographic disparities in PET use by medicare benefi-
    ciaries with cancer. *Journal of American College of Radiology, 9*(9), 635–642.

Parcel, G., & Baranowski, T. (1981). Social learning theory and health education. *Health Education, 12*, 14–18.

Parcel, G., & Baranowski, T. (2002). How individuals, environments, and health behavior interact: Social cognitive theory. In K. Glanz, B. Rimer & F. Lewis (Eds.), *Health behavior and health education: Theory, research and practice* (pp. 165–184). San Francisco, CA: Jossey-Bass.

Ross, C. E., & Mirowsky, J. (2010). Why education is the key to socioeconomic differentials in health. In C. E. Bird, P. Conrad, A. M. Fremont & S. Timmermans (Eds.), *Handbook of medical sociology* (5th ed.). Nashville, TN: Vanderbilt University Press.

Schnittker, J., & McLeod, J. D. (2005). The social psychology of health disparities. *Annual Review of Sociology, 31*, 75–103.

Smedley, B. D., Stith, A. Y., & Nelson, A. R. (Eds.). (2003). *Unequal treatment: Confronting racial and ethnic disparities in health care.* Institute of Medicine. Washington, DC: National Academies Press.

Takeuchi, D. T., Walton, E., & Leung, M. (2010). Race, social contexts and health: Examining geographic spaces and places. In C. E. Bird, P. Conrad, A. M. Fremont & S. Timmermans (Eds.), *Handbook of medical sociology* (5th ed.). Nashville, TN: Vanderbilt University Press.

Truman, B. I., Smith, C., Smith, K., Roy, K., Chen, Z., Moonesinghe, R., … Zaza, S. (2011, January 14). Rationale for regular reporting on health disparities and inequalities, United States. *Morbidity and Mortality Weekly Report (Supplements), 60*(1), 3–10.

U.S. Department of Health and Human Services. (2000, November). *Healthy people 2010* (2nd ed.), Vols. 1-2: *With understanding and improving health and objectives for improving health.* Washington, DC: U.S. Government Printing Office.

U.S. Department of Health and Human Services. (2013). *Healthy People 2020.* Retrieved from http://www.healthypeople.gov/2020/about/disparitiesAbout.aspx. Accessed on March 1, 2013.

Wennberg, J., & Gittelsohn, A. (1973). Small area variations in health care delivery: A population-based health information system can guide planning and regulatory decision-making. *Science, 182*, 1102–1108.

Wennberg, J. E. (1984). Dealing with medical practice variations: A proposal for action. *Health Affairs, 3*(2), 6–32.

.

PART 2
GEOGRAPHICAL AND PLACE
FACTORS AND DISPARITIES

ADDRESSING HEALTH DISPARITIES: UNDERSTANDING PLACE IN THE ROLE OF SOCIAL DETERMINANT INTERVENTIONS

Anne M. Hewitt

ABSTRACT

Purpose – *Recent national policy adoptions of the social determinants of health approach present enormous challenges to practitioners designing health promotion programs aimed at eliminating health disparities. This chapter provides a framework for understanding the social determinant rationale embedded in* Healthy People 2020 *and introduces the concept of* place *as an important consideration.*

Methodology/Approach – *This chapter presents a conceptual explanation of social determinant thinking and describes the potential impact for traditional health promotion activities that target the at-risk populations.*

Findings – *Two major resources, the Health Impact Assessment Toolkit and the HHS Disparities Action Plan, have emerged as frameworks for developing a* health in all policies *approach that will enable health practitioners to enhance their social determinant interventions.*

Social Determinants, Health Disparities and Linkages to Health and Health Care
Research in the Sociology of Health Care, Volume 31, 23–39
Copyright © 2013 by Emerald Group Publishing Limited
All rights of reproduction in any form reserved
ISSN: 0275-4959/doi:10.1108/S0275-4959(2013)0000031004

Research limitations/implications – *Current social determinant approaches and models need to be strategically tailored to interventions aiming to reduce health disparities. Additional research focusing on how these approaches are integrated within the existing health promotion program frameworks is required.*

Practical implications – *Very few health practitioners have had the opportunity to integrate a social determinant approach that emphasizes the concept of* place *and explores the consequences of using a* health in all policies *approach. This chapter serves as a practical introduction and outlines the major challenges.*

Originality/value of paper – *The tipping point for the inclusion of social determinants of health in addressing health disparities occurred with the publication of* Healthy People 2020. *As this innovation begins to diffuse throughout the country, health practitioners will benefit by reviews and applications of the new rationale and model.*

Keywords: Social determinants of health; health disparities; health policy; health promotion; place; health in all policies approach

In today's technologically advanced, socially connected, and medically sophisticated society, health disparities remain America's primary, public health embarrassment. The underlying construct of health disparities is simply that an undesirable difference exists between and among different populations within our country. These health differences manifest themselves in some of the most costly and debilitating diseases challenging our health care system (Joint Center for Political and Economic Studies, 2010). According to several major reports, disparities are evident in health care (IOM, 2002), human services infrastructure and workforce (IOM, 2004), general health, safety, and well being (CDC, 2011), and in scientific knowledge and innovation (IOM Subcommittee, 2009). Community health textbooks routinely list the six most common areas of health disparities as: infant mortality, cancer screening and management, cardiovascular disease, diabetes, HIV/AIDS, and adult/child immunizations (McKenzie, Pinger, & Kotecki, 2012). The quality of life impact attributed to health disparities continues to be studied, researched, and debated with new national initiatives produced on a regular basis.

Yet, despite decades of Surgeon General Reports (US DHEW, 1979), renewed commitment to Healthy People goals (US DHHS 2000; US DHHS,

2010), and the Institute of Medicine's future projections (IOM, 2002; IOM, 2011), health disparities remain stubbornly entrenched within certain sub-populations. These at-risk populations remain familiar to anyone involved in solving our current health dilemma as they include minorities, immigrants, women, and lower socioeconomic groups (National Prevention Strategy, 2010). Over time, popular explanations for health disparities among these vulnerable populations have included variations of three main approaches. These three explanatory frameworks collectively emphasize: (a) unusual or excessive exposures to risk-factors, (b) lack of access to preventive and primary health services, and (c) social determinant factors as a root cause for health inequities (Smith, Orleans, & Jenkins, 2004; Williams & Sternthal, 2010; Wright & Perry, 2010).

The purpose of this chapter is to briefly review contributions of medical sociologists to the general racial–ethnic disparities dialog with special attention paid to the emergence of the social conditions as an important factor on health status. It further examines the recent policy adoption and prominence of social determinant approaches including the key component of *place* and its relationship to health promotion interventions and explores the future challenges of a *health in all policies* strategic framework. The chapter concludes with two practitioner-friendly recommendations for implementing a social determinant approach to reduce health disparities.

ESTABLISHING CONTEXT FOR SOCIAL DETERMINANT APPROACHES

The enigma of health disparities within American society presents daily challenges to clinical professionals who provide delivery of healthcare, health policy makers who strive to develop inclusive mandates that will eliminate health inequities, and medical sociologists who actively search for theories to explain and remediate the impact of this undesirable dilemma. In a recent article, Williams and Sternthal (2010) succinctly articulate four major sociological contributions to this important, national dialog. They conclude that medical sociologists have framed the racial/ ethnic disparity discussion by (a) challenging society's understanding of race, (b) highlighting the important role of social structure and context on health determinants, (c) broadening our understanding of how racism can affect health, and (d) underscoring the dynamics of changing populations (migration) on health status. These authors also provide compelling evidence of the continued existence of racial differences in health status over time by citing works from W.E.B. DuBois and recent studies focusing on Hispanic/Latino migration (Williams & Sternthal, 2010). These contributions provide a conceptual underpinning for three commonly cited and most familiar explanations for health equities: limited access to health services, risk-factor exposure, and social determinants as primary causes of health disparities.

Limited Access to Health Services

Multiple studies have documented that a common barrier facing minority populations is the ability to access both prevention-based and primary care health services (AHRQ, 2012). Results from specific research on maternal/child outcomes (Lu & Halfon, 2003), diabetes prevention (Lutfey & Freese, 2005), and cancer prevention screenings (AHRQ, 2012) continue to highlight the discrepancy in opportunities for vulnerable populations to receive appropriate care and disease management services. Over the years, medical sociologists have helped researchers identify, articulate, and analyze the delivery variance for these types of health services. Today, health policy makers have a better understanding of the biased distribution of health services, how those inequalities can then impact the health service organization itself, and most importantly, how the quality of healthcare from these organizations directly impacts minority health status (Wright & Perry, 2010). Although remedial policies to increase healthcare service access show important positive outcomes, inequity gaps still remain. Even Canada, with universal access to health services through national health insurance, also reports inequalities of healthcare utilization among vulnerable groups (Lasser, Himmelstein, & Woolhandler, 2006). This finding suggests that other important factors have mediating influences on health status.

Risk-Factor Exposure Approach

Different experts, interested in studying the health inequity phenomenon, support the exposure to risk-factor explanation for health status variation among populations instead of the health policy perspective emphasizing access to health services (Smith et al., 2004). For several years, the dominant environmental model view held that exposure to disease-causing risks, such as pollution, toxins, and unsanitary living conditions, would account for health inequities. With the recent focus on chronic disease and the recognition that many risk factors are behavioral and life-style embedded, current emphasis has shifted to modifying individual activities, habits, and decision-making processes (Koh, Piotrowski, Kumanyika, & Fielding, 2011). In addition, other research has also identified that many minority and underserved groups make up the majority of individuals who participate in risky behaviors, whether it be smoking, over-eating, or unprotected sexual activity (Healthy People 2020, 2010). It appears that any current explanation for health inequality cannot be understood or solutions developed without an examination of social conditions as fundamental causes in modifying risk-factor behavior.

Implications of Social Conditions on Health

The importance of understanding racial inequalities and their relationship to social constructs such as socioeconomic status (SES) remains essential for creating any potential solutions to this embedded American problem. Medical sociology research on the fundamental causes of health inequities has evolved over the last twenty years with special attention being focused on social conditions as the root causes of the current health disparity environment. Link and Phelan (2010) explain how the risk-factor model of health inequalities does not fully describe or account for the impact of social conditions on health status. The authors alternatively suggest that the primary component inherent in the fundamental cause theory, the access to resources essential to avoid disease, is a more forceful argument for understanding health inequities. The fundamental cause theory forces health professionals to view the health environment not simply based on a population's racial/ethnic status or access to healthcare services, but instead on addressing root causes of health inequities inherent in social conditions that have the potential to impact their total environment.

Using the social determinant approach requires an understanding of several streams of research all focused on identifying factors that serve as fundamental causes of health disparity. Editors of the 6th edition of the *Handbook of Medical Sociology* devote several chapters to investigating social contexts and health disparities (Bird, Conrad, Fremont, & Timmerans, 2010). Prominent chapter authors address the impact of social capital (Kawachi, 2010) and social supports (Lovasi, Adams, & Bearman, 2010), education (Ross & Mirowsky, 2010), gender (Rieker, Bird, & Lang, 2010), life-course (Robert, Cagney, & Weden, 2010), migration (Dubowitz, Bates, & Acevedo-Garcia, 2010), and race in relation to geographic spaces and places (Takeuchi, Walton, & Leung, 2010). It is the relationship between race/ethnicity and geographic location that is of current interest to health policy makers and their recent policy solutions to eliminate health inequities.

Health policy makers are well aware that social determinants often lead to and exacerbate health disparities (CDC, Social Determinants of Health, 2012), and primary stakeholders also recognize that social determinants are inextricably linked to community quality of life. These social sources of disparities, often directly related to race, are embedded within an individual community and include residential segregation, place stratification, and constrained life choices impacting education, income, and housing (Takeuchi et al., 2010). The latest emphasis on social determinants within the community is reflected in federal policy that highlights the role of *place* and all the variables inherent in both the social and physical environment.

POLICY ADOPTION AND THEORETICAL ROLE OF *PLACE* IN SOCIAL DETERMINANT APPROACHES

Policy experts, researchers, and epidemiologists have long known that health disparities are caused by complex social factors (Carter-Pokras & Baquet, 2002; Marmot, 2000; US DHHS, 2000). Social ecological factors most often linked to health disparities include: social, physical, economic, and political influences that interrelate within an individual's environment (Bronfenbrenner, 1979). Current health policy documents often refer to these factors using a catch-all phrase – socialeconomic status, although other factors are also implicated. As Bandura (1986, 2001) postulated in his social cognitive theory, these collective factors construct an environment that not only interacts with the individual, but can also be influenced by the individual's behavior. This three-way dynamic interaction between individual, environment, and behavior is known as reciprocal determinism, and it has also served as a theoretical rationale for integrating social ecology approaches into population health improvement efforts. The inclusion of the environment as part of the social ecological approach also provided a conceptual framework for the development of health education (Parcel & Baranowski, 1981, 2002). While social ecological theory emphasizes a holistic approach to environmental factors, newer social determinant approaches recognize that these elements are part of a system that also includes medical care and that the community or *place* is extremely important.

The World Health Organization (WHO) developed the definitive interpretation of social determinants of health by observing that "the circumstances in which people are born, grow up, live, work, and age, as well as the systems put in place to deal with illness, do impact their health and that these circumstances can be additionally impacted by economics, social policies, and politics" (2008). This definition underscores the importance of economics (income), policy development, and politics, but also supports that the concept of *place* as environment is crucial for understanding determinants of health. The WHO Board then adopted a resolution with three main priorities: "(1) improve living conditions including environmental circumstances, (2) tackle the inequitable distribution of power, money, and resources, and (3) measure and understand the problem and assess the impact of action" (WHO, Commission on Social Determinants of Health, 2008). WHO clearly believes that health inequities are avoidable inequalities?

The latest American health policy document, *Healthy People 2020*, prioritizes the role of social determinants by including it as one of the four goals for the next 10 years (Healthy People, 2010). The *Healthy People 2020* strategic plan similarly describes social determinants of health as the "environments in which people are born, live, learn with wide range of health, functioning, and quality-of-life outcomes and risks" (Healthy People 2020, 2010). A recent article traces over time the role and importance of social determinants within the four iterations of Healthy People (Koh et al., 2011). Although *Healthy People 2020* does differentiate between social and physical health determinants, the document comprehensively addresses for the first time such factors as poverty, education, and other influential dimensions of social structure. These are the same factors medical sociologists have directly linked to racial inequalities (Link & Phelan, 2010). Green and Allegrante (2011) suggest that social determinants of health were subsumed in previous Healthy People objectives. However, they acknowledge that a growing awareness and recognition of health disparities and inequities served as a reinforcing factor during the development of *Healthy People 2020*. Table 1 shows the relationship between the generic social ecology perspective, the WHO social determinants of health definition, and the *Healthy People 2020* policy perspective.

The social determinant approach is a logical extension and enhancement of the social ecological model as it focuses on the discrete components of the original all-encompassing ecological perspective.

Table 1. Social Ecological Model Dimensions → WHO Perspective → Healthy People Social Determinant Approach.

Social Ecological Model Dimensions	WHO Determinants of Health	Healthy People 2020 Social Determinants of Health
Environmental factors that influence an individual and their behavior. Social factors	Individual circumstances where people are born, grow up, live, work, and age (micro-level concept of place) Systems put in place to deal with illness (micro-level concept of health care)	Individual circumstances where people are born, grow up, live, learn, work, play, worship, and age (micro-level concept of place) *Social determinants:* Availability to resources to meet daily needs Access to educational, economic, and job opportunities Access to health care services Quality of education and job training Availability of community-based resources in support of community living and opportunities for… Transportation options Public safety Social support Social norms and attitudes (e.g., discrimination, racism, and distrust of government) Exposure to crime, violence, and social disorder (e.g., presence of trash and lack of cooperation) in addressing Also stress conditions that accompany socioeconomic condition Residential segregation

		Language/Literacy
		Access to mass media and emerging technologies (e.g., cell phones, the internet, and social media)
		Culture
		Physical determinants:
		Natural environment (green space/ weather)
		Build environment
Economic factors	Economics (macro-level)	Worksites, schools, and recreational settings
		Housing and community design
		Exposure to toxic substances
		Physical barriers (for people with disabilities)
		Aesthetic elements (lighting, trees, benches)
Political factors	Social policies (macro-level)	
Physical factors	Politics (macro-level)	

Sources: Bronfenbrenner (1979), WHO, Commission on Social Determinants of Health (2008), Healthy People 2020 (2010), Healthy People (2010).

INTERVENTIONAL ROLE OF SOCIAL
DETERMINANTS: THE CHALLENGE OF *PLACE*

One of *Healthy People 2020*'s significant contributions is the delineation of social and physical factors directly linked to *place*. *Place* denotes the underlying acceptance that social determinants of health are specific to a location. Examples of social *place* indicators focus on access to education, economic opportunities, jobs, health care, transportation, and the role of mass media. All of these community indicators have been repeatedly linked to racial/ethnic inequalities in health status. Physical determinants that exemplify the *place* perspective include both natural and manmade environment with emphasis on green space, aesthetic elements, and sustainability. The detailed delineation of social and physical determinants of health in *Healthy People 2020* suggests the need for tailoring health promotion and disease prevention interventions to *place* as part of any social determinant approach. For those interested in mitigating and eliminating health inequities, the issue of *place* within the social determinant approach is primary.

Faced with designing a complex health promotion intervention based on *Healthy People 2020*, most researchers and health practitioners focused on eliminating racial inequalities might need to create their own definition of *place*. As in the past, this step would typically be accomplished by identifying a geographical area, a population, or even a disease state, such as individuals receiving cancer treatment in a particular facility. With the addition of the social determinant approach to *Healthy People 2020*, interventionists should examine variables outlined in Table 1 and alter them to represent the issues particularly relevant such as racism, segregation, and community constraint on choices. For example, an exercise program for inner city minority or senior residents should be coupled with companion initiatives focusing on green space, community safety, and a reduction in social disorder. A recent study examining the relationship between race, place, and obesity reported that community racial/ethnic composition is an important correlate of obesity risk (Kirby, Liang, Chen, & Wang, 2012). This finding reinforces the link between community-level mediating factors and *place* as important in eliminating risk factors for vulnerable populations. Regardless of whether a community or city approach is adopted, using a social determinant approach provides a stronger framework for intervention design. Health interventions that follow a social determinant approach with an emphasis on *place* should have stronger positive outcomes.

APPLICATIONS FOR SOCIAL
DETERMINANT-BASED PRACTICE

Two primary challenges both health researchers and intervention practitioners face are:

(1) How do you facilitate a social determinant approach as part of health promotion initiative that is inclusive of *place*?
(2) Where are the opportunities for tailoring these interventions to achieve health and racial/ethnic equity within the community?

One solution to these two practical questions is outlined in the health policy document, *Healthy People 2020*. Based on the World Health Assembly's policy efforts to reduce health inequities using actions on social determinants and similar Australian policy mandates, US policy makers are now encouraging that every policy initiative must consider the health impact on the local community (Commission on U.S. Federal Leadership in Health and Medicine: Charting Future Directions, 2009; Puska & Stahl, 2010). *Healthy People 2020* also supports the use of a *health in all policies* approach when addressing health inequalities. This approach simply recognizes that social determinants impact health status and that the root causes of health inequalities can be addressed by coordinating policies that address housing, environment, agriculture, and education (Commission on U.S. Federal Leadership in Health and Medicine: Charting Future Directions, 2009). To help healthcare professionals using the social determinant approach in their conventional health promotion interventions, two important frameworks are available for linking with a *health in all policies* strategy.

The first strategy available to both public and nonprofit health practitioners is to utilize a Health Impact Assessment (HIA). HIAs refer to a "combination of procedures, methods, and tools by which a policy, program, or project may be judged as to its potential effects on the health of a population, and the distribution of those effects within the population" (Gothenburg Consensus Statement, 1999). The HIA is an objective framework that helps to evaluate the positive health outcomes of any proposed project in concert by assessing the impact of the project using a system-wide perspective. The six steps involved in the HIA process include:

- Screening to identify HIA utility
- Scoping to select which health effects to consider
- Assessing risks and benefits
- Developing recommendations

- Reporting to decision makers
- Evaluating the initiative

An HIA is recommended by the US Department of Health and Human Services as a planning option for *Healthy People 2020* initiatives. The steps provided here can be tailored to match any community whether urban, rural, or suburban setting. This planning activity will help health planners create interventions that enhance policy goals and potentially improve health outcomes. Several consumer-friendly HIA sites and toolkits are now available on the web including *The Health Impact Project* sponsored by the collaboration between the Robert Wood Johnson Foundation and the PEW Charitable Trust (The Health Impact Project, 2009).

The second resource, available for health stakeholders specifically interested in improving current health and ethnic disparities, is the recent HHS Action Plan to Reduce Racial and Ethnic Inequalities (2011). This report, *A Nation Free of Disparities in Health and Health Care*, focuses not only on health disparities associated with race and ethnicity, but also addresses related disparities for underserved and vulnerable subpopulations as well. The primary goals of this document are accompanied by coordinated strategies and actions applicable to health care organizations and agencies looking for guidance in implementing a social determinant approach as part of their intervention plan. This action plan also recommends in Strategy III the adoption of a *health in all policies* approach and suggests the use of a health disparity impact assessment for proposed policies and programs. The unique contribution of this framework is that the suggested strategies already emphasize the importance of *place* whether working with a local community health center, obtaining a health professional opportunity grant, or seeking funds for community transformation grants. The plan covers the major provisions of the Affordable Care Act that address health disparities and which offer a plethora of *place*-specific opportunities including:

- The HRSA Community Health Center Program
- Health Professional Opportunity Grants
- Maternal, Infant, and Early Childhood Home Visitation Programs
- The National Health Service Corps and Prevention
- Public Health Funds: Community Transformation Grants

(HHS Action Plan, Appendix A, 2011)

Together, these two documents offer frameworks for integrating the social determinant approach into health education and health promotion planning and practice. The leap to a health in all policies within a public health context will be the primary challenge for the next decade.

IMPLICATIONS AND NEXT STEPS

Several recent articles, texts, and blogs have been published using the phrase "The New Public Health" (Halpin, Morales-Suárez-Varela, & Martin-Moreno, 2010; RWJF, 2011; Tulchinsky & Varavikova, 2009). This phrase is an attempt to differentiate in American minds the public health impetus of the 20th century, which focused on successfully improving health through basic sanitation and vaccination strategies, from the public health of the 21st century which will increase health promotion efforts by addressing social, economic, and environmental factors and take on the challenge of reducing chronic disease in America. The Kaiser Family Foundation refers to this current initiative as a "groundswell of activity in local communities to support healthier lifestyles" (KFF, 2011).

All national health initiatives require a solid basis in theory, research, and subsequent practice. The CDC lists four steps for reframing current health promotion programs using the social determinants approach:

• Familiarize and partner with the CDC and other national agencies and organizations to provide leadership and set agendas for further discussion
• Create relevant metrics for social determinants of health and develop adequate data systems to inform future decision-making
• Enhance local capacity-building efforts and build traditional and nontraditional partnerships to further funding efforts and identification of at risk populations
• Focus on participatory prevention research based on engaging community members

(CDC - FAQ, 2012)

The immediate impact of this initiative for health care providers, policy makers, and practitioner will be a challenge for all to integrate social determinants of healthcare into their conceptual thinking. For those involved in eliminating health inequalities, the additional requirement of tailoring interventions to meet the barriers of racism will also need to be recognized. Fortunately, research findings from medical sociology studies outline important themes for consideration. The next major thrust will be to develop pilot programs that demonstrate effective best practices linking evidence-based practices with HIAs. Finally, the third major challenge will be to tailor these guided interventions and reach those at-risk populations who suffer from health disparities and inequities without stigmatizing them or their communities.

Koh and colleagues (2011) state that *Healthy People 2020* and other recent policies serve as avenues for a shared responsibility to achieve health equity and they also underscore the importance for integrating social determinants via a *health in all policies* approach. As stated by the Commission to Build a Healthier America, "The health of America depends on the health of all Americans" (Commission, 2009).

REFERENCES

Agency on Healthcare Research and Quality (AHRQ). (2012). *National healthcare disparities report*. Retrieved from http://www.ahrq.gov/qual/nhdr11/nhdr11.pdf. Accessed on March 15, 2012.

Bandura, A. (1986). *Social foundations of thought and action*. Englewood Cliffs, NJ: Prentice Hall.

Bandura, A. (2001). Social cognitive theory: An agent perspective. *Annual Review of Psychology, 52*, 1–26.

Bird, C. E., Conrad, P., Fremont, A. M., & Timmerans, S. (Eds.). (2010). *Handbook of medical sociology*. Nashville, TN: Vanderbilt University Press.

Bronfenbrenner, U. (1979). *The ecology of human development: Experiments by nature and design*. Cambridge, MA: Harvard University Press.

Carter-Pokras, O., & Baquet, C. (2002). What is a "health disparity? *Public Health Reports, 117*(5), 426–434.

Centers for Disease Control and Prevention (CDC). (CDC). CDC health disparities and inequalities report, United States, 2011. *MMWR, 60*(Supplement), 1–114.

Centers for Disease Control and Prevention (CDC). (2012). *Social determinants of health: FAQ*. Retrieved from http://www.cdc.gov/socialdeterminants/FAQ.html. Accessed on January 15, 2012.

Commission on U.S. federal leadership in health and medicine: Charting future directions. (2009). In S. J. Blumenthal & D. A. Cortese (Eds.), *New horizons for a healthy America: Recommendations to the new administration*. Center for the Study of the Presidency and Congress.

Commission to Build a Healthier America. (2009). *Breaking through on the social determinants of health and health disparities*. Robert Wood Johnson Foundation. Retrieved from http://www.commmissiononhealth.org. Accessed on January 25, 2012.

Dubowitz, T., Bates, L. M., & Acevedo-Garcia, D. (2010). The latino health paradox: Looking at the intersection of sociology and health. In C. Bird, P. Conrad, A. Fremont & S. Timmerans (Eds.), *Handbook of medical sociology* (pp. 106–552). Nashville, TN: Vanderbilt University Press.

Gothenburg Consensus Statement. (1999). *Health impact assessment*. Retrieved from http://www.euro.who.int/en/what-we-do/health-topics/environmental-health/health-impact-assessment. Accessed on January 14, 2012.

Green, L. W., & Allegrante, J. P. (2011). Healthy people 1980–2020: Raising the ante decennially or just the name from public health education to health promotion to social determinants? *Health Education and Behavior, 38,* 558–562.

Halpin, H. A., Morales-Suárez-Varela, M. M., & Martin-Moreno, J. M. (2010). Chronic disease prevention and the new public health. *Public Health Reviews, 32,* 120–154.

Healthy People. (2010). *Social determinants of health.* Objectives. Retrieved from http://healthypeople.gov/2020/topicsobjectives/overview.aspx?topicid=39. Accessed on February 2, 2012.

Healthy People 2020. (2010). *Healthy people 2020: Topics and objectives.* Retrieved from http://www.healthypeople.gov/2020/topicsobjectives2020/default.aspx. Accessed on February 1, 2012.

HHS Action Plan to Reduce Racial and Ethnic Health Disparities (2011). *A Nation free of disparities in health and health care.* Retrieved from http://minorityhealth.hhs.gov/npa/files/Plans/HHS/HHS_Plan_complete.pdf. Accessed on January 15, 2012.

Institute of Medicine (IOM). (2002). *Unequal treatment: Confronting racial and ethnic disparities in health care.* Washington, DC: The National Academies Press.

Institute of Medicine (IOM). (2004). *In The Nation's compelling interest: Ensuring diversity in the health care workforce.* Washington, DC: The National Academies Press.

Institute of Medicine (IOM). (2011). *Leading health indicators for healthy people 2020.* Washington, DC: National Academies Press.

Institute of Medicine (IOM) Subcommittee on Standardized Collection of Race/Ethnicity Data for Healthcare Quality. (2009). *Race, ethnicity, and language data: Standardization for health care quality improvement.* Washington, DC: The National Academies Press.

Joint Center for Political and Economic Studies. (2010). *Patient protection and affordable care act of 2010: Advancing health equity for racially and ethnically diverse populations.* Washington, DC.

Kaiser Family Foundation (KFF). (2011, June 10). *Preventing chronic disease: The new public health.* Retrieved from http://www.kff.org/ahr061011video.cfm. Accessed on January 18, 2012.

Kawachi, I. (2010). Social capital and health. In C. Bird, P. Conrad, A. Fremont & S. Timmerans (Eds.), *Handbook of medical sociology* (pp. 18–32). Nashville, TN: Vanderbilt University Press.

Kirby, J. B., Liang, L., Chen, H. J., & Wang, Y. (2012). Race, place, and obesity: The complex relationships among community racial/ethnic composition, individual race/ethnicity, and obesity in the United States. *American Journal of Public Health, 102*(8), 1572–1578. doi:10.2105/AJPH.2011.300452

Koh, H. K., Piotrowski, J. J., Kumanyika, S., & Fielding, J. E. (2011). Healthy people: A 2020 vision for the social determinants approach. *Health Education and Behavior, 38,* 551–557.

Lasser, K. E., Himmelstein, D. U., & Woolhandler, S. (2006). Access to care, health status, and health disparities in the United States and Canada: Results of a cross-national population-based survey. *American Journal of Public Health, 96*(7), 1300–1307.

Link, B., & Phelan, J. (2010). Social conditions as fundamental causes of health inequalities. In C. Bird, P. Conrad, A. Fremont & S. Timmerans (Eds.), *Handbook of medical sociology* (pp. 13–17). Nashville, TN: Vanderbilt University Press.

Lovasi, G. S., Adams, J., & Bearman, P. S. (2010). Social support, sex, and food: Social networks and health. In C. Bird, P. Conrad, A. Fremont & S. Timmerans (Eds.), *Handbook of medical sociology* (pp. 75–91). Nashville, TN: Vanderbilt University Press.

Lu, M. C., & Halfon, N. (2003). Racial and ethnic disparities in birth outcomes: A life-course perspective. *Maternal and Child Health Journal, 7*(1), 13–30.

Lutfey, K., & Freese, J. (2005). Toward some fundamentals of fundamental causality: Socioeconomic status and health in the routine clinic visit for diabetes. *The American Journal of Sociology, 110*, 1326–1372.

Marmot, M. (2000). Social determinants of health: From observation to policy. *The Medical Journal of Australia, 172*(8), 379–382.

McKenzie, J. F., Pinger, R. R., & Kotecki, J. E. (2012). *An introduction to community health*, (7th ed). Chapter 10–community health and minorities, (pp. 271–306). Sudbury, MA: Jones & Bartlett Learning.

National Prevention Strategy. (2010). *Factsheet*. Retrieved from http://www.surgeongeneral. gov/initiatives/prevention/strategy/national-prevention-strategy-fact-sheet.pdf. Accessed on July 15, 2013.

Parcel, G., & Baranowski, T. (1981). Social learning theory and health education. *Health Education, 12*, 14–18.

Parcel, G., & Baranowski, T. (2002). How individuals, environments, and health behaviour interact: Social cognitive theory. In K. Glanz, B. Rimer & F. Lewis (Eds.), *Health behavior and health education: Theory, research and practice* (pp. 165–184). San Francisco, CA: Jossey-Bass.

Puska, P., & Stahl, T. (2010). Health in all policies – the Finnish initiative: Background, principles and current issues. *Annual Review of Public Health, 31*, 315–318.

Rieker, P., Bird, C. E., & Lang, M. E. (2010). Understanding gender and health: Old patterns, new trends, and future directions. In C. Bird, P. Conrad, A. Fremont & S. Timmerans (Eds.), *Handbook of medical sociology* (pp. 52–74). Nashville, TN: Vanderbilt University Press.

Robert, S. A., Cagney, K. A., & Weden, M. M. (2010). A life-course approach to the study of neighborhoods and health. In C. Bird, P. Conrad, A. Fremont & S. Timmerans (Eds.), *Handbook of medical sociology* (pp. 124–143). Nashville, TN: Vanderbilt University Press.

Robert Wood Johnson Foundation (RWJF). (2011, March 29). *Thenewpublichealth*. Retrieved from http://blog.rwjf.org/publichealth/category/welcome/. Accessed on January 18, 2012.

Ross, C. E., & Mirowsky, J. (2010). Why education is the key to socioeconomic differentials in health. In C. Bird, P. Conrad, A. Fremont & S. Timmerans (Eds.), *Handbook of medical sociology* (pp. 33–51). Nashville, TN: Vanderbilt University Press.

Smith, T. W., Orleans, C. T., & Jenkins, C. D. (2004). Prevention and health promotion: Decades of progress, new challenges and an emerging agenda. *Health Psychology, 23*(2), 126–131.

Takeuchi, D. T., Walton, E., & Leung, M. (2010). Race, social contexts, and health: Examining geographic spaces and places. In C. Bird, P. Conrad, A. Fremont & S. Timmerans (Eds.), *Handbook of medical sociology* (pp. 92–105). Nashville, TN: Vanderbilt University Press.

The Health Impact Project. (2009). *A collaboration of the Robert Wood Johnson Foundation and the Pew Charitable Trusts*. Retrieved from http://www.healthimpactproject.org/. Accessed on July 15, 2013.

Tulchinsky, T. H., & Varavikova, E. A. (2009). *The new public health: An introduction for the 21st century* (2nd ed.). UK: Elsevier Pub.

U.S. Department of Health, Education and Welfare. (1979). *Healthy people: Surgeon general's report on health promotion and disease prevention.* Washington, D.C: Office of Disease Prevention and Health Promotion.

U.S. Department of Health and Human Services. (2000). *Healthy people 2010* (2nd ed.). Washington, DC: Office of the Assistant Secretary for Health.

U.S. Department of Health and Human Services. (2010). *Healthy people 2020.* Retrieved from http://www.healthypeople.gov/2020/about/DOHAbout.aspz. Accessed on January 15, 2012.

Williams, D. R., & Sternthal, M. (2010). Understanding racial-ethnic disparities in health: Social contributions. *Journal of Health and Social Behavior, 51*(1), S15–S27.

World Health Organization (WHO), Commission on Social Determinants of Health. (2008). *Closing the gap in a generation: Health equity through action on the social determinants of health.* Retrieved from http://www.who.int/social_determinants/thecommission/final report/key-concepts/en/index. Accessed on January 14, 2012.

Wright, E. R., & Perry, B. L. (2010). Medical sociology and health services research: Past accomplishments and future policy challenges. *Journal of Health and Social Behavior, 51,* S107–S115.

THE IMPACT OF NEIGHBORHOOD COHESION ON OLDER INDIVIDUALS' SELF-RATED HEALTH STATUS

Neale R. Chumbler and Tamara Leech

ABSTRACT

Purpose – *The purpose of this chapter is to advance the medical sociology literature on the relationship between social cohesion and SRHS on an individual level. There is little information about how neighborhood social characteristics affect seniors' SRHS. Guided by tenets of the collective efficacy theory, this chapter hypothesized that older individuals who perceived that their neighborhood has high levels of social cohesion around elderly issues will have better SRHS. A secondary hypothesis investigates whether the relationship was attenuated once their neighbors' actual, self-reported attitudes toward seniors were taken into account.*

Methodology – *Data come from a telephone survey of Indianapolis, Indiana residents, court data, and census information.*

Findings – *Logistic regression analyses indicated that both social cohesion and low income are statistically significant predictors of poor*

Social Determinants, Health Disparities and Linkages to Health and Health Care
Research in the Sociology of Health Care, Volume 31, 41–55
Copyright © 2013 by Emerald Group Publishing Limited
All rights of reproduction in any form reserved
ISSN: 0275-4959/doi:10.1108/S0275-4959(2013)0000031005

self-rated health status. Although both are statistically significant, the protective association between cohesion and poor SRHS (−0.69 log odds) is of similar magnitude to the risky association between income and poor health (−0.64 log odds).

Research implications – *Consistent with the classic work of Durkheim who found that individuals who were more socially integrated with society had lower rates of suicide, our study found a significant association between social cohesion and SRHS.*

Value of paper – *Future research is needed to target other health status outcomes in other geographical locations. Even though the body of research exploring the predictors of SRHS among older individuals is quite robust, this chapter adds to a more recent growing body of research, which has articulated the importance of the social environment in which an individual lives, especially community-dwelling older adults, is associated with their health status.*

Keywords: Older adults; social cohesion; health status

INTRODUCTION

It is well documented that self-rated health status (SRHS) is a key marker of health status. In fact, SRHS is a strong predictor of disability, mortality, and health care utilization, and these findings are even more pronounced among those at older ages (Cagney, Browning, & Wen, 2005; Liang et al., 2010). Even though the body of research exploring the predictors of SRHS among older individuals is quite robust, a more recent growing body of research has articulated the importance of the social environment in which an individual lives and their health. There are collective characteristics of communities and societies that are associated with population health status (Kawachi & Berkman, 2000). For instance, the association between place and health has been found to vary by geographic unit (Cagney et al., 2005). The neighborhood where individuals reside, especially in the context of America's poor, has been found to contribute to health (Browning & Cagney, 2002). This chapter extends previous research by exploring the extent to which social cohesion around elderly issues is associated with older individuals' SRHS. Social cohesion represents the level of connectedness and integration among groups in society (Kawachi & Berkman, 2000).

To our knowledge, there have been no studies that examined the association between elderly individuals' perceptions about how elderly specific issues are treated and viewed in the neighborhood context and SRHS. We hypothesize that older individuals who perceived that elderly neighbors in general are integrated into their neighborhood will have better SRHS. And, second we explore if such a relationship is attenuated once older respondents' level of education and income and neighbors' self-reported attitudes toward seniors are taken into account. Our investigation is guided by collective efficacy theory (Sampson, Raudenbush, & Earls, 1997). This standpoint, which is discussed in greater detail below, under-scores the salience of social resources and neighborhood-based economic factors in enhancing individual health (Cagney et al., 2005).

THEORETICAL PERSPECTIVES

The theoretical underpinnings of social cohesion and the extent to which it can be applied in this context could be traced back to specific contentions made by Emile Durkheim in his classic work on social integration. In his book, *The Rules of Sociological Method* (1895, 1964), Durkheim recognized that "society is not a mere sum of individuals. Rather, the system formed by their association represents a specific reality which has its own characteristics ... . The group thinks, feels, and acts quite differently from the way in which its members would were they isolated" (1895, 1964, pp. 103–104). Further, in one of Durkheim's other classic, *Suicide* (1897, 1997), he demonstrated that a society's suicide rate is correlated with its degree of social integration. More specifically, societies who had a high degree of social integration were inversely associated with suicide rates, suggesting that social integration can enhance population well-being (Kawachi, Kennedy, & Glass, 1999).

Social cohesion refers to the level of connectedness and solidarity among groups in society and can be traced back to the work of Durkheim in *Suicide* (1897, 1997). Durkheim contended that a cohesive society is one denoted by a richness of "mutual moral support, which instead of throwing the individual on his own resources, leads him to share in the collective energy and supports his own when exhausted" (Durkheim 1897, 1997, p. 210; also see Kawachi & Berkman, 2000). More specifically, Kawachi and Berkman (2000) offer more specific and detailed conceptual clarifications of social cohesion by articulating that it refers to two broad, entwined aspects of society: (1) the lack of suppressed social conflict (i.e., in the form of income inequality); and (2) the manifestation of fervent social relations as assessed by the degrees of trust and standards of reciprocity. A related, but conceptually distinct from social cohesion is social capital, defined as features of social structures (e.g., perception of trust and reciprocity through norms, values, and attitudes), which function as reserves for individuals and enable collective action (Engstrom, Mattsson, Jarleborg, & Hallqvist, 2008; Kawachi & Berkman, 2000; Subramanian, Kim, & Kawachi, 2002). In other words, the presence of social capital is evident when individuals are linked to one another via trusting networks and shared values (Putnam, 2000, p. 312). The benefits of social capital have been examined in several lines of inquiry and the theoretical contribution from a study in the field of criminology is especially relevant to the present study. A study of 8,782 residents of 343 Chicago neighborhoods by Sampson et al. (1997) found that mutual trust and altruism among neighbors and their preparedness to mediate when they witnessed children being unruly were significantly associated with less crime. A neighborhood's *collective efficacy* (a concept that integrates social cohesion, trust and informal social control and measured by items such as "people in this neighborhood can be trusted") was a stronger predictor of and inversely associated with neighborhood violence than SES. Findings from this study underscore the fact that individuals' choices and behaviors are strongly influenced by their neighbors (Putnam, 2000).

Still, yet an additional study that examined the effects of social capital, aggregated at the state level, on individual SRHS (Kawachi et al., 1999). Kawachi et al. (1999) operationalized social capital with items assessing interpersonal trust and norms of reciprocity (measured as whether or not people are considered to be helpful) and found that individuals (ages 18 and older) who resided in states with low social capital were at increased risk of poor self-rated health. Kawachi et al. (1999) further found that those with the lowest income and the oldest age (individuals 65 years and older) had the strongest associations with self-rated fair or poor health. These findings coupled with other evidence that found that social engagement and participation is related to improved health functioning and a reduction in mortality (Cramm, Van Dikj, Lotters, van Exel, & Niboer, 2011) underscore the importance of examining seniors' views of social cohesion, and the extent to which older individuals perceive social cohesion in their neighborhood is associated with SRHS.

Social Cohesion in the Context of Socialization to Aging

Older individuals not only affect society, but are also affected by it. Theoretically speaking, as older individuals' age, they experience issues and challenges of social roles as they socialize into being a senior (Rosow, 1974). The major premise of Rosow's (1974) landmark book *Socialization to Old Age* was that "people are not effectively socialized to old age" (p. xii). According to Rosow's (1974) adult socialization theoretical perspective, aging establishes a special circumstance of socialization to an undervalued status, thereby making facilitation to old age being contingent upon appropriate social integration (see also Barron's [1953] work that served as a precursor to this work of Rosow). If the appropriate social integration does not occur, then distressing consequences can transpire including stereotyping (Rosow, 1974). Stereotypes are a subset of attitudes and affect intergroup relations by biasing information processing concerning in-group and out-group members, thereby facilitating self-fulfilling prophecies (Stephan et al., 1993). Research studies demonstrate that many people have stereotypical and negative perceptions about elderly individuals (see Ron, 2007). Rosow (1974) argued that older persons even have negative views toward their senior elderly counterparts. However, more recent findings have indicated that attitudes of elderly people toward their own age group are more positive than the attitudes of young individuals toward them (O'Hanlon, Camp, & Osofsky, 1993; Ron, 2007). Seniors spend more time in their neighborhood than younger adults (Krause, 1996) and therefore may experience greater social cohesion. One possible explanation for this phenomenon is social cohesion. Since older adults report greater residential stability and spend many hours of the day at home, it is possible to expect that they are impacted by their neighbors and their neighborhood surroundings (Cramm, van Kikj, & Nieboer, 2013; Mohnen, Groenewegen, Volker, & Flap, 2011). When older people experience and perceive more support from their neighbors, they experience high levels of neighborhood senior attachment. Thus, older individuals' social interactions are crucial for elders. Previous research found that reduced social interactions have been associated with lower self-rated health (Subramanian, Kubzansky, Berkman, Fay, & Kawachi, 2006).

Further, existing studies concerning older adults have been limited by the way in which they have failed to adjust for the influence of socioeconomic factors. This void in the literature could lead to biased outcomes and inferences regarding the effect of social cohesion and social capital on older individuals' SRHS. In this chapter, we aim to determine if older adults' social cohesion (i.e., measured by seniors' views of social cohesion around neighborhood issues concerning elderly residents and thereby perceiving that their elderly neighbors are integrated into their neighborhood) is associated with better SRHS. And, second, we examined if such a relationship remained stable after considering relevant individual characteristics (e.g., older respondents' level of education and income and neighbors' attitudes toward seniors).

DATA AND METHODS

The data used to test these hypotheses comes primarily from a survey of Indianapolis, Indiana residents, court data, and census information. Survey responses were collected via telephone interviews in October and November of 2009. The Survey Research Center at Indiana University–Purdue University Indianapolis used random digit dialing to contact residents and solicit participation. Those agreeing to participate spent 10 to 15 minutes answering questions and were compensated with a gift card.

In total, 603 residents (a 65% response rate) from 92 census block groups participated in the larger study. The analyses in this chapter rely primarily on information garnered from the 156 respondents who were between the ages of 65 and 92. Two of the variables in the analyses – neighbors' level of comfort interacting with seniors and neighbors' beliefs that it is important to visit with the elderly – are derived from the responses from the 447 other respondents aggregated to the neighborhood level.

Dependent Variables

The primary variable of interest is elderly respondents' levels of self-rated physical health. The survey posed the question, "How would you rate your physical health?" Respondents answered on a scale of 1–5: 1 "poor," 2 "fair," 3 "Good," 4 "Very Good," and 5 "Excellent." In line with existing literature, we recoded the responses into a binary variable. Our final measure can be understood as whether the respondent is in fair to poor health, with 1 representing poor health and 0 representing good, very good, or excellent health.

Independent Variables

Three predictors were of particular conceptual importance in the analyses. The variable "elderly social cohesion" is intended to measure seniors' views of social cohesion around neighborhood issues that are particularly salient to elderly residents. It presents the mean of responses to the following questions on a 1–5 likert scale ranging from strongly disagree to strongly agree, or very unlikely to very likely.

- People on this block watch out for each other and help out when they can
- You have a strong sense of community with the people on this block
- The specific block you live on is a close knit block
- People on this block check in on elderly neighbors during bad weather
- If he/she needed it, what is the likelihood that a neighbor would assist someone with a cane or walker to cross the street
- If he/she needed it, what is the likelihood of a neighbor reading the newspaper to someone with poor eyesight

The Cronbach's alpha for this scale is 0.83.

We were also interested in neighbors' self-reported feelings about elderly neighbors. We measured this with two separate questions. These questions were not highly correlated with each other (-0.40), so we are left with two measures. Neighbors' social unease toward older adults is based on responses to the statement "I don't feel comfortable around the elderly," and neighbors' attitudes toward interacting with older adults are based on responses to the statement "It is important to visit with elderly neighbors." Level of agreement with each of these statements was rated on a 1–5 scale and then aggregated to the neighborhood level. These measures were included in the database according to neighborhood, so they represent elderly participants' neighbors' responses.

Control Variables

The control variables introduced were seniors' study respondents' education, income, race, age, and gender. Two demographic control variables were coded as dichotomous measures of race (1 = Black; 0 = others) and gender (1 = female). Income included six different categories (ranging from under $10,000 to > $120,000) and was adjusted based on multiple imputation to account for the 35 missing cases. The imputation was based on respondents' level of education, race, gender, and the median household income of their neighborhood. We also controlled for respondents' education attainment, which was entered in the model in three categories: less than high school, high school diploma, and any higher education (as the referent category). The study respondent's age was also included as a continuous measure. We controlled for these variables because previous research has found that each have been associated with SRHS in the senior population (Clark & Maddox, 1992; Ferraro, 1993; Ferraro & Farmer, 1996; Lima-Costa, De Oliveira, Macinko, & Marmot, 2012; Wolinsky et al., 2008).

Analytic Strategy

Using Stata/IC 11.1, we ran multivariate logistic regressions to model associations. To account for the conceptual model, we implemented a nested design. The first model includes all control variables and the social cohesion measure. The other independent measures are added incrementally in Models 2 and 3. Separate analyses indicate that there is little reason to be concerned about multicollinearity in the models.

RESULTS

Table 1 reports the descriptive statistics of the dependent variable, the three key independent variables, and the five control variables. As shown in Table 1, the respondents have diverse background characteristics. The mean age for respondents is 74 years old. The sample is fairly even split according to race: 48% is Black and 50% is White. The majority of respondents are female (69%) and have at least some college education, though educational levels range from less than high school to post graduate degrees. Annual income levels are dispersed between less than $10,000 and over $120,000 per year. Although not represented in the table, the average median family income in these seniors' neighborhoods is nearly $48,000. Overall, 28.7% of individuals reported their health as poor (17.8% as "fair" and 10.8% as "poor"), whereas 71.3% reported their health as being excellent (16.6%), very good (28%), or good (26.7%).

Table 2 reports the results of the multiple logistic regression analysis. Model I indicates that education and income are significantly associated with SRHS. The higher the respondent's income, the less likely s/he is to report poor health. Similarly, people with some college education are less likely to report poor SRHS than those with less than a high school diploma or a high school diploma, respectively. Furthermore, seniors' perception of strong elderly cohesion among neighbors is inversely related to poor health. The protective association between cohesion and poor health (−0.69 log odds) is of a similar magnitude to the risky association between low income

Table 1. Descriptive Characteristics of Participants ($N = 156$).

	Percent (%)
Race	
Black or African American	48.1
White	50.32
Some other race	1.27
Gender	
Female	69.43
Male	30.57
Age	
65–70 years	29.94
71–75 years	30.57
76–80 years	19.1
81–85 years	11.46
86–90 years	7.01
91 + years	1.91
Education	
Less than High School	13.46
High School Graduate	28.21
Some College	17.31
Technical School	3.21
College Graduate	12.82
Post Graduate	25.00
Income	
Under $10,000	14.88
More than $10,000 but less than $30,000	33.06
More than $30,000 but less than $60,000	36.36
More than $60,000 but less than $90,000	9.92
More than $90,000 but less than $120,000	1.65
More than $120,000	4.13
Rating of physical health	
Excellent	16.56
Very Good	28.03
Good	26.75
Fair	17.83
Poor	10.83

and poor health (-0.64 log odds). These variables explain about one-fifth of the variance in poor health among the older respondents (R-squared $= 0.22$).

Model II introduces the first indicator of neighbors' attitudes toward seniors. The results for education and income are similar to those in

Table 2. Nested Logistic Regression of Self-Reported Poor Health on Individual and Neighborhood Characteristics ($N = 156$).

	Model I Coefficient (S.E.)	Model II Coefficient (S.E.)	Model III Coefficient (S.E.)
Constant	−2.69	−3.26	−4.14
	(2.90)	(2.94)	(4.23)
Senior Cohesion	−0.69*	−0.69*	−0.70*
	(0.27)	(0.27)	(0.27)
<High School Education	1.90**	2.29***	2.30***
	(0.61)	(0.65)	(0.65)
High School Education	1.16*	1.12*	1.13*
	(0.47)	(0.49)	(0.49)
Income	−0.64*	−0.67*	−0.67*
	(0.26)	(0.27)	(0.27)
Race	0.09	0.04	0.04
	(0.44)	(0.45)	(0.45)
Age	0.27	0.04	0.04
	(0.32)	(0.03)	(0.03)
Gender	−0.48	−0.17	−0.18
	(0.48)	(0.50)	(0.50)
Unease Around Seniors[a]	–	1.43*	1.33
		(0.67)	(0.73)
Interact with Seniors[a]	–	–	0.24
			(0.83)
Pseudo R^2	0.2184	0.2458	0.2463

Note: *$p < .05$; **$p < .01$; ***$p < .001$.
[a]Based on direct, aggregate reports from neighbors.

Model I. Additionally, neighbors' reports of high social unease toward older adults is significantly associated with seniors' poor health. However, unease around elderly does not explain away the association between neighborhood cohesion and seniors' health: the measure of social cohesion retains statistical significance. Adding the measure of social unease increase the explained variance slightly (R-squared increases to 0.25). Finally, Model III indicates that the association between poor health and seniors' views of neighborhood cohesion remains significant and strong even when neighbors' self-reported feelings about visiting elderly are added into statistical models. This measure is not associated with senior's reports of poor SRHS. Furthermore, when it is added to the model, the association between social unease and poor SRHS loses statistical significance.

DISCUSSION AND CONCLUSION

The primary purpose of this chapter was to test the association between neighborhood cohesion and older individuals' self-rated health status. Hypotheses were grounded in theories with original underpinnings from the classic work of Durkheim, and in turn, culminated in more contemporary perspectives surrounding social connectedness, collective efficacy, and aging. This chapter employed data that reflected the responses of a race–ethnic and socioeconomically diverse sample of community dwelling elders, a segment of society where such information related to the link of neighborhood cohesion and health is scarce. This void in the literature is particularly striking due to the demographic reality of the United States aging population.

Even though the United States presently has a smaller segment of older persons than many of the developed countries, there will soon be demographic challenges. Today, there are over 40 million individuals who are 65 years of age and older and this number is projected to more than double to 89 million by 2050, with most of this increase occurring by 2030. Moreover, those who are 85 and older will number 19 million by 2050, translating into one-fifth of the total population ageing 65 and older (Jacobson, Kent, Lee, & Mather, 2011). This continued increase in life expectancy will offer distinct challenges of keeping older individuals active and maintaining their health status.

Results supported our primary hypothesis. We found that older respondents' perception of strong neighborhood cohesion around issues of particular concern to the senior population was inversely and strongly associated with poor SRHS. This significant association was not attenuated and was of similar magnitude even after adjusting for the participants' neighbors' direct responses regarding their social unease around seniors and their attitudes toward interacting with seniors. In other words, the health of the elderly participants in our study is less dependent on their neighbors' instrumental actions to visit with them or spend time with them. It is more dependent on the neighborhood's willingness to act as a group to address concerns or issues that could have a considerable effect on the elderly population.

These findings are consistent with a growing body of literature on the theoretical link between social cohesion and health status (e.g., see Browning & Cagney, 2002; Cagney et al., 2005; Cramm et al., 2013). However, our study makes several unique contributions to the literature. First, in contrast to many of the previous studies, our study developed and implemented a social cohesion and measure specifically tailored for and related to older adults' residential experience. This elderly-specific cohesion measure has not been previously developed, but shows good internal consistency. Our contribution, therefore, advances the measurement literature on collective efficacy, especially in an older adult population. Second, whereas many of the previous studies have used a state-level analysis, we were able to focus on a different unit of analysis (i.e., individual-level measure) that enables examination of unique contextual effects of socioeconomic factors.

A secondary purpose of the study was to examine if the effect between older adults' social cohesion and SRHS exists despite accounting for two relevant socioeconomic indicators (respondents' income and level of education). With reference to these significant associations regarding income and education, our findings are similar to previous research. For instance, the work of Subramanian and colleagues (2006) investigated the independent relationship between neighborhood context (i.e., age structure; economic conditions) and SRHS among elders in one US city, and found an individual-level relationship between education and income and poor SRHS among elders. More specifically, Subramanian et al. (2006) found that not having a high school diploma and having an income less than \$10,000 (in 1985) were correlated with a greater likelihood of reporting poor health.

We acknowledge the following caveats specific to the present study. First, our data consists exclusively on self-report information regarding the neighborhood environment and health status at the individual level. There are several methods available for the measurement of neighborhood conditions. For instance, administrative data sources such as US Census data provides objective assessments, as does the measurement of neighborhoods by independent, trained observers (Pruitt, Jeffe, Yan, & Schootman, 2012). However, the self-reported perceived neighborhood social relations and social processes and conditions that our chapter focused on could arguably be only collected via self-report and not by outside observers. In fact, our new and novel measure of "elderly social cohesion" had remarkably high internal consistency (Cronbach's alpha = 0.83). And, this notion has been supported by a recent study, which found that self-reported neighborhood conditions demonstrated satisfactory validity and test–retest reliability in urban populations (Pruitt et al., 2012). At any rate, however, a more comprehensive approach that considers not only individual characteristics, but also older people's neighborhood contexts (e.g., homicide rate for the neighborhood) is warranted to better understand factors associated with SRHS (Bjornstrom, 2011; Cramm et al., 2011, 2013).

Second, it should be pointed out that we did not collect information on elders' social networks and social support, or information on the extent to which the elderly respondents were part of civic associations. Previous research has found that social networks and social support are key characteristics in neighborhoods, especially for elderly individuals, and are correlated with health status (Kawachi et al., 1999; Putnam, 2000; Subramanian et al., 2006). Future research should employ measures of elders' social networks and social support as parallel independent variables in examining the association between "elderly social cohesion" and elders' health status. Despite the fact that we employed a novel item that assessed the elderly respondents' perception of social unease toward the elderly and our social cohesion measure that no study previously used, other research has used an explicit item of social trust as a measure that has some operational overlap. Based on data from the Los Angeles Family and Neighborhood Survey, Bjornstrom (2011) found that distrust in neighbors was significantly associated with fair or poor SRHS. Future research could incorporate Bjornstrom's (2011) single item that assessed trust in neighbors along with the same variables as our study to more comprehensively investigate the link between social cohesion and SRHS.

Third, our sample was from a survey of Indianapolis, IN residents. Due to the unique nature of our sample and its relatively small size ($n = 156$), it is unclear how generalizable our findings are to a broader population of older adults. However, a strength of our sample is that it contained a hetero-geneous group of older adults in terms of race/ethnicity, gender, SRHS, and socioeconomic characteristics. Fourth, our dependent variable, SRHS, is a fundamental measure of health status employed in the sociological and public health literature. It has been found to have high predictive and concurrent validity with several key outcome variables including (morbidity, mortality, and utilization of health services) (Idler & Benyamini, 1997; Idler, Russell, & Davis, 2000). However, at least a couple of studies have found that the reliability of SRHS is worse for disadvantaged socio-demographic groups (e.g., those with lower education and lower income) (Dowd & Zajacova, 2007; Zajacova & Dowd, 2011). Future research should use other self-rating measures of health status in addition to SRHS. Indeed future research should use measures of well-being and measures of mental health (Cramm et al., 2013).

Despite these limitations, this chapter makes contributions in the disciplines of both public health and sociology which has found the link between social environment of local residential neighborhoods and poorer physical health (see Pruitt et al., 2012; Robert, 1999). We can conclude that social cohesion is beneficial to the health status of older adults. These findings are particularly important given the US movement of "active aging," a process of optimizing opportunities for social participation and well-being for community-dwelling seniors (Cramm et al., 2013).

REFERENCES

Barron, M. (1953). Minority group characteristics of the aged in American society. *Journal of Gerontology, 8*, 447–482.

Bjornstrom, E. E. S. (2011). The neighborhood context of relative position, trust, and self-rated health. *Social Science and Medicine, 73*, 42–49.

Browning, C. R., & Cagney, K. A. (2002). Neighborhood structural disadvantage, collective efficacy, and self-rated physical health in an urban setting. *Journal of Health and Social Behavior, 43*, 383–399.

Cagney, K. A., Browning, C. R., & Wen, M. (2005). Racial disparities in self-rated health at older ages: What difference does the neighborhood make? *Journal of Gerontology: Social Sciences, 60*, S181–S190.

Clark, D. O., & Maddox, G. L. (1992). Racial and social correlates of age-related changes in functioning. *Journals of Gerontology: Social Sciences, 47*, S222–S232.

Cramm J. M., van Kijk, H., Lotters, F., van Exel, F., & Nieboer, A. P. (2011). *Evaluating an integrated neighborhood approach to improve well-being of frail elderly in a Dutch community: A study protocol.* BMC Research Notes, 4, 532. Biomedcentral.com/1756-0500/4/532.

Cramm, J. M., van Dikj, H. M., & Nieboer, A. P. (2013). The importance of neighborhood social cohesino and social capital for the well being of older adults in the community. *The Gerontologist, 53*(1), 142–152. doi:10.1093/geront/gns052

Dowd, J. B., & Zajacova, A. (2007). Does the predictive power of self-rated health for subsequent mortality risk vary by socioeconomic status in the US? *International Journal of Epidemiology, 36*, 1214–1221.

Durkheim, E. (1895, 1964). In G. E. G. Catlin (Ed.), *The rules of sociological method* (S. A. Solovay & J. H. Mueller, Trans.) (8th ed.). New York, NY: Free Press.

Engstrom, K., Mattsson, F., Jarleborg, A., & Hallqvist, J. (2008). Contextual social capital as a risk factor for poor self-rated health: A multilevel analysis. *Social Science and Medicine, 66*, 2268–2280.

Ferraro, K. F. (1993). Are black older adults health-pessimistic? *Journal of Health and Social Behavior, 34*, 201–214.

Ferraro, K. F., & Farmer, M. M. (1996). Double jeopardy, aging as a leveler or persistent health inequality? A longitudinal analysis of white and black Americans. *Journals of Gerontology: Social Sciences, 51*, S319–S328.

Idler, E. L., & Benyamini, Y. (1997). Self-rated health and mortality: A review of twenty-seven community studies. *Journal of Health and Social Behavior, 38*, 21–37.

Idler, E. L., Russell, L. B., & Davis, D. (2000). Survival, functional limitations, and self-rated health in the NHANES I Epidemiologic follow-up survey. *American Journal of Epidemiology, 152*, 874–883.

Jacobson, L. A., Kent, M., Lee, M., & Mather, M. (2011). America's aging population. *Population Bulletin, 66*(1).

Kawachi, I., & Berkman, L. (2000). Social cohesion, social capital, and health. In L. Berkman & I. Kawachi (Eds.), *Social epidemiology* (pp. 174–190). New York, NY: Oxford University Press.

Kawachi, I., Kennedy, B. P., & Glass, R. (1999). Social capital and self-rated health: A contextual analysis. *American Journal of Public Health, 89*, 1187–1193.

Krause, N. (1996). Neighborhood deterioration and self-rated health in later life. *Psychology and Aging, 11*, 342–352.

Liang, J., Quinones, A. R., Bennett, J. M., Ye, W., Xu, X., Shaw, B. A., & Ofstedal, M. B. (2010). Evolving self-rated health in middle and old age: How does it differ across black, hispanic, and white americans? *Journal of Aging and Health, 22*, 3–26.

Lima-Costa, M. F., Oliveria, C., Jacinko, J., & Marmot, M. (2012). Socioeconomic inequalites in health in older adults in Brazil and England. *American Journal of Public Health, 102*, 1535–1541.

Mohnen, S. M., Groenewegen, P. P., Volker, B., & Flap, H. (2011). Neighborhood social capital and individual health. *Social Science and Medicine, 72*, 660–667.

O'Hanlon, A. M., Camp, C. J., & Osofsky, H. J. (1993). Knowledge of and attitudes toward aging in young, middle aged and older college students. *Educational Gerontology, 19*, 753–766.

Pruitt, S. L., Jeffe, D. B., Yan, Y., & Schootman, M. (2012). Reliability of perceived neighborhood conditions and the effects of measurement error on self-rated health across urban and rural neighborhoods. *Journal of Epidemiology and Community Health, 66*, 342–351.

Putnam, R. D. (2000). *Bowling alone.* New York, NY: Simon & Schuster.

Robert, S. A. (1999). Socioeconomic position and health: The independent contribution of community socioeconomic context. *Annual Review of Sociology, 25*, 489–516.

Ron, P. (2007). Elderly people's attitudes and perceptions of aging and old age: The role of cognitive dissonance? *International Journal of Geriatric Psychiatry, 22*, 656–662.

Rosow, I. (1974). *Socialization to old age.* Berkeley, CA: University of California Press.

Sampson, R. J., Raudenbush, S. W., & Earls, F. (1997). Neighborhoods and violent crime: A multilevel study of collective efficacy. *Science, 227*, 918–923.

Stephan, W. G., Stephan, C. W., Stefanenko, T., Ageyev, V., Abalakina, M., & Coates-Shrider, L. (1993). Measuring stereotypes: A comparison methods using Russian and American samples. *Social Psychology Quarterly, 56*, 54–64.

Subramanian, S., Kim, D., & Kawachi, I. (2002). Social trust and self-rated health in US communities: A multilevel analysis. *Journal of Urban Health, 79*(4 Suppl. 1), 21–34.

Subramanian, S., Kubzansky, L., Berkman, L., Fay, M., & Kawachi, I. (2006). Neighborhood effects on self-rated health of elders: Uncovering the relative importance of structural and service related neighborhood environments. *Journal of Gerontology: Social Sciences, 61*, S153–S160.

Wolinsky, F. D., Miller, T. R., Malmstrom, T. K., Miller, J. P., Schootman, M., Andresen, E. M., & Miller, D. K. (2008). Self-rated health: Changes, trajectories, and their antecedents among African Americans. *Journal of Aging and Health, 20*, 143–158.

Zajacova, A., & Dowd, J. B. (2011). Reliability of self-rated health in US adults. *American Journal of Epidemiology, 174*, 977–983.

STRUCTURAL AND HIDDEN BARRIERS TO A LOCAL PRIMARY HEALTH CARE INFRASTRUCTURE: AUTONOMY, DECISIONS ABOUT PRIMARY HEALTH CARE, AND THE CENTRALITY AND SIGNIFICANCE OF POWER

Christopher R. Freed, Shantisha T. Hansberry and Martha I. Arrieta

ABSTRACT

Purpose – *To examine a local primary health care infrastructure and the reality of primary health care from the perspective of residents of a small, urban community in the southern United States.*

Methodology/approach – *Data were derived from 13 semistructured focus groups, plus three semistructured interviews, and were analyzed inductively consistent with a grounded theory approach.*

Social Determinants, Health Disparities and Linkages to Health and Health Care
Research in the Sociology of Health Care, Volume 31, 57–81
Copyright © 2013 by Emerald Group Publishing Limited
All rights of reproduction in any form reserved
ISSN: 0275-4959/doi:10.1108/S0275-4959(2013)0000031006

Findings – Structural barriers *to the local primary health care infrastructure include transportation, clinic and appointment wait time, and co-payments and health insurance.* Hidden barriers *consist of knowledge about local health care services, nonphysician gatekeepers, and fear of medical care. Community residents have used home remedies and the emergency department at the local academic medical center to manage these structural and hidden barriers.*

Research limitations/implications – *Findings might not generalize to primary health care infrastructures in other communities, respondent perspectives can be biased, and the data are subject to various interpretations and conceptual and thematic frameworks. Nevertheless, the structural and hidden barriers to the local primary health care infrastructure have considerably diminished the autonomy community residents have been able to exercise over their decisions about primary health care, ultimately suggesting that efforts concerned with increasing the access of medically underserved groups to primary health care in local communities should recognize the centrality and significance of power.*

Originality/value – *This study addresses a gap in the sociological literature regarding the impact of specific barriers to primary health care among medically underserved groups.*

Keywords: Structural and hidden barriers; local primary health care infrastructure; autonomy; decisions; power; health disparities

INTRODUCTION

In 2000, former United States Secretary of Health and Human Services Donna E. Shalala and former Assistant Secretary for Health and Surgeon General David Satcher challenged the nation to accomplish the agenda set forth in *Healthy People 2010*, an ambitious array of health-related objectives and focus areas intended to increase the life quality and expectancy among all Americans by 2010 and to entirely eliminate health disparities. Diversity is one of the country's most important attributes, Shalala and Satcher declared, but it also presents an enormous challenge with respect to improving the health of the American population, in particular "the principle that – regardless of age, gender, race or ethnicity, income, education, geographic location, disability, and sexual orientation – every person in every community across the Nation deserves equal access to comprehensive, culturally competent, community-based health care systems that are committed to serving the needs of the individual and promoting community health" (U.S. Department of Health and Human Services, 2000, p. 16).

That *Healthy People 2010* sought to ensure equal access to community-based health care systems for "every person in every community across the Nation" reconfirmed that a substantial portion of Americans confronted numerous barriers to health care in their local community, this despite myriad efforts since the mid-19th century to reduce such barriers (see Dell & Whitman, 2011; U.S. Department of Health and Human Services, 1990; Williams & Sternthal, 2010). As we detail shortly using data that convey the long-term relevance of this *Healthy People 2010* principle, less pronounced in the current *Healthy People 2020* report (U.S. Department of Health and Human Services Office of Disease Prevention and Health Promotion, n.d.), barriers to health care in local communities have included transportation (e.g., Ahmed, Lemkau, Nealeigh, & Mann, 2001; Carr, Ibuka, & Russell, 2010; Horton & Johnson, 2010; Pesata, Pallija, & Webb, 1999; Rittner & Kirk, 1995; Silver, Blustein, & Weitzman, 2012), wait time for medical care (e.g., Carr et al., 2010; Green et al., 2008; Kaplan et al., 2006; Pesata et al., 1999; Rust et al., 2008), treatment costs and inadequate or no health insurance (e.g., Ahmed et al., 2001; Horton & Johnson, 2010; Seccombe & Amey, 1995; Snead & Cockerham, 2002; Stevens & Keigher, 2009), scarce information about health services (e.g., Ahmed et al., 2001; Kirby & Kaneda, 2006; Silver et al., 2012; Thiede, 2005; Umberson & Montez, 2010), run-ins with nonphysician staff at community clinics (e.g., Arber & Sawyer, 1985; Barr & Wanat, 2005; Ford, Tilson, Smurzynski, Leone, & Miller, 2008; Hughes, 1989; Kaplan et al., 2006), and the unintended consequences of medical diagnoses (e.g., Darby, Davis, Likes, & Bell, 2009; Ford et al., 2008; Green et al., 2008; Jutel, 2009; Martin et al., 2010). The research literature has of course covered how race, ethnicity, and socioeconomic status can act as barriers to health care (e.g., Barr, 2008; Budrys, 2010; Cockerham, 2007; Eiser & Ellis, 2007; Hoberman, 2012; Horton & Johnson, 2010; Kasper, 2000; Kirby & Kaneda, 2005; Kronenfeld, 2005, 2010; Lichtenstein, 2003; Link & Phelan, 1995; Lutfey & Freese, 2005; Martin et al., 2010; Mechanic, 2002; Williams, 2012; Williams & Collins, 1995; Williams & Sternthal, 2010) as well as methods utilized to handle these barriers (e.g., Boyd, Taylor, Shimp, & Semler, 2000; Brown & Segal, 1996; Eiser & Ellis, 2007; Koenig, McCullough, & Larson, 2001; Malone, 1995; Martin et al., 2010; Rust et al., 2008; Shippee, Schafer, & Ferraro, 2012; Walls, Rhodes, & Kennedy, 2002).

Barriers to health care in local communities, however, do not simply limit access to health care in general. More to our focus, barriers to health care in local communities limit access to local systems of health care clinics and hospital services that comprise a local primary health care infrastructure. One route to better understand barriers to a local primary health care infrastructure, including the broader significance of these barriers to the individuals who confront them, is to consider the perspectives of community residents whom the infrastructure should serve. Indeed, a "micro-community" approach is suited to capture "local level" perspectives (Channing, 2011, p. vii–viii) about barriers to health care (U.S. Department of Health and Human Services, 2000). Community-specific data can expose local barriers to a primary health care infrastructure and strategies local residents use to manage these barriers (see Shah, Whitman, & Benjamins, 2011).

In this chapter, we examine a local primary health care infrastructure from the perspective of residents from seven different zip codes of a small, urban community in the southern United States. What we conceptualize as *structural barriers* to the local primary health care infrastructure include transportation, clinic and appointment wait time, and co-payments and health insurance. *Hidden barriers* to the local primary health care infrastructure consist of knowledge about local health care services, nonphysician gatekeepers, and fear of medical care. Residents we spoke to have used home remedies and the emergency department at the local academic medical center to manage these structural and hidden barriers. Berger and Luckmann (1966) contend that "everyday life presents itself as a reality interpreted by men and subjectively meaningful to them as a coherent world" (p. 19). To understand this reality, "account must be taken of its intrinsic character" (Berger & Luckmann, 1966, p. 19). The reality of primary health care from the perspective of community residents is that the structural and hidden barriers to the local primary health care infrastructure have limited the access they and other community members have to primary health care. More intrinsically, however, the structural and hidden barriers to the local primary health care infrastructure have considerably diminished the autonomy community residents have been able to exercise over their decisions about primary health care, ultimately suggesting that efforts concerned with increasing the access of medically underserved groups to primary health care in local communities should recognize the centrality and significance of power.

METHODS

Data for this chapter are derived from 13 semistructured focus groups with three to nine respondents in each, plus three semistructured interviews (due to unforeseen respondent scheduling matters) conducted by study personnel with experience in qualitative methods between March 2006 and September 2006. To promote the study, we displayed posters about the research at the local academic medical center and at the medical center's adjacent health care clinic that identified recruitment sites, explained recruitment procedures, and listed the location of focus groups. We also distributed flyers with this information in the emergency department waiting area of the local academic medical center and in the waiting area of the medical center's adjacent health care clinic. To be included in the study, respondents needed to reside in one of seven zip codes that comprise the focus area of the Excellence in Partnerships for Community Outreach and Research on Disparities in Health and Training (EXPORT), an initiative sponsored by the National Institutes of Health that encourages collaboration among academic and community groups. Individuals younger than 19 years of age, persons with a psychiatric diagnosis, and residents of the EXPORT focus area who did not speak English were excluded from the study.

We recruited a total of 75 respondents: 39 respondents at two Federally Qualified Health Centers (FQHCs) and at the local academic medical center's adjacent health care clinic that both served the uninsured and underinsured, 21 respondents at a local not-for-profit social service agency for the disadvantaged, including the uninsured and underinsured, and 15 respondents at a church and a public library. Each respondent provided informed consent and received $15.00 for participating in the research. To preserve the anonymity of respondents since over half of the study participants (52%) were recruited at the two FQHCs or at the local academic medical center's adjacent health care clinic where they had visited and could visit again, we did not record their names or identifying background or demographic information, although based on observations almost all respondents were African-American and the vast majority were female (M. I. Arrieta, personal communication, June 22, 2012). Throughout the chapter we do identify by code, where appropriate, the focus group or interview from which data were derived: FG = focus group and I = interview. The number adjacent to these codes represents the order in which the focus groups and interviews were conducted. The University of South Alabama Office of Research Compliance and Assurance approved the study protocol.

Four focus groups were conducted at the FQHCs, three focus groups and the three interviews were conducted at a public library neighboring the local academic medical center's adjacent health care clinic, and six focus groups were conducted at the not-for-profit social service agency, the church, or the public library where we recruited a portion of respondents. Each focus group and interview was tape-recorded and 45 minutes to two hours in duration to elicit the perspectives of respondents about the local primary health care infrastructure, in particular perspectives about infrastructure services, primary health care needs in the EXPORT focus area, and what it means to have a primary health care provider. In 2006, the local primary health care infrastructure consisted of 18 health care clinics and six hospitals, but usually respondents talked about a more select group of facilities, mainly those clinics with which they were most familiar, that to protect the location of the study we do not identify by name.

Consistent with a grounded theory approach (e.g., Glaser & Strauss, 1967/ 2006; Grbich, 2007; Liamputtong, 2011), we analyzed the focus group and interview data inductively using the qualitative analysis program Atlas.ti to organize the information. In the course of reading each focus group and interview transcript, the lead analyst (CRF) followed an open coding scheme to identify phrases, sentences, and segments of focus group and interview text that yielded 15 emerging analytic categories. These categories were "agency and autonomy," "context," "continuity," "cost," "elderly," "emergency room," "fear," "gatekeeping," "homeless," "home remedy," "knowledge," "solutions," "transportation," "treatment and insurance," and "wait time." Next, the lead analyst reexamined each of the coded focus group and interview transcripts to confirm the accuracy of these analytic categories. During this stage of analysis the lead analyst also coded additional phrases, sentences, and segments of focus group and interview text missed during the first level of open coding. These data corresponded to one or more of the original 15 analytic categories, exposed new analytic categories, and, following an axial coding scheme to reach thematic saturation, required that some of the first-level analytic categories be combined under an existing or renamed thematic code or be omitted from the analysis altogether because of insufficient data. With consensus from the research team, the lead analyst then reorganized the focus group and interview data under 10 main thematic categories: "community context," "cost," "fear," "gatekeeping and mis-treatment," "home remedies," "hospital emergency department," "knowl-edge," "solutions," "transportation," and "wait time." These thematic categories provide the conceptual and organizational basis for the chapter and point to a link between structural and hidden barriers to the local primary health care infrastructure and autonomy over decisions about primary health care.

THE EXPORT FOCUS AREA: COMMUNITY DEMOGRAPHICS AND HEALTH-RELATED CHALLENGES

Before we present the structural and hidden barriers to the local primary health care infrastructure that respondents identified, we should first describe the basic demographic composition of residents who lived in the EXPORT focus area in 2006 and, briefly, specific health-related challenges that respondents reported area residents confront.

African-Americans comprised between 41% and 99% of the total population of each EXPORT focus area zip code (U.S. Census Bureau, 2000a). Approximately 88% of residents in the EXPORT focus area were employed, the median household income was $21,033, and 20%–51% of the total population of each EXPORT focus area zip code lived below poverty (U.S. Census Bureau, 2000b). Thirty-one percent of residents in the EXPORT focus area had earned a high school diploma while another 30% did not complete high school (U.S. Census Bureau, 2000c). Between 2004 and 2007, nearly 85% of residents from the EXPORT focus area who were admitted to the local academic medical center for treatment were uninsured or relied on Medicaid or Medicare to pay for health care (Gulati, Mohammad, & Arrieta, 2009; see Table 1 for more information). Correspondingly, 80% of the respondents in this study were recruited at sites that served the uninsured or underinsured (see above).

Respondents described their neighbors as "very sick" and neighborhoods in the EXPORT focus area as "infested" (FG-8) with high blood pressure, high cholesterol, and diabetes. "Lifestyle [and] bad diets," "eating habits," "the way you prepare your food," and "lack of exercise" (I-2) have contributed to these conditions. In addition, "a lot of people will opt for medication other than doing what it takes to try to [be healthy]" (I-2) whereas others, as we explain later in the chapter, "are just treating themselves … because they can't see anybody [a primary care provider] because they don't have the funds" (FG-11). One informant argued that "a health care problem … could consist of … something that was a risk to everybody's health." For example, "I live right on the corner where the ditch forever holds water," this informant described, "and that water is

Table 1. EXPORT Focus Area Zip Code Delimited Population by Poverty, Race, and Insurance Status.

Zip Code	Total Population	Below Poverty[a,b,c]	White[a,c]	African-American[a,c]	Insurance Status[d,e]						
					Uninsured	Medicaid	Medicare	Private	Military	Other	Unknown
-02	867	22.3	54.8	42.0	0.3	0.3	0.2	0.0	0.0	0.2	0.0
-03	12,526	50.6	6.1	92.6	3.0	3.8	3.2	0.3	0.0	0.3	0.7
-04	11,533	26.6	44.6	53.0	2.3	1.7	1.2	0.3	0.1	0.2	0.4
-05	33,471	28.1	36.4	61.1	5.9	7.7	4.0	1.7	0.2	0.5	1.2
-06	19,007	19.9	56.5	40.5	2.9	2.0	2.0	0.7	0.1	0.3	0.8
-10	19,717	49.1	2.8	96.3	9.3	11.0	6.4	1.3	0.1	0.2	1.6
-17	16,158	30.3	0.8	98.5	5.2	6.4	6.1	1.4	0.2	0.3	2.1

[a]Source: U.S. Census Bureau (2000a, 2000b).
[b]Among individuals for whom poverty status is determined.
[c]% of total population.
[d]% of admissions (N = 1,510) to local academic medical center, 2004–2007 (based on the latest encounter) (M. I. Arrieta, personal communication, February 20, 2011). Percentages do not total 100 due to rounding.
[e]Source: Gulati et al. (2009).

a breeding ground for mosquitoes, rodents, and other little pests that will come in your house" (I-3). Focus groups discussed neighborhood violence and identified "gunshot wounds" and "stabbing" (FG-2B) as familiar reasons for emergency medical care. "I just see [my neighbors] get shot and [the] ambulance ... takes them out," one respondent stated. "I try not to associate with anybody ... so I won't be in none of that trauma" (FG-2A). Indeed, residents in some EXPORT focus area zip codes "don't seek health care" because they are "scared to get out" (I-2).

STRUCTURAL BARRIERS TO THE LOCAL PRIMARY HEALTH CARE INFRASTRUCTURE

Transportation

Respondents seldom mentioned access to private transportation to get to and from medical facilities of the local primary health care infrastructure. They did, however, frequently criticize public bus transportation. The wait for the public bus was a source of frustration as was the distance between bus stops and homes and local clinics. Other problems with public bus transportation included travel time to, and personal safety in, some of the areas where health care clinics were located. The following statements illustrated the disadvantages of public bus transportation:

> If you don't have a car and you have to wait for the bus, it kind of makes you mad (FG-12).

> The bus don't [drop] you off in your community (FG-9).

> I had to walk 10 blocks from the bus stop. It hard to be traveling to these clinics (FG-9).

> They [the bus] always go way over here somewhere or over there somewhere .... You might as well get ready to be on a bus for an hour (FG-10).

> It's still a kind of problem with the bus because of security. The bus is still a barrier. The problem is the area getting off the bus getting to the doctor (FG-9).

Elderly residents too frail to ride the public bus, as well as their family members, have dealt with additional transportation challenges. "Some people might not have anybody to help them" (FG-12) such as "an older lady [with] Alzheimer's [who] says that there is never no one around to take her to [the] doctor" (FG-3). As it happens, younger relatives have moved from the local area. Family members who do live close to aging loved ones have had to miss work to make certain older relatives promptly receive the primary care they need. The comments below typified these challenges, and uncertainty about who is responsible for health care for the elderly:

> Some of them [elderly residents] just can't get around. Their relatives, children's children's, have moved out (FG-9).

> My aunts and all of us are taking off from work to … make sure they get to the doctor's…. So that's kind of hard (FG-4).

> You may have where the family member can't … take them, so maybe they won't go that time. They will go eventually, but not like when they need [to] (I-1).

> I am thinking responsibility for care to the elderly. I am wondering who that falls to (FG-4).

Clinic and Appointment Wait Time

Long wait times for medical care at clinics in the local primary health care infrastructure were common. Focus groups attributed long waits to physician staffing shortages. One clinic, for instance, "only have two doctors, so it take like all day to get waited on." This clinic opened at 8:00 am, but one of its physicians "only get there like at 9:00 or 9:15. And then he [the physician] have like 20 people up in there waiting." At another clinic, "it just takes a long time [to see the physician] because it's only him and he got like a few trained people who are helping him" (FG-3). Wait times in excess of three to four hours have persuaded area residents to delay primary health care. "Some of them will get up and leave" after deciding "[I] ain't going to stay no longer" (FG-12). This decision can be permanent:

> I'm not going to go to a doctor when I'm sick, because I can't wait (I-3).

> I am not coming back (FG-12).

Fixed appointment times have not reduced long waits, especially if "you got 30 people coming in for one appointment" (FG-7). Moreover, long gaps between appointments have made preexisting medical conditions such as chronic arthritis worse. Consider the following:

> I had an appointment like 7 o'clock in the morning. I don't leave up out of [the clinic] until 4 o'clock in the evening. I have six kids. I have to be home to get my kids off the bus. I have to let my kids in the house. And that just makes it very hard on me (FG-2A).

> Once you do call and try to make an appointment, your appointment is so far away (FG-12).

They [the clinic] say, "We want to see you in six months," [but] they won't make you no appointment. If he [the physician] want to see you [in] three months, they will not make appointments. They will tell you to call them. But when you call back, they will put you off.... I swells up sometimes. I can't turn over. I can't move.... I make myself deal with the pain, but it's not right (FG-11).

Co-Payments and Health Insurance

To reiterate, in 2006 the median household income in the EXPORT focus area was $21,033. In one EXPORT focus area zip code, 51% of residents lived below poverty. "People in the community ... don't go to the doctor because they don't have the money. They would like to go, but they don't have the money" (FG-11). Co-payments particularly discouraged respondents from seeking care through the local primary health care infrastructure. Furthermore, some infrastructure facilities refused to treat patients without the required co-payment:

You would go if you could get in there – if they will just accept you without the co-pay (FG-7).

Sometimes that $5.00 can add up by me going regular like I should instead [of only] on the days that I can (FG-10).

Once they bring you up, they will ask you for your money. [Without the co-payment], you can't be seen (FG-2B).

If I don't have the co-pay, they might just say, "The doctor can't see you today" (FG-12).

Respondents also saw a connection between health insurance and the quality of medical care, from the speed with which services were rendered to the treatment patients received. They expressed considerable frustration, directed at physicians, about health care costs and about health insurance in general. Amid the comments in reference to these issues were:

Somebody comes in and they don't have any insurance, nor do they have Medicaid. They [the primary care facility] wait on them more slower (I-3).

I got two kids. One got Blue Cross and one has Medicaid. The one that got Blue Cross, they put him in a private room. The one with Medicaid, they want to put him in a different one. I said, "No, I want them in the same room".... It look like the one with Medicaid got treated a little bit better when he was in the room with the good insurance. It's a difference (FG-4).

I was watching the animal program one day and the dog couldn't have the operation because the lady didn't have the money to pay for it.... They had to put the dog to sleep.

I think we are about the same way. When we don't have our insurance, I think they [physicians] would put us to sleep too. But they don't put us to sleep because they have to take a Hippocratic Oath. They just put us on the bottom end (I-3).

HIDDEN BARRIERS TO THE LOCAL PRIMARY HEALTH CARE INFRASTRUCTURE

Knowledge about Local Health Care Services

A number of respondents reported that their neighbors lacked information about the services offered through the local primary health care infrastructure: what facilities to go to for primary health care, the nature of the assistance offered, and the cost of medical treatment. For example, when an informant identified a health care clinic whose pharmacy dispensed free medication, "I know that," said someone in the same focus group, "but everybody don't" (FG-6). It seems that communication and networking among area residents about health-related issues have rarely occurred. Typical remarks about these matters included:

They don't know what places to go to [for primary health care] (FG-2B).

[They] don't know that you can go places where [medical care] is affordable or even free (I-2).

The other day this man was talking. He didn't go [to a clinic] because he didn't have any money. They don't know about the benefits they could get.... I think that people would go more if they knew (I-3).

[Health care] is not really nothing that you have a conversation about .... I really never had a conversation with anybody about where you go.... Just never thought about bringing it up, or nobody ever talked about [it].... We don't never sit and talk about [the] doctor. We don't never say, "Who your doctor?"... We don't dwell on that conversation (I-3).

Nonphysician Gatekeepers

Gatekeepers "grant or withhold benefits on behalf of the employing institution that possesses and disburses them" (Freidson, 1986, p. 167). Nonphysician staff, mostly in health care clinics, have acted as gatekeepers vis-à-vis the authority they have to "put [you] on the back burner" (I-3). To be sure:

You just have some, ... they want to take control and take over. They think they own the place (FG-12).

Those ladies that be sitting out there in the front desks, they sit out there [and] run their mouth. They would not call you for nothing. They sit up there and talk about who went to bed with who, who dated who, what happened last week (FG-12).

You out there standing two or three hours ... [while] they are back there gossiping (FG-11).

A receptionist at one clinic ignored a patient who could not afford high blood pressure treatment. "She [the patient] didn't see a doctor. The receptionist stopped it cold" (FG-11). At a different clinic, a respondent waited "practically three hours" for care. "My doctor had to go to the emergency room. I blame the nurses and the people in the back that didn't let me know" (I-3).

In the medical profession, support staff seek to reduce obstacles that interfere with their carrying out assigned tasks (Freidson, 1970). Patients who nonphysician gatekeepers perceived as troublesome or otherwise difficult, therefore, occasionally experienced disrespect. This happened to one informant at the very clinic where we conducted one of the focus groups:

Yesterday, because they changed my appointment, I came in here [irritated].... The security guard grab me. He bruised my arm.... [I said], "If he put his hands on me I was going to kick his [expletive]" .... Came in here today and the man out there told me if *he* [italics added] had been here yesterday, "What happened yesterday wouldn't have happened".... He had no business saying nothing to me. You have some people up in here that are so nasty. They think ... just because they work behind the desks that we are supposed to take all the mess that they want to issue out (FG-12).

The confrontation that ensued after a respondent asked a clinic staff member for a doctor's note ended just as badly. "It was the way that the lady spoke to me.... Her and I had words and then the receptionist jumped in and said, 'You need to take your trashy butt on out of here'" (FG-11). One informant remembered when a staff member at a local facility suggested that the side-effects of the medication he was prescribed were no excuse for "a man" to miss work:

One lady, one time, had pulled my sleeve up. She said, "You see them muscles you got there? You can work." I said, "Madame, these papers say for me not to drive, not to work, not to operate no machine, or nothing. You see all this medicine here? If I take this medicine now, I won't be able to do nothing." [She said], "But you are able now to do something. You are [a] man. You are not a woman. You are not wearing a dress".... I mean, really, this is what I was told (FG-9).

We cannot assume that racial prejudice provokes these types of attitudes. Indeed:

A lot of times it be some of our race ... that does it towards us (FG-6).

It don't have to be somebody White that's doing it towards somebody Black. We go against our own race (FG-6).

Fear of Medical Care

Occasionally, respondents mentioned rather familiar fears about medical care such as "the thought of having to stick a needle in me" (FG-11). More commonly, however, they expressed fears about receiving an adverse medical diagnosis. One informant, for instance, raised the topic of HIV-AIDS. "As long as a person don't know that they got something, life goes on. Once they know about these things, it kills them. The body and the mind just deteriorate" (FG-9). Still broader comments related to fears about receiving an adverse medical diagnosis included the following:

They may tell me something that I don't want to hear (FG-7).

I don't want to know something that's going to make me scared (FG-7).

They may make matters worse (FG-7).

A lot of people fear what is wrong ... [because they] just can't afford it.... They don't have any insurance (FG-7).

A respondent in one focus group experienced "a lot of incidents [as a child] where I did not go to the doctor. I slammed my fingers in an iron door and [my mother] wouldn't take me to the hospital." Participants in the same focus group explained. "If her mom would have taken her to the hospital, they [hospital staff] might have said, ... 'Who slammed your finger in the door? ... Did your mom slam your finger in the door?'" In short, "they want to report you to [child protective services]" (FG-4). An informant and her brother had to contend with a situation like this when she was a young girl. As this informant recalled:

We were playing in the backyard and he [the informant's brother] dislocated his elbow. When he got to the hospital he kept saying, "My sister did it.... We were just playing." But when my mom left out of the room for a minute, the police asked my brother, "Who really did this? Did your mom do it?" He kept saying, "My sister made a mistake.... We were just playing".... [The police] would wait a few minutes and then come back in and ask him to see if he was telling the same thing (FG-4).

Not surprisingly, fear of being accused of child abuse has posed serious health consequences. In one especially alarming case that a respondent cited:

I know this lady [with] two small children. [One child's] skin had broke out real bad and [the lady] come knock on my door. And I was like, "I don't know you," but she [the child] had an allergic reaction to something. I was like, "Go on and take her to the hospital." [The lady] was like, "Oh no, no, no" and she kept putting it off. Fifteen minutes later she come beating on my door talking about, "Let me use your phone. My baby is over there having [a] seizure" (FG-4)!

The lasting emotional effects of racial oppression have also generated fear of medical care. According to one informant, "all the Black people are a little bit afraid of White people, and that from slavery – all older Black people in their 70s and 80s." In fact, "the majorities [of Black people] are fearful [of White doctors]," this informant continued. "My mother ... was afraid to go to them and her condition had got severe – too severe" (I-3).

STRATEGIES TO MANAGE THE STRUCTURAL AND HIDDEN BARRIERS

Home Remedies

For some respondents, one strategy to manage the structural and hidden barriers to the local primary health care infrastructure has been to "treat their own selves" (I-3) with home remedies. "You don't need to go running to the doctor [when] you don't feel good" (I-1) because, as one informant asserted, "whoever at home ... [can] tell you what to take, and you get cured at home sometimes" (FG-2B). Home remedies have included "green water and juice" for the chicken pox, "the yoke from inside the raw egg" for a boil (FG-8), and "turpentine and sugar" (FG-9) for the common cold. A respondent suffering from back pain "just deal[s] with it" to which someone else replied, "that's a home remedy" (FG-4). In addition:

When I was a little girl I stepped on some nails in a block and it went through my feet. My mom did not take me to the hospital. She took me upstairs, got a hammer, and beat the palm of my feet ... to get [the] bad blood out (FG-4).

Everything is, "Take a laxative." If your stomach hurts, "Take a laxative." If your back [or] ... your head hurts, "You just need to be cleaned out" (FG-4).

We got a "neighborhood doctor".... He ain't really no licensed practiced doctor. We go to him under the table when [we] can't afford a doctor (FG-9).

"Older people think the home remedy is going to fix it all" (FG-4). One informant told us about a toothache his father once had. "He wouldn't go to the dentist. He would take something like 'oral gel'" (I-2). A respondent's grandfather with severe calluses on the bottom of his feet refused repeatedly to see a podiatrist. "He just say, 'I'll just put some lotion on it'.... I keep telling him if it gets any worse, you can lose your feet" (FG-4). Residents in the local area have also looked to spiritual faith as a home remedy. One informant's grandfather apparently died because of his spiritual faith. "He wasn't supposed to believe that God was going to let him get sick because, 'God don't do no evil'.... He died with cancer because he wouldn't go to the doctor" (FG-8). Other statements about prioritizing spirituality over primary health care were:

> You got people that believe, "Nothing is wrong with me and I don't care ... if [the physician] believe any different. I believe in Jesus Christ".... They won't go [to the doctor] for that reason (FG-8).

> [You] really don't have to take any medicine. All you have to do is give it some time and eat right and your body will cure itself. That's the way God made it (FG-8).

> Can't anybody cure but Jesus (FG-7).

The Emergency Department at the Local Academic Medical Center

At about the time this study was conceived, 61% of emergency department visits at the local academic medical center were for conditions that could have been managed in a primary care setting (Arrieta & Mulars, 2006). "Some people think everything is [an emergency]" (FG-4) including, as respondents listed, a headache, coughing, cramps, diarrhea, and gas. "I got my toenail removed," one informant acknowledged, "because it was in trauma" (FG-2B). Others described the emergency department, especially at the local academic medical center, as a "fellowship" (FG-9) that "a lot of the people think ... is funny. 'There goes Ms. Jones going to the emergency room again'.... [However], they don't look down on them" (I-1).

Indeed, area residents have not stigmatized individuals who have taken advantage of emergency department services, and have themselves sought primary health care from the emergency department at the local academic medical center, knowing that neither cash nor health insurance is needed to receive treatment. But more than this, for a majority of emergency department patients at the local academic medical center, as many as 77% of whom once had a primary care provider (Arrieta & Mulars, 2006), the emergency department has been "the best resource" (FG-2B) for primary health care compared to the alternative:

> If I'm sick, I'm not going [to the doctor] just to sit (I-3).

> Say you're not in dire, dire need but you feel like you need to be checked on. That's the time your doctor's office may be closed.... [In] the emergency room, [you] find out tonight (I-1).

When you call the doctor and tell them you are having problems, ... they will tell you they don't have any openings, so you might as well go to the emergency room (FG-6).

I call my doctor and he doesn't call me back. I go to the hospital for just about anything (FG-3).

AUTONOMY, DECISIONS ABOUT PRIMARY HEALTH CARE, AND POWER

The general sentiment among respondents was that they and other area residents "wait until they get to their weakest point" before they seek primary health care, or claim "I ain't sick, it will pass, it will go away" (FG-12) to avoid primary health care altogether. These decisions reflect the reality of primary health care for respondents. Berger and Luckmann (1966) contend that "everyday life presents itself as a reality interpreted by men and subjectively meaningful to them as a coherent world" (p. 19). To understand this reality, "account must be taken of its intrinsic character" (Berger & Luckmann, 1966, p. 19). The reality of primary health care from the perspective of respondents is that the structural and hidden barriers to the local primary health care infrastructure have limited the access they and other area residents have to primary health care. More intrinsically, however, the structural and hidden barriers to the local primary health care infrastructure have considerably diminished the autonomy respondents and other area residents have been able to exercise over their decisions about primary health care. "Power has to do with whatever *decisions* [italics added] men make about the arrangements under which they live" (Mills, 1958, p. 29). Respondents and other area residents have suffered "a feeling that have them down where they just can't do anything about [primary health care]" (FG-4).

To illustrate, we can revisit the structural and hidden barriers to the local primary health care infrastructure and speculate, where appropriate, about links between these barriers and some of the health-related challenges local residents have confronted. For example, neighborhood violence and concerns for personal safety in areas where health care clinics are located have forced respondents and other residents to decide whether or not to travel – by public bus or otherwise – for primary health care. Violence and safety concerns have also compelled local residents to disassociate from one another, a decision that might explain the reported lack of communication and networking about health-related issues. Perhaps we should not attribute the decision elderly residents have had to make to delay or do without primary health care to their transportation challenges per se but to a corresponding and equally compulsory decision second and third generation relatives have made – their "children's children's" (FG-9) who maybe once provided transportation – to move to communities that are not a "breeding ground" (I-3), to repeat one informant, for emergency medical care or poor health and disease (see, e.g., Klinenberg, 2002; Wilson, 1987). Family members who remain in the area have had to choose work or offer this transportation, a decision possibly imposed by a rigid day-to-day schedule dictated by the constraints of underemployment (indicated by high employment rates in the EXPORT focus area but a low median household income) and the threat of job loss from what is likely a surplus pool of low-wage workers (see, e.g., Newman, 1999; Wilson, 1996). To miss work can mean less money for these family members to pay for their own primary health care and thus less autonomy over their own primary health care decisions.

It seems fairly clear how public bus transportation, long wait times for medical care and appointments at local clinics, and unaffordable co-payments as well as inadequate or no health insurance coverage can all unduly influence decisions about primary health care. Remember one respondent, for instance, who "had to walk 10 blocks from the bus stop" (FG-9) to a local clinic, a focus group member who was "not coming back" (FG-12) to a clinic because of long waits, or the informant who felt "on the bottom end" (I-3) of health care priorities due to costs and no insurance coverage. We should also reiterate that nonphysician gatekeepers, in the course of exercising authority as the agents of administrative and medical leadership, have required respondents and other area residents to wait extensively and sometimes needlessly for treatment, have disrespected patients, including other African-Americans, and have exploited, at least in one reported case, gender stereotypes, each of which might trigger a decision to postpone or forgo primary health care. And recall fear of medical care: as one respondent acknowledged, medical care, particularly receiving an adverse medical diagnosis, "comes with that fear because … [it is] going to add up to a responsibility" (FG-12). But how can respondents and other area residents fulfill this responsibility – that is, self-assuredly decide to "seek *technically competent* help … and to *cooperate* … in the process of trying to get well" (Parsons, 1951, p. 437) – and thereby reduce their fear of medical care if burdened by primary health care costs or accusations of child abuse by hospital staff, state officials, or local law enforcement (especially against minority women), or by worries of racism that elements of American medical science have fueled among African-Americans since slavery (e.g., Hoberman, 2012; Jones, 1981; Skloot, 2010; Washington, 2006).

We should not be surprised if home remedies or the emergency department at the local academic medical center have provided respondents and other area residents with a measure of autonomy over their decisions about primary health care. Reconsider, for example, how some respondents and area residents have decided to put home remedies, from laxatives to spiritual faith, before primary health care, or the account from one informant about how area residents have not stigmatized individuals who have taken advantage of emergency department services, this perhaps signaling that community members have recognized inherent value in incorporating the emergency department into decisions about primary health care despite the drawbacks of emergency department treatment (e.g., Moskop, Sklar, Geiderman, Schears, & Bookman, 2009a, 2009b). Autonomy over primary health care decisions could also increase, respondents might propose, if local clinics established a "first come, first serve" (I-3) policy, if all infrastructure facilities "[saw] people whether they have money or not" (FG-11), or if local officials organized "health fairs" (FG-11) to educate the public about fit lifestyles and primary care options.

The point is this: the structural and hidden barriers to the local primary health care infrastructure that have necessitated these strategies and stimulated these ideas from respondents in the first place, compounded by health-related challenges that stem from broader social issues such as urban violence, urban disrepair, intra-urban migration (e.g., Brown & Moore, 1970), and underemployment that we allude to in this discussion, have not simply limited access to primary health care but have also considerably diminished the autonomy – the power – that respondents and other area residents have been able to exercise over their decisions about primary health care. Accordingly, because "freedom requires access to the means of decision" (Mills, 1958, p. 31), and because health disparities will diminish only when individuals become empowered with full access to health care (U.S. Department of Health and Human Services, 2000), it would seem that efforts concerned with increasing the access of medically underserved groups to primary health care in local communities, whether initiated by elements of a local primary health care infrastructure, locally "elected corporate people" (FG-9), or even state or federal decree, for instance, local implementation of the new Patient Protection and Affordable Care Act (see One Hundred Eleventh Congress of the United States of America, 2010), should give practical thought and due standing to the centrality and significance of power.

CONCLUSION

This study has several limitations. The research sample was purposive to elicit the perspectives of focus group and interview respondents about the services of the local primary health care infrastructure, primary health care needs in the EXPORT focus area, and what it means to have a primary health care provider. In other words, our findings and interpretations might not generalize to local systems of health care clinics and hospital services that comprise a local primary health care infrastructure in other small, urban communities. Respondent perspectives, of course, can be biased: area residents more satisfied with the local primary health care infrastructure may well have been disinclined to participate in the study. Correspondingly, because we recruited a number of respondents ($n = 39$) at two FQHCs and at the local academic medical center's adjacent health care clinic, we cannot be certain that these respondents represented those in the local area most vulnerable to the structural and hidden barriers to the local primary health care infrastructure. Four focus groups ($n = 26$) were conducted at the FQHCs during operating hours. No representatives of these facilities, including caregivers or gatekeepers, were present during the focus groups and study personnel reminded the respondents in these focus groups about the freedom they had to candidly express their perspectives about the local primary health care infrastructure. We grant, however, that having conducted focus groups on the premises of the FQHCs could have reduced the comfort level of these respondents to speak openly. Missing background information from respondents limited conclusions we could draw about demographic variables and the local primary health care infrastructure while, by and large, focus group and interview data are subject to various interpretations and conceptual and thematic frameworks. Lastly, research that asks disempowered groups to identify the sources of their disempowerment risks increasing the vulnerability of these groups to injustice or maltreatment. We have no evidence to indicate any respondents experienced this outcome, but we feel this is an important caveat to mention.

These limitations notwithstanding, "the goal of creating a healthier, more productive community is not dependent on sophisticated clinical interventions but on understanding the community and its needs" (Channing, 2011, p. vii–viii). Having set out to understand the reality of primary health care from the perspective of residents in the EXPORT focus area, we argue that the structural and hidden barriers to the local primary health care infrastructure have not only limited the access of respondents and other area residents to primary health care but have also considerably diminished their autonomy over primary health care decisions, ultimately suggesting that efforts concerned with increasing the access of medically underserved groups to primary health care in local communities should recognize the centrality and significance of power. Indeed, to give practical thought and due standing to the concept of power is to more fully comprehend, and to thereby draw nearer to appreciably diminishing and eventually eliminating, health disparities. We hope this chapter can make a small contribution toward achieving these worthy objectives.

ACKNOWLEDGMENTS

Funding for this project was made possible by 1P20MD0002314 from the National Center on Minority Health and Health Disparities. The views expressed in written materials or publications and by program coordinators do not necessarily reflect the official policies of the Department of Health and Human Services, nor does mention by trade names, commercial practices, or organizations imply endorsement by the U.S. Government.

REFERENCES

Ahmed, S. M., Lemkau, J. P., Nealeigh, N., & Mann, B. (2001). Barriers to healthcare access in a non-elderly urban poor American population. *Health and Social Care in the Community, 9*(6), 445–453.

Arber, S., & Sawyer, L. (1985). The role of the receptionist in general practice: A "dragon behind the desk"? *Social Science & Medicine, 20*(9), 911–921.

Arrieta, M. I., & Mulars, A. (2006, June). Pilot study on barriers to health care among patients admitted to the USA Medical Center for ambulatory care sensitive conditions. Poster session presented at the meeting of the International Society on Hypertension in Blacks, Atlanta, GA.

Barr, D. A. (2008). *Health disparities in the United States: Social class, race, ethnicity, and health.* Baltimore, MD: The Johns Hopkins University Press.

Barr, D. A., & Wanat, S. F. (2005). Listening to patients: Cultural and linguistic barriers to health care access. *Family Medicine, 37*(3), 199–204.

Berger, P. L., & Luckmann, T. (1966). *The social construction of reality: A treatise in the sociology of knowledge.* New York, NY: Doubleday.

Boyd, E. L., Taylor, S. D., Shimp, L. A., & Semler, C. R. (2000). An assessment of home remedy use by African Americans. *Journal of the National Medical Association, 92*(7), 341–353.

Brown, L. A., & Moore, E. G. (1970). The intra-urban migration process: A perspective. *Geografiska Annaler, Series B, Human Geography, 52*(1), 1–13.

Brown, C. M., & Segal, R. (1996). The effects of health and treatment perceptions on the use of prescribed medication and home remedies among African American and white American hypertensives. *Social Science & Medicine, 43*(6), 903–917.

Budrys, G. (2010). *Unequal health: How inequality contributes to health or illness* (2nd ed.). Lanham, MD: Rowman & Littlefield Publishers, Inc.

Carr, D., Ibuka, Y., & Russell, L. B. (2010). How much time do Americans spend seeking health care? Racial and ethnic differences in patient experiences. In J. J. Kronenfeld (Ed.), *Research in the sociology of health care: The impact of demographics on health and health care: Race, ethnicity and other social factors* (Vol. 28, pp. 71–98). Bingley, UK: Emerald Group Publishing Limited.

Channing, A. H. (2011). Preface. In S. Whitman, A. M. Shah & M. R. Benjamins (Eds.), *Urban health: Combating disparities with local data* (pp. vii–viii). New York, NY: Oxford University Press.

Cockerham, W. C. (2007). *Social causes of health and disease.* Cambridge, UK: Polity Press.

Darby, K., Davis, C., Likes, W., & Bell, J. (2009). Exploring the financial impact of breast cancer for African American medically underserved women: A qualitative study. *Journal of Health Care for the Poor and Underserved, 20*(3), 721–728.

Dell, J. L., & Whitman, S. (2011). A history of the movement to address health disparities. In S. Whitman, A. M. Shah & M. R. Benjamins (Eds.), *Urban health: Combating disparities with local data* (pp. 8–30). New York, NY: Oxford University Press.

Eiser, A. R., & Ellis, G. (2007). Viewpoint: Cultural competence and the African American experience with health care: The case for specific content in cross-cultural education. *Academic Medicine, 82*(2), 176–183.

Ford, C. L., Tilson, E. C., Smurzynski, M., Leone, P. A., & Miller, W. C. (2008). Confidentiality concerns, perceived staff rudeness, and other HIV testing barriers. *The Journal of Equity in Health, 1*(1), 7–21.

Freidson, E. (1970). *Profession of medicine: A study of the sociology of applied knowledge.* New York, NY: Dodd, Mead & Company.

Freidson, E. (1986). *Professional powers: A study of the institutionalization of formal knowledge.* Chicago, IL: The University of Chicago Press.

Glaser, B. G., & Strauss, A. L. (2006). *The discovery of grounded theory: Strategies for qualitative research.* New Brunswick, NJ: Aldine Transaction. (Original work published 1967).

Grbich, C. (2007). *Qualitative data analysis: An introduction.* London: SAGE Publications Ltd.

Green, A. R., Peters-Lewis, A., Percac-Lima, S., Betancourt, J. R., Richter, J. M., Janairo, M.-P. R., ... Atlas, S. J. (2008). Barriers to screening colonoscopy for low-income Latino and White patients in an urban community health center. *Journal of General Internal Medicine, 23*(6), 834–840.

Gulati, A., Mohammad, F. A., & Arrieta, M. I. (2009). Hospitalizations for ambulatory care sensitive conditions at the University of South Alabama Medical Center, 2004–2007 [Abstract]. *Journal of Investigative Medicine, 57*(1), 333.

Hoberman, J. (2012). *Black & blue: The origins and consequences of medical racism.* Berkeley, CA: University of California Press.

Horton, S., & Johnson, R. J. (2010). Improving access to health care for uninsured elderly patients. *Public Health Nursing, 27*(4), 362–370.

Hughes, D. (1989). Paper and people: The work of the casualty reception clerk. *Sociology of Health & Illness, 11*(4), 382–408.

Jones, J. H. (1981). *Bad blood: The Tuskegee syphilis experiment.* New York, NY: The Free Press.

Jutel, A. (2009). Sociology of diagnosis: A preliminary review. *Sociology of Health & Illness, 31*(2), 278–299.

Kaplan, S. A., Calman, N. S., Golub, M., Davis, J. H., Ruddock, C., & Billings, J. (2006). Racial and ethnic disparities in health: A view from the South Bronx. *Journal of Health Care for the Poor and Underserved, 17*(1), 116–127.

Kasper, J. D. (2000). Health-care utilization and barriers to health care. In G. L. Albrecht, R. Fitzpatrick & S. C. Scrimshaw (Eds.), *Handbook of social studies in health and medicine* (pp. 323–338). London: SAGE Publications.

Kirby, J. B., & Kaneda, T. (2005). Neighborhood socioeconomic disadvantage and access to health care. *Journal of Health and Social Behavior, 46*(1), 15–31.

Kirby, J. B., & Kaneda, T. (2006). Access to health care: Does neighborhood residential instability matter? *Journal of Health and Social Behavior, 47*(2), 142–155.

Klinenberg, E. (2002). *Heat wave: A social autopsy of disaster in Chicago.* Chicago, IL: The University of Chicago Press.

Koenig, H. G., McCullough, M. E., & Larson, D. B. (2001). *Handbook of religion and health.* New York, NY: Oxford University Press.

Kronenfeld, J. J. (Ed.). (2005). *Research in the sociology of health care: Health care services, racial and ethnic minorities and underserved populations: Patient and provider perspectives* (Vol. 23). Amsterdam: Elsevier Ltd.

Kronenfeld, J. J. (2010). Social factors leading to differences in health and health care: The influence of factors such as race/ethnicity, geography, and gender. In J. J. Kronenfeld (Ed.), *Research in the sociology of health care: The impact of demographics on health and health care: Race, ethnicity and other social factors* (Vol. 28, pp. 3–17). Bingley, UK: Emerald Group Publishing Limited.

Liamputtong, P. (2011). *Focus group methodology: Principles and practice.* London: SAGE Publications Ltd.

Lichtenstein, B. (2003). Stigma as a barrier to treatment of sexually transmitted infection in the American deep South: Issues of race, gender and poverty. *Social Science & Medicine, 57,* 2435–2445.

Link, B. G., & Phelan, J. (1995). Social conditions as fundamental causes of disease. *Journal of Health and Social Behavior, 36*(Extra Issue), 80–94.

Lutfey, K., & Freese, J. (2005). Toward some fundamentals of fundamental causality: Socioeconomic status and health in the routine clinic visit for diabetes. *American Journal of Sociology, 110*(5), 1326–1372.

Malone, R. E. (1995). Heavy users of emergency services: Social construction of a policy problem. *Social Science & Medicine, 40*(4), 469–477.

Martin, S. S., Trask, J., Peterson, T., Martin, B. C., Baldwin, J., & Knapp, M. (2010). Influence of culture and discrimination on care-seeking behavior of elderly African Americans: A qualitative study. *Social Work in Public Health, 25*(3), 311–326.

Mechanic, D. (2002). Disadvantage, inequality, and social policy. *Health Affairs, 21*(2), 48–59.

Mills, C. W. (1958). The structure of power in American society. *The British Journal of Sociology, 9*(1), 29–41.

Moskop, J. C., Sklar, D. P., Geiderman, J. M., Schears, R. M., & Bookman, K. J. (2009a).
    Emergency department crowding, part 1 – Concepts, causes, and moral consequences.
    Annals of Emergency Medicine, 53(5), 605–611.
Moskop, J. C., Sklar, D. P., Geiderman, J. M., Schears, R. M., & Bookman, K. J. (2009b).
    Emergency department crowding, part 2 – Barriers to reform and strategies to overcome
    them. *Annals of Emergency Medicine, 53*(5), 612–617.
Newman, K. S. (1999). *No shame in my game: The working poor in the inner city.* New York,
    NY: Vintage Books.
One Hundred Eleventh Congress of the United States of America. (2010). *The patient protection
    and affordable care act.* Retrieved from http://www.gpo.gov/fdsys/pkg/BILLS-111hr
    3590enr/pdf/BILLS-111hr3590enr.pdf. Accessed on July 15, 2012.
Parsons, T. (1951). *The social system.* New York, NY: The Free Press.
Pesata, V., Pallija, G., & Webb, A. A. (1999). A descriptive study of missed appointments:
    Families' perceptions of barriers to care. *Journal of Pediatric Health Care, 13*(4), 178–182.
Rittner, B., & Kirk, A. B. (1995). Health care and public transportation use by poor and frail
    elderly people. *Social Work, 40*(3), 365–373.
Rust, G., Ye, J., Baltrus, P., Daniels, E., Adesunloye, B., & Fryer, G. E. (2008). Practical
    barriers to timely primary care access: Impact on adult use of emergency department
    services. *Archives of Internal Medicine, 168*(15), 1705–1710.
Seccombe, K., & Amey, C. (1995). Playing by the rules and losing: Health insurance and the
    working poor. *Journal of Health and Social Behavior, 36*(2), 168–181.
Shah, A. M., Whitman, S., & Benjamins, M. R. (2011). The importance of local data. In
    S. Whitman, A. M. Shah & M. R. Benjamins (Eds.), *Urban health: Combating disparities
    with local data* (pp. 31–35). New York, NY: Oxford University Press.
Shippee, T. P., Schafer, M. H., & Ferraro, K. F. (2012). Beyond the barriers: Racial
    discrimination and use of complementary and alternative medicine among Black
    Americans. *Social Science & Medicine, 74*(8), 1155–1162.
Silver, D., Blustein, J., & Weitzman, B. C. (2012). Transportation to clinic: Findings from a
    pilot clinic-based survey of low-income suburbanites. *Journal of Immigrant and Minority
    Health, 14*(2), 350–355.
Skloot, R. (2010). *The immortal life of Henrietta Lacks.* New York, NY: Broadway Paperbacks.
Snead, M. C., & Cockerham, W. C. (2002). Health lifestyles and social class in the deep
    south. In J. J. Kronenfeld (Ed.), *Research in the sociology of health care: Social
    inequalities, health and health care delivery* (Vol. 20, pp. 107–122). Amsterdam: Elsevier
    Science Ltd.
Stevens, P. E., & Keigher, S. M. (2009). Systemic barriers to health care access for U.S. women
    with HIV: The role of cost and insurance. *International Journal of Health Services, 39*(2),
    225–243.
Thiede, M. (2005). Information and access to health care: Is there a role for trust? *Social
    Science & Medicine, 61*(7), 1452–1462.
Umberson, D., & Montez, J. K. (2010). Social relationships and health: A flashpoint for health
    policy. *Journal of Health and Social Behavior, 51*(S), S54–S66.
U.S. Census Bureau. (2000a). *Profile of general demographic characteristics, Mobile County,
    Alabama. U. S. Census 2000.* Washington, DC: Author.
U.S. Census Bureau. (2000b). *Profile of selected economic characteristics, Mobile County,
    Alabama. U. S. Census 2000.* Washington, DC: Author.

U.S. Census Bureau. (2000c). *Profile of selected social characteristics, Mobile County, Alabama. U. S. Census 2000.* Washington, DC: Author.

U.S. Department of Health and Human Services. (1990). *Healthy people 2000: National health promotion and disease prevention objectives.* Washington, DC: U.S. Government Printing Office.

U.S. Department of Health and Human Services. (2000). *Healthy people 2010: Understanding and improving health* (2nd ed.). Washington, DC: U.S. Government Printing Office.

U.S. Department of Health and Human Services Office of Disease Prevention and Health Promotion. (n.d.). *Healthy people 2020.* Retrieved from http://healthypeople.gov/2020/default.aspx. Accessed on May 8, 2012.

Walls, C. A., Rhodes, K. V., & Kennedy, J. J. (2002). The emergency department as usual source of medical care: Estimates from the 1998 National Health Interview Survey. *Academic Emergency Medicine, 9*(11), 1140–1145.

Washington, H. A. (2006). *Medical apartheid: The dark history of medical experimentation on Black Americans from colonial times to the present.* New York, NY: Doubleday.

Williams, D. R. (2012). Miles to go before we sleep: Racial inequities in health. *Journal of Health and Social Behavior, 53*(3), 279–295.

Williams, D. R., & Collins, C. (1995). US socioeconomic and racial differences in health: Patterns and explanations. *Annual Review of Sociology, 21,* 349–386.

Williams, D. R., & Sternthal, M. (2010). Understanding racial-ethnic disparities in health: Sociological contributions. *Journal of Health and Social Behavior, 51*(S), S15–S27.

Wilson, W. J. (1987). *The truly disadvantaged: The inner city, the underclass, and public policy.* Chicago, IL: The University of Chicago Press.

Wilson, W. J. (1996). *When work disappears: The world of the new urban poor.* New York, NY: Vintage Books.

THE EFFECTS OF RESIDENTIAL ADVANTAGES UPON RURAL RESIDENTS' SELF-REPORTED PHYSICAL HEALTH AND EMOTIONAL WELL-BEING

James W. Grimm, D. Clayton Smith, Gene L. Theodori and A. E. Luloff

ABSTRACT

Purpose – *This chapter assesses the effects of two rural community residential advantages – economic growth and availability of health services – upon residents' health and emotional well-being.*

Methodology/approach – *A de facto experimental design divided communities into four analytical types based on their economic growth and health services. Household survey data were gathered via a drop-off/ pickup procedure and 400 randomly selected households were surveyed in each location. Physical health was measured with a subset of items from the Medical Outcomes Study's 36-item short form. A 10-item emotional well-being index was used. Beyond sociodemographic items, questions concerned household assets, medical problems, social supports, and*

Social Determinants, Health Disparities and Linkages to Health and Health Care
Research in the Sociology of Health Care, Volume 31, 83–107
Copyright © 2013 by Emerald Group Publishing Limited
All rights of reproduction in any form reserved
ISSN: 0275-4959/doi:10.1108/S0275-4959(2013)0000031007

community ties. Nested regression analyses were used to assess the effects of residential advantage upon health, net of potentially confounding factors.

Findings – *Contrary to expectations, both residential advantages were necessary for improved health. The most important negative net effect on health was aging. Beyond household assets and community economic expansion, miles commuted to work was the next most important factor enhancing physical health. In all types of communities, residents' emotional well-being scores were independent of age, but positively related to household income and religious involvement.*

Research limitations/implications – *Obviously the study is limited by geography and by the small number of communities in each residential type. While we could measure the effects of household members not being able to address all health needs, we could not assess the effects of such problems on anyone else in the households beyond the respondents. Our survey approach is also unable to address the effects of rural residents being unable to meet their health needs over time.*

Originality/value of study – *Ours is the first study that we know of applying a de facto natural experimental design to assess community residential effects. The interrelated effects of residential community resources for residents' health suggests that more studies like this one should be done.*

Keywords: Health; emotional well-being; household assets; social supports; community ties; and religiosity

Previous research has focused insufficiently upon the interrelatedness of residential effects that influence the health of rural residents. Many inquiries have been limited in focusing upon whether mortality and morbidity is higher or lower in rural areas than in their urban counterparts. Studies that have dealt primarily with provider issues (accessibility, for example) have often found rural rates of morbidity and mortality somewhat higher than those of urban areas (Johnson, 2004; Jones, Parker, & Ahearn, 2009; Morton, 2004; Stern et al., 2010; Szreter, 1997; Wallace, Grindeanu, & Cirillo, 2004). Studies that have dealt primarily with support issues (family unity and helpful friends, for example) have often found rural rates of morbidity and mortality to be a bit lower than those of urban areas

(House et al., 2000; Kitagawa & Hauser, 1973; Laditka, Laditka, Olatosi, & Elder, 2007; Smith, Anderson, Bradham, & Longino, 1995). The preponderance of these types of inquiries have not addressed how the confluence of residential effects in rural areas explains residents' health patterns. That such effects are numerous and may be in opposition is suggested by the inconsistency of the outcomes of previous studies.

Diverse and divergent residential effects upon rural residents' health also are suggested by the substantial differences in health in different types of rural areas. Residents in rural areas that ring urban counties are often healthier than those in rural areas more distant from regional medical centers. Rural residents with greater access to urban health centers and urban public health programs can probably meet and deal with their health problems (Grigsby & Goetz, 2004; Meng et al., 2009; Morton, 2004; Wallace et al., 2004). Yet, beyond health providers and services being more available in or near rural residence, other research shows that mere availability of health services need not mean that health care is affordable or used (Dussault & Franceschini, 2006). Obviously, more stagnant versus growing rural areas differ in both the provision of outpatient services for less serious health needs, in various screens and the centers of care that give them, and in the number and types of providers (Stern et al., 2010). Some rural areas are losing providers and centers of service while others are not (Morton, 2004; Wallace et al., 2004). Economic activity including traditional types of employment place many rural workers in more dangerous work environments that increase health problems (such as meat packing) (Wallace et al., 2004). Traditional farm employment also limits health insurance benefits and increases costs for the self-employed (Jones et al., 2009). If and how the positive effects of higher levels of social supports and family unity in many rural areas offset the negative rural influences upon health is not well understood (Beggs, Haines, & Hurlbert, 1996; House, Landis, & Umberson, 1988; Laditka et al., 2007; Smith et al., 1995).

Another shortcoming in previous research upon the patterns of rural residents' health is the general failure to include household resource effects and countywide indices of resources. Previous research including our own clearly establishes that socioeconomic status is related positively to both physical health (Grimm, Smith, Theodori, & Luloff, 2009; Lutfey, & Freese, 2005; Mackenzie, Wallace, & Weeks, 2010; Mirowsky & Ross, 2003; Phelan, Link, Diez-Roux, Kawachi, & Levin, 2004) and mental health (Clark, Marshall, House, & Lantz, 2011; Grimm et al., 2009; Miech & Shanahan, 2000; Schieman, Van Gundy, & Taylor, 2001). Yet, the net effects of rural residents' income and their other sources of economic security, as well as having health insurance or not, remain unclear (Hummer, Pacewicz, Wang, & Collins, 2004). Household economic disparity is just as important to consider in explaining rural residents' health as it is for Americans overall.

The purpose of this chapter is to decipher the effects of various household and residential effects upon the self-reported health and emotional well-being scores of rural residents. The data used here come from samples of residents in four different types of rural communities in Pennsylvania. These communities were part of a larger study of residential areas in that state (Luloff et al., 2000; Steele et al., 2001; Theodori, 1999, 2001). We have previously used these data to study household effects upon rural residents' self-reported health status (Grimm et al., 2009). Here, we expand our analytical focus to include the important differences in residential features among the four types of rural communities. Such differences were used to create strata in the stratified sampling design used to collect the data in the Summer of 1998. The two stratification criteria used originally to sample and that we use here to compare different residential effects upon health are whether the counties were growing in size and whether health care services were widely available (Luloff et al., 2000; Theodori, 1999, 2001).

The stratification criteria employed in selecting the residents of different types of rural municipalities gave us the chance to conduct research using a de facto natural experimental design. The original sampling design first selected two rural counties: County A had experienced economic growth during the two decades before data were collected, while the opposite was true of county B. Within each county two contrasting localities were selected (towns, townships, and/or boroughs). The first type (A1, B1) were those places with high availability of health and social services and the second type (A2, B2) were those places with low availability of such services (Luloff et al., 2000). These combinations allowed us to compare residents' self-reported health scores to assess the combined and separate effects of development and health services as well as their absence.

In this study, we had two working hypotheses. The first was the expectation that economic and population growth and availability of services each would have independent positive effects upon residents self-reported health statuses. We grounded the first part of this hypothesis in the work including our own that has found socioeconomic status to positively influence physical health (Grimm et al., 2009; MacKenzie et al., 2010; Meng et al., 2009; Mirowsky & Ross, 2003; Warren, 2009). The second part of the hypothesis was grounded in the studies showing rural areas with more providers have residents with better health (Morton, 2004; Stern et al., 2010; Young, 2004). In testing our first hypothesis, we sought to take into account the respondents' demographic characteristics, household effects, and a variety of household resources (economic and social supports) known to influence health and utilization of healthcare options. Such controls helped guard against the ecological fallacies that might have influenced area comparisons without them.

Several specific corollaries of the first working hypothesis were examined. First, it was expected that positive net residential effects would be most evident among residents in Type 1 communities (economic growth/high availability of health and social services) and least apparent among those living in Type 4 areas (economic decline/low availability of health and social services). Under the assumption that the residential advantages of growth and service provision could operate independently, it was also expected that while residents in Type 2 (economic growth/low availability of health and social services) and Type 3 (economic decline/high availability of health and social services) communities might exhibit fewer positive residential effects upon health than those in Type 1 areas, they would likely have more such effects than people residing in Type 4 communities.

A second hypothesis, contingent upon the first, was that residents in communities with fewer residential advantages would be more likely to evidence household resource effects (economics and supports) on their self-reported health scores. This reflected the idea that the absence of growth and services being widely available locally would make those residents in households with economic resources and social supports, including community ties, better able to deal with their health needs. That is, following the results of earlier research using these data, we already knew respondents living in households in which all members' health needs could be afforded were healthier (Grimm et al., 2009). We also grounded this expectation in studies that have found that socioeconomic status is related to better physical and mental health (Clark et al., 2011; Miech & Shanahan, 2000; Warren, 2009; Yang, 2007). Based on our previous work (Grimm et al., 2009), we believed different household effects would be important for physical health and emotional well-being, but since we were primarily interested in the net effects of residential advantages, we applied the same two basic hypotheses to both of our self-reported health status indices.

METHODS

Data

The data employed in this study were collected as part of a larger research project on rural economic development and individual well-being (Luloff et al., 2000; Theodori, 1999, 2001). The selection of study sites began at the county level. Using US Census of Housing and Population data, each county in the Commonwealth of Pennsylvania was classified with respect to its history of population change for the period 1950–1990. From this empirical classification, two northern-tier counties – McKean and Tioga – both of which contained numerous rural communities were selected. Between 1950 and 1990, Tioga County experienced approximately a 17% increase in population. During that same period, the population in McKean County declined by approximately 14%.

The use of 1970 to 1990 United States Census of Population and Housing data, as well as field observations of each municipality within Tioga and McKean Counties, aided in the identification and selection of sites at the community level. Four sites – two in each county – were selected to represent contrasting economic trends (i.e., growth or decline) and how available health and social services were (dichotomized as high availability of services and low availability of services). This facilitated comparisons among sites with differing levels of recent economic performance and availability of health and social services.

The four sites selected included a central place and an aggregate of several contiguous surrounding municipalities. Clusters of minor civil divisions were used to reflect centre-hinterland relationships within the sites. Previous work with similar ecological clustering revealed that the units used were meaningful for respondents (Bourke, Jacob, & Luloff, 1996; Claude & Luloff, 1995; Luloff, Bourke, Jacob, & Seshan, 1995; Theodori, Luloff, & Willits, 1998).

The first type (economic growth/high availability of services) was represented by the Wellsboro area of Tioga County. This area consisted of Wellsboro Borough and Delmar Township. The second type (economic growth/low availability of services) was represented by the Blossburg area of Tioga County. This area included Blossburg and Liberty Boroughs and Bloss, Hamilton, Liberty, and Union Townships. The third type (economic decline/high availability of services) was represented by the Bradford area of McKean County. This site consisted of Bradford City, Lewis Run Borough, and Bradford and Foster Townships. The fourth type (economic decline/low availability of services) was represented by the Port Allegany area of McKean County. This area included Port Allegany Borough and Annin, Ceres, Liberty, and Norwich Townships.

Household survey data were gathered via a drop-off/pick-up question-naire procedure (Steele et al., 2001). During the summer of 1998, survey questionnaires were hand-delivered to 400 randomly selected households in each study site and picked-up within a few days of delivery. To obtain a representative sample of individuals within households, response was requested from the adult who had celebrated the most recent birthday. The survey instrument, organized as a self-completion booklet, contained 61 questions and required approximately 30 minutes to complete. After adjusting for nondeliverables, deceased respondents, bad addresses and the like, the overall response rate was 72%, resulting in 1,265 completed questionnaires across the four sites (Wellsboro, $n = 215$; Blossburg, $n = 224$; Bradford, $n = 200$; and Port Allegany, $n = 213$).

Table 1 presents selected sample distributions and comparable Census data from 1990 and 2000. As can be seen in the table, the sample is more educated than the general population in the study areas, both in the number of individuals with a high school degree or higher and those holding a BA or higher degree. In addition, the sample is also older. Nevertheless, large majorities of respondents at all sites were less than 65 years old.

Table 1. Selected Sample Distributions Compared with 1990 and 2000 Census Data.

	Census 1990	Sample 1998	Census 2000
Percent of population 25 years and older with high school or higher degree			
Wellsboro	77.9	90.2	83.2
Blossburg	71.5	87.1	81.0
Bradford	76.8	93.4	83.4
Port Allegany	71.1	90.3	83.4
Percent of population 25 years and older with bachelor's degree or higher			
Wellsboro	20.0	31.1	20.7
Blossburg	11.4	23.8	12.8
Bradford	13.8	26.2	17.6
Port Allegany	8.4	21.4	12.6
Percent of population 65 years and older			
Wellsboro	19.9	24.0	24.6
Blossburg	15.9	29.7	24.2
Bradford	18.1	30.4	23.5
Port Allegany	14.0	25.3	20.7

Note: Information from Census 1990 taken from Theodori (1999) and information from Census 2000 drawn from American Fact Finder (US Census Bureau 2008).

Physical and Emotional Well-being Measures

We used a subset of physical functioning items from the Medical Outcomes Study's 36-item short form (Ware & Sherbourne, 1992). The seven items included some activities of daily living (ADLs) such as traversing stairs, kneeling or stooping, lifting or carrying objects less than ten pounds, and using hands and fingers. The remaining items included instrumental activities of daily living (IADLs) such as seeing (even with glasses), hearing, and walking. Following traditional procedures, respondents could choose from among three answer alternatives as they indicated the extent (if any) of the difficulty they had doing the activities: none (3), some (2), a great deal (1). When summed, the respondents' scores reflected the extent of their physical well-being by the absence of difficulty completing items. The reliability and validity of this scale has been described previously (Grimm et al., 2009).

Ten questions were asked about respondents' emotional status and outlooks on life. They were used to index emotional well-being; five response options ranged from "almost always true" to "never true." Following previous analyses (Grimm et al., 2009; Theodori, 2001), one item, "I am bothered by noise," was removed from the analysis based on factor and reliability analyses. The remaining items were reverse coded to reflect almost always true (5) for positively worded items (e.g., "I generally feel in good spirits") and never true (5) on items that were negatively phrased (e.g., "Things seem hopeless"). Respondents were asked about how true the items were concerning their emotional state and their general outlook on life. The latter included items like "I feel down in the dumps" and the former included things like "I feel depressed." Emotional well-being scores reflect the summation of the factor weighted scores of the nine items. Our scoring meant that scores increased with emotional well-being. Again, the reliability and validity of the index has been previously described (Grimm et al., 2009).

Individual Characteristics

Several respondent traits that are known to influence health status – age (measured in years), gender (female = 1), marital status, educational attainment, and employment status – were incorporated as controls. Marital status was measured with two variables – married and widowed – which are dichotomous indicator variables (0 = no, 1 = yes). The comparison category is anyone not married or widowed. Educational attainment was measured as a five-category variable (1 = did not complete high school to 5 = Graduate or professional training beyond college degree). Employment status was a three-category variable (1 = Not employed currently, 2 = Employed part time, 3 = Employed full time).

Driving distance (in miles) and commuting time (in minutes) from the respondents' homes and their work were also measured. Both variables were severely positively skewed. To improve their normality, the inverse of both variables were calculated. Therefore, a large value means a shorter driving distance and a shorter commuting time, respectively.

Household Characteristics

Household context was indicated by items dealing with household size as well as household composition – number of members less than five years old, six to 18 years old, and numbers of the household more than 65 years of age. In addition, change in household size over the past year was also measured (0 = Decreased, 1 = Stayed the same, 2 = Increased).

Household Assets Measures

We used a variety of household asset indicators. Two were global indicators – total household income and home ownership – but others were specific measures of liquidity (e.g., business income, investment income, social security payments, and retirement pensions) that could be used to address health care needs and costs. Household income was measured using a set of ten ordered categories (1 = under \$9,999 to 10 = \$90,000 or more). Home ownership was measured as a dichotomy (1 = yes, 0 = no), as were the other specific measures of liquidity.

Household Medical Profile

Several factors related to household access to medical care were measured including a set of dichotomous items dealing with household members having unmet health care needs – a member of the household unable to get medical help, dental help, or prescriptions filled – were included (1 = yes, 0 = no). Whether all household members had health insurance (1 = yes, 0 = no), the time since last seeing a dentist (on a five-point scale from 1 = "Less than 1 year ago" to 5 = "never"), the distance to local medical care (on a five-point scale from 1 = "Less" than 5 miles to 5 = "more than 40 miles"), and overall rating of local medical care (on a five-point Likert scale from 1 = "completely dissatisfied" to 5 = "Completely satisfied') were also measured.

Social Supports

We included an interaction measure that consisted of items such as interacting with close friends and neighbors (Cronbach's $\alpha = .65$). In addition, we created a perceived assistance index consisting of items dealing with having access to people able to help with household tasks, to care for the house when the residents were gone, to care for members of the household who were unwell, and having access to someone capable of providing a ride when necessary (Cronbach's $\alpha = .89$). Higher scores on both indices indicated more interaction and support.

Community Ties Measures

Community orientation measures used included length of residence (in years), religious attendance (on a six-point scale from 0 = "Never" to 5 = "More than once a week"), the proportion of adults in the community the respondents' knew (on a four-point scale from 1 = "None of them" to 4 = "Most or all of them"), and the respondents' ratings concerning their community as a place to raise a family (on a five-point Likert scale from 1 = "completely" dissatisfied to 5 = "Completely satisfied"). In addition, a community embeddedness index was created which consisted of items measuring community interest, community activeness, level of belonging to community clubs, hours spent in community activities, and participation in cooperative building/funding raising (Cronbach's $\alpha = .75$). Length of residence (in years) was moderately positively skewed and it was transformed by taking the square root of the length of residence. Still, higher numbers on all these variables indicate increased levels of community ties.

Analysis

Nested regression techniques were used to build a statistical model of variation in respondents' physical and emotional well-being scores. In model-building we first entered the control variables: respondents' sociodemographics and household context indicators. Then, we introduced sets of items about financial assets, supports, aspects of healthcare for household members, and community viewpoints/ties. The net effects of types of household assets and other influences were assessed in terms of their contribution to the total model across the stepwise regression procedure. The outcome of each final model for each community type consisted of only the statistically meaningful determinants (Reduced model). Doing this enabled us to draw conclusions about which net effects upon respondents' self-reported physical and emotional well-being were statistically important in each of the four types of communities in the analyses.

RESULTS

Results of the net effects upon the self-reported physical health scores of residents in the four different types of communities appear in Table 2. Communities are arranged from Type 1 to Type 4, left to right. In discussing the results in Table 2, we will only be using the reduced model for respondents in each of the rural areas. The comparisons of the reduced models include only the net effects of the statistically significant differences that remained after controlling for all other variables. As we proceed with our discussion of results, we compare the size and direction of net influences upon physical health and emotional well-being scores of residents in each of the four types of rural communities.

Results in Table 2 provide only limited evidence for the first hypothesis that growth and service availability would have positive net effects upon respondents' self-reported physical health scores. As compared with other residents in all other communities, those living in Type 1 communities reported higher health scores, in household members being able to deal with dental needs (+ .13) and prescription needs (+ .15), as well as in ratings of local medical services (+ .19) and our community involvement index (+ .18). Less evidence than was expected came from residents in Type 2 and Type 3 areas, however. Like those respondents living in Type 1 communities, those in Type 3 areas (with more available services) evidenced the positive net effect upon health of all households members being able to get their prescriptions filled (+ .13), but not the positive benefits of being able to deal with dental needs. In fact, time since last dental screen negatively affected (−.18) Type 3 residents' health scores, as did distance to providers' clinics (−.13). Those health needs that are more difficult to obtain may contribute to declining health. Our findings clearly show that the increased availability

Table 2. Betas and Coefficients of Determination for Independent and Control Variables on Physical Well-Being.

	Wellsboro		Blossburg		Bradford		Port Allegany	
	Full	Reduced	Full	Reduced	Full	Reduced	Full	Reduced
Individual characteristics								
Age	-.32**	-.30***	-.44***	-.48***	-.47***	-.42***	-.24*	-.36***
Gender	-.03		.07		-.06		.05	
Married	.03		-.04		.08		-.19*	-.15*
Widowed	.13		.16		.18*	.15**	-.10	
Education	-.10		.01		.13		.02	
Employed	.02		.21		.21		.19	
Minutes to work (Inverse)	-.20	-.27***	.22		.48		.45	
Miles to work (Inverse)	-.05		-.25	-.26***	-.41	-.18**	-.45	-.16*
Household characteristics								
Household size	-.19		-.04		-.24		-.02	
No. in hhold under 5	.01		.11		.13		.15	
No. in hhold between 6–18	.13		.17		.13		-.05	
No. in hhold over 65	.20*		.10		.05		.02	
Change in hhold size	-.01		-.09		-.04		.07	
Household assets								
Total hhold income ($)	.14		.12		.01		.16	.18*
Own home (y/n)	-.03		.10		-.01		.12	.16*
Business income (y/n)	.03		-.13*		-.07		-.09	
Investment income (y/n)	.05		.13*	.12*	.17*	.19**	.15*	.15*
Social security income (y/n)	-.39**		-.20		-.07		-.12	
Pension income (y/n)	.13		.29***	.20**	.04		.09	

Household medical profile							
Unable to get MD help	.05		-.03			.17**	.18**
Unable to get dental help	.09	.13*	.05		-.02	.05	
Unable to fill prescriptions	.11	.15**	.04		.11	.13*	.02
Everyone in hhold insured	-.03		-.04		-.02		.09
Time since last dental screen	.00		-.04		-.12	-.18**	-.10
Distance to doctor/clinic	-.08		.05		-.13*	-.13*	.03
Rating of medical services	.15*	.19***	-.04		-.07		.02
Social supports							
Interaction with friends/neighbors index	.05		-.01		-.08		-.03
Perceived assistance index	.09		.11	.13*	.08		.02
Community ties							
SQRT length of residence	.06		.09		-.14	-.16*	-.01
Religious attendance	.08		.21**	.24**	.07		.03
Proportion of adults known	-.10		.00		.03		.00
Rating as place to raise family	.00		.07		.15*		.10
Embeddedness index	.13	.18**	-.08		.00		-.08
Adjusted R^2	.32	.32	.31	.31	.38	.39	.27	.27
F-test	4.00***	17.73****	3.99****	17.51***	4.75***	17.06***	3.33***	12.24***
N	215	215	224	224	200	200	213	213

Note: $^*p<.05$, $^{**}p<.01$, $^{**}p<.001$.

of health services does not necessarily mean that they are readily available or affordable for many residents in nondeveloping rural areas. In contrast, when increased services are coupled with economic development, health is increased in many important respects. The positive effects of economic growth upon rural resident health insurance options may be one reason (cf. Jones et al., 2009).

While there is limited support for service availability positively affecting health scores, apart from economic growth, the reverse clearly was not true. No evidence exists of any positive net effects upon health among Type 2 communities in household members being able to meet all their health needs. The results suggest economic viability in rural areas is not a sufficient cause of residents' improved health. Moreover, the greater net effects of household members being able to deal with their health needs expected in community Types 2 and 3, vis-a-vis those living in Type 4 areas, were not found. In fact, residents of Type 4 communities health scores were positively affected by all household members being able to deal with their health needs ($+.18$). Overall, both economic growth and services being available were necessary conditions for there to be positive net effects upon rural residents' health scores. Lacking more widely present health services, community development alone does not lead to improvements in health. One reason for this may be that many rural residents in developing countries only have access to regional hospitals and health centers rather than to local providers (cf. Stern et al., 2010).

Results in Table 2 provide considerable evidence for our second hypotheses that without residential advantages of their communities, rural residents' health scores would primarily be enhanced by household resources. These results include being widowed in Type 3 areas ($+.15$), being married ($-.15$), household income ($+.18$), and home owning ($+.16$) in Type 4 communities, pension payments ($+.20$), having people to assist with household concerns ($+.13$), and religious attendance ($+.24$) among residents in Type 2 communities. The most consistent evidence in support of our second hypothesis about differences in physical health scores by community areas are those that show household investment income positively affects physical health scores among Type 2 ($+.12$), 3 ($+.19$), and 4 ($+.15$) communities.

Two other issues are evident in the results reported in Table 2. First, neither community effects nor household resources offset the sizable negative impact of aging on health. Neither residential advantages of localities nor the advantages of more available household resources affect the declining effects upon physical health as rural residents age. Given that large majorities of respondents in all types of communities studied were less than 65 years old, our results indicate the ongoing lower levels of health with aging among residents in general in all types of rural communities. Second, it is ironic the results consistently indicate that commuters (minutes to work in Type 1 communities and miles to work in all other areas) have higher physical health scores (negative signs due to the use of inverse indicators). This makes the impact of health care usage upon health much more contingent upon being able to get employment outside the communities where people and their families live, where healthcare opportunities and benefits are greater. Such benefits may be much better for and more accessible to commuters than by the more limited and more costly benefits of direct-purchase insurance self-employed rural residents have (Jones et al., 2009).

There is very little support for our expectations about the positive residential context effects upon respondents' emotional well-being scores. Few, if any, net impacts of health care usage indicators support our predictions with respect to enhanced emotional well-being. Even among residents in Type 1 communities, only the rating of local health services is related to enhanced well-being (+ .17). Such scores are enhanced (+ .16) by all household members being able to deal with dental needs (in Type 2 areas) and by all members being able to deal with all their prescription needs in Type 3 (+ .18) and Type 4 (+ .12) communities. Those who live in Type 4 areas have enhanced well-being scores (+ .15) in relation to their ratings of local providers.

Household income enhanced respondents' well-being scores in all types of rural municipalities studied. The same was true of respondents having people in their communities who would assist them with household concerns including travel to providers. Except for residents in Type 4 areas, respondents' rating of their localities as places to raise a family were positively related to well-being scores. And, except for residents in Type 1 communities, residents of all other areas had higher well-being scores in relation to church attendance. Residents in Type 2 areas had higher well-being scores in relation to interaction with others in their communities. That household resources are more important than residential effects in relation to well-being scores also is evident among Type 1 residents, where being married enhances well-being (+ .15), but household size does not (−.23). Similarly, among residents of Type 3 areas, being widowed enhances well-being while the number of youth in the household does not (−.14). While interpreting the reasons for these differences in household contexts regarding well-being scores is beyond the scope of this chapter, results

Table 3. Betas and Coefficients of Determination for Independent and Control Variables on Emotional Well-Being.

	Wellsboro		Blossburg		Bradford		Port Allegany	
	Full	Reduced	Full	Reduced	Full	Reduced	Full	Reduced
Individual characteristics								
Age	-.03		.07		.14		.16	.19**
Gender	-.01		-.04		.01		.07	
Married	.12	.19**	.08		-.01		-.02	
Widowed	-.06		.18*		.13	.14*	-.07	
Education	.00		-.02		.05		-.14	
Employed	-.06		-.19		.08		.20	
Minutes to work (Inverse)	.11		.13		.15		.50	
Miles to work (Inverse)	-.19		-.30		-.16		-.37	
Household characteristics								
Household size	-.38***	-.23***	-.03		.06		-.19	
No. in hhold under 5	.06		.01		.09		.08	
No. in hhold between 6–18	.08		.09		-.16	-.14*	.11	
No. in hhold over 65	.13		.11		-.06		-.07	
Change in hhold size	-.05		-.05		.06		.09	
Household assets								
Total hhold income ($)	.24**	.28****	.15	.13*	.18*	.25***	.21*	.17**
Own home (y/n)	.15*		.02		-.05		-.02	
Business income (y/n)	.01		.01		.01		.06	
Investment income (y/n)	.08		.08		.06		.03	
Social security income (y/n)	.02		-.15		-.13		-.03	
Pension income (y/n)	-.13		.06		.11		.09	

	(1)	(2)	(3)	(4)	(5)	(6)	(7)	(8)
Household medical profile								
Unable to get MD help	-.07		-.04		-.08		-.01	
Unable to get dental help	.07		.14*	.16**	.12		.06	
Unable to fill prescriptions	.04		.05		.16*	.18**	.12	.12*
Everyone in hhold insured	-.08		-.02		.12	.13*	-.03	
Time since last dental screen	.05		.00		.01		.02	
Distance to doctor/clinic	-.12		.05		.00		-.05	
Rating of medical services	.20**	.17**	.00		.05		.12	.15*
Social supports								
Interaction with friends/neighbors index	-.03	.17*	.17*	.17**	.00		.08	
Perceived assistance index	.24***	.24***	.24***	.24***	.25***	.30***	.21**	.28***
Community ties								
SQRT Length of residence	-.07		-.08		.00		.12	
Religious attendance	.07	.20**	.20**	.24***	.19***	.23***	.16*	.16*
Proportion of adults known	.06		.04		.04		-.13	
Rating as place to raise family	.13*	.14*	.14*	.13*	.17*	.20***	.08	.16*
Embeddedness index	.09		.03		.09		.07	
Adjusted R^2	.32	.33	.26	.29	.37	.39	.21	.23
F-test	4.04***	17.83***	3.30***	15.34***	4.39***	16.39***	2.69***	11.36***
N	210		217		191		209	

Note: $*p < .05$, $**p < .01$, $***p < .001$.

clearly show that well-being is positively affected by household resources and negatively affected by some aspects of household composition.

Overall, results presented in Table 3 provide very little support for our expectations about rural residential effects being important for enhancing well-being. Instead, aspects of general rural living and household resources enhance well-being the most. These results are consistent with recent research suggesting that mental illness patterns over lifetimes are primarily affected by successful ongoing social roles and supports (Clark et al., 2011). In rural areas having the resources and supports to deal with more health problems may play an important role in explaining why aging per se is not associated with declining emotional well-being (Blanchflower & Oswald, 2008; Yang, 2007).

DISCUSSION

Several important conclusions about residential effects upon rural residents' self-reported health status are evident from the results of our study. First, neither community economic growth nor more health and social services being available in communities by themselves are important as independent enhancements of residents' physical health. With few exceptions, our results indicate that these residential advantages being present together are important in enhancing respondents' health scores. The only exceptions are the enhanced physical health scores among commuters in all communities, the enhanced health scores of residents in Type 3 areas where all members of household can meet their prescription needs, and among residents in Type 4 areas where all household members can see providers they need. These results suggest that affordability effects become more important when both types of residential advantage are not present (Dussault & Franceschini, 2006). For example, affordability effects with respect to dental care decrease health in Type 3 areas, where providers are more available. Overall, then, rural residents' health generally is most enhanced in growing communities with more and better providers. In communities without both these residential advantages, health is much more dependent upon households being able to afford health care that they need. Our results suggest that affordability issues are particularly important regarding providers such as dentists that are less likely to be covered by health insurance (Hummer et al., 2004). The same is true for rural residents being less likely to be able to afford outpatient care including doctor visits or visits to emergency rooms (Stern et al., 2010).

Economic disparity affects physical health most among residents in rural municipalities without economic and provider advantages. Residents in households with higher investment income were healthier in Type 2, 3, and 4 communities. Those residents in Type 4 areas with higher income and who owned their homes were healthier. Likewise, fewer household resources explained the poorer physical health of married people in Type 4 communities. Beyond these disparity effects upon physical health differences, the results also clearly showed that the most important influence upon the physical health of all rural residents was aging. Our results showed that despite the residential advantages of their community and disparity in household resources, rural residents, overall, experienced significant declines in health as they aged. One possible reason for this might be the cumulative effects of rural residents being less able to deal with all their health needs (Ferraro & Shippee, 2009).

The most obvious conclusion about our results concerning differences among rural residents' emotional well-being scores as a function of where they reside is how different they are compared with the differences in physical health found. For example, aging effects were absent from differences in emotional well-being scores. Where differences were found by age, (among residents in Type 4 communities), the effect was positive! Contrary to the residential effects upon higher physical health scores, emotional well-being scores were much more related to household effects among residents in communities with fewer residential advantages. Being able to deal with all household members' dental needs (Type 2 residents), being able to deal with all members' prescription needs (Type 3 and 4 residents) and everyone being insured (among Type 3 residents) are examples. Other household effects enhancing respondents' emotional well-being scores were household income (in all types of areas), interaction rates with others in the community (among Type 2 residents), having people who can assist with household concerns (all types of communities), respondents positively evaluating the community as a place to raise a family (people residing in Type 1, 2, and 3 areas), and religion attendance (in Types 2, 3, and 4 areas). These findings support the positive roles of supports and social connectivity in enhancing mental health (Schieman et al., 2001). These results are less supportive of the idea that in rural areas aging is related to fatalism and declining aspirations (Blanchflower & Oswald, 2008).

Overall, the differences in emotional well-being scores found among respondents depended mostly upon household effects including marital status and household size. This is clear in residents in Type 1 communities, those with the most residential advantages. Among such residents, being married enhanced well-being while household size reduced it. Similar results were uncovered for residents in Type 3 communities in being widowed (+) and the number of youth residing in the household (–). Household income was as generally important in enhancing emotional well-being scores among our respondents as aging in negatively affecting their physical health. Our results clearly showed that conclusions about the mental health of rural residents were independent of inferences about the state of their physical health. These findings also suggest the importance of resources and ongoing social roles for better mental health (Schieman et al., 2001). They also suggest that it is not aging per se but the survival and coping aspects of the life cycle that explain mental well-being (Yang, 2007).

The most important reasons for the disconnect between rural residents' physical health and emotional health might be associated with key and pervasive features of rural living. Rural life is often family-centered and is marked by closer supports and other ties through churches and community organizations. These things enhance emotional well-being, beyond differences in health status or age (House et al., 2000; Kitagawa & Hauser, 1973; Laditka et al., 2007). However, there is some irony in these results. Americans living in diverse rural areas have numerous health problems, including those related to aging, yet are often happy people. It is hoped that the positive effects of rural living upon residents' emotional well-being can be better matched by increasing access to health services for their physical health needs, especially as they age. Better provision of health services for rural residents' needs is obviously needed to more closely match their physical and mental health.

These results suggest some important considerations in the quest to improve health care for rural residents. First, efforts to improve the economic well-being of rural communities either may not necessarily improve local health care provision or contribute to residents being better able to meet their health needs. We found very little evidence that without more widely accessible health services, social services and economic development were themselves related to better health. Oddly, we found that rural residents who commuted also reported better health. Our study suggests that economic development in rural areas should be accompanied by the development of public health programs that increase rural health services and make them more affordable to residents in all localities. Moreover, efforts to provide incentives for health care providers to locate in all types of rural areas would help provide health services that are sufficient for meeting all residents healthcare needs. In particular, public health programs to assist those in need to see more distant providers, including dentists, are needed (Jones et al., 2009).

One of the clearest results of our study is that neither differences in economic development and population increases nor the increased avail- ability of providers diminish the very general and significant decline in rural residents' health as they age. The magnitude of the aging effects that we found suggests that the higher morbidity and mortality in rural areas may result from increased health problems across residents' life cycles rather than because rural populations have more elderly members (Ferraro & Shippee, 2009). Our findings point to the need for determining what it is about rural residence that negatively affects the overall health of residents as they age. This objective should be pursued particularly with respect to the unmet health care needs of rural residents throughout their life cycles. In particular, our results indicate such factors may be related to people being unable to deal with all their health needs due to insurance limitations, affordability problems, and accessibility problems, especially as distance to providers increases (Jones et al., 2009). A possible explanatory perspective suggested by our results is that rural residents are less healthy because many of them cannot address or deal with all their health problems. In turn, this contributes to their ongoing declines in health and their being unable to afford dealing with them (Mechanic, 2004). Moreover, this means more complex and costly health problems of older rural residents (Laditka et al., 2007). Our study also suggests that the least advantaged rural residents might be most positively affected by enhanced public health programs (Meng et al., 2009).

The overall scope of our results also suggests that residential effects upon the physical and emotional health of rural residents does in fact involve at least two opposing general forces. First, many aspects of rural residence – such as having others who can help with household problems, religious involvement, and positive feelings about locality as a place to raise a family – have positive effects upon residents' emotional well-being and outlooks on life. How these generally positive frames of emotional reference interact with the health problems many residents cannot deal with remain important topics to be pursued in future research. Our results suggest that it may not be fatalism that sustains the outlooks of less healthy rural residents, but the positive and proactive features of rural living that with many types of supports better enable them to cope with their ongoing health problems. How generally good mental health can be better combined with dealing with all health needs is a vitally important public policy goal in rural areas. Conversely, finding out more about the cumulative effects of stress and the inability to confront health problems on rural residents' health will be very important in future research (Ferraro & Shippee, 2009).

Our results suggest that rural development without separate and ongoing efforts to increase the number and accessibility of providers and health services merely accentuates the effects of household resource disparities. More people and more jobs, as our results show, may merely mean that some rural residents have the benefits of employment that enable them to deal with their health needs; many others do not. How to develop public health programs in rural areas that give all residents affordable ways to deal with their health needs will be a key public policy goal (Meng et al., 2009). Attracting employers and increasing the number of people in the rural labor force will not automatically mean residents have the means and opportunity to deal with their health needs. Our results suggest programs to help ensure the affordability of prescriptions and assistance in travel to more distant providers, including dentists, would help improve residents' health. These could well be grounded in the existent and important support networks in most rural communities.

Ironically, one of our most consistent findings is that increased employment opportunity for rural residents may give them the means and opportunity to deal with their health needs in work locations to which they commute, while economic development may not necessarily provide the means and opportunity for rural residents to get healthcare in their communities. Local economic development may allow others to do so, if they take better jobs some distance from where they live. Overall, lacking development in more stagnant rural areas, it is important to better understand the forces that increase residents' opportunities to seek and find the health care that they need in locations more distant from where they live. Our results suggest that such forces include employment that involves commuting, supportive others to help with traveling to more distant providers, and the supportive effects of religious involvement in dealing with health needs and less accessible health care. Better and more pervasive ways of overcoming distance effects will be of primary importance in helping the more disadvantaged rural dwellers better deal with their health problems (Stern et al., 2010).

CONCLUSION

Rural residents continue to have health problems and difficulties in reaching health providers to deal with their health needs. Problems with respect to variance in health and health care vary by community context and household resources. A key conclusion sustained by the results of our study, however, is that economic revitalization in rural communities will not by itself improve most residents' health. More and increasing variety of services available for the range of needs all community residents have also will be necessary. Services that are more available to commuters who live in rural areas (and appear to get medical care closer to or in their workplaces) must be supplemented by services for the needs of all rural residents including those who do not commute or who are elderly. Beyond availability of more providers and health services, our results suggest that pervasive aspects of rural living, such as close-ties supports and church involvement could and should be used to help all rural residents with health needs to get to the services of more distant providers should they need them. If these pervasive aspects of rurality associated with enhanced emotional well-being can be used to ensure that residents can use all the providers and services available to them in their communities and beyond, then general health status of the rural population will be increased. And, public health programs must be infused with the resources to provide travel access for those in need – such as travel to providers and the means of allowing providers to travel to many rural residents who need them but otherwise would not see them.

REFERENCES

Beggs, J. J., Haines, V. A., & Hurlbert, J. S. (1996). Revisiting the rural-urban contrast: Personal networks in nonmetropolitan and metropolitan settings. *Rural Sociology, 61,* 306–325.

Blanchflower, D. G., & Oswald, A. J. (2008). Is well-being u-shaped over the life cycle? *Social Science and Medicine, 66*(8), 1733–1749.

Bourke, L., Jacob, S., & Luloff, A. E. (1996). Response to Pennsylvania's agricultural preservation programs. *Rural Sociology, 61,* 606–629.

Clark, P., Marshall, V., House, J., & Lantz, P. (2011). The social structuring of mental health over the adult life course: Advancing theory in the sociology of aging. *Social Forces, 89,* 1287–1314.

Claude, L. P., & Luloff, A. E. (1995). *Comparative case studies: Coudersport, austin, liberty, emporium.* Agricultural Economics and Rural Sociology Research Report 252. Department of Agricultural Economics and Rural Sociology, The Pennsylvania State University, University Park, PA.

Dussault, G., & Franceschini, M. C. (2006). Not enough there, too many here: Understanding geographic imbalances in the distribution of the health workforce. *Human Resources for Health, 4,* 1–16.

Ferraro, K. F., & Shippee, T. P. (2009). Aging and cumulative inequality: How does inequality get under the skin? *The Gerontologist, 49*(3), 333–343.

Grigsby, W., & Goetz, S. J. (2004). Telehealth: What promise does it hold for rural areas? In N. Glasgow, L. W. Morton & N. E. Johnson (Eds.), *Critical issues in rural health* (pp. 237–250). Ames, IA: Blackwell Publishing.

Grimm, J. W., Smith, D. C., Theodori, G. L., & Luloff, A. E. (2009). Effects of household assets upon rural residents' self-reported physical and emotional well-being". In J. J. Kronenfeld (Ed.), *Social sources of disparities in health and health care and linkages to policy, population concerns and providers of care (Research in the sociology of health care)* (Vol. 27, pp. 277–300). Bingley, UK: Emerald Group Publishing Limited.

House, J. S., Landis, K. R., & Umberson, D. (1988). Social relationships and health. *Science, 214,* 540–545.

House, J. S., Lepkowski, J. M., Williams, D. R., Mero, R. P., Lantz, P. M., Robert, S. A., & Chen, J. (2000). Excess mortality among urban residents: How much, for whom and why? *American Journal of Public Health, 90,* 1898–1904.

Hummer, R. A., Pacewicz, J., Wang, S., & Collins, C. (2004). Health insurance coverage in nonmetropolitan America. In N. Glasgow, L. W. Morton & N. E. Johnson (Eds.), *Critical issues in rural health* (pp. 197–209). Ames, IA: Blackwell Publishing.

Johnson, N. E. (2004). Spatial patterning of disabilities among adults. In N. Glasgow, L. W. Morton & N. E. Johnson (Eds.), *Critical issues in rural health* (pp. 27–36). Ames, IA: Blackwell Publishing.

Jones, C. A., Parker, T. S., & Ahearn, M. (2009). Taking the pulse of rural health care. *Amber Waves, 7*(3), 10–15. Retrieved from http://www.ers.usda.gov/amberwaves/september09/features/RuralHealth.htm. Accessed on September 18, 2011.

Kitagawa, E. M., & Hauser, P. M. (1973). *Differential mortality in the United States: A study of socioeconomic epidemiology.* Cambridge, MA: Harvard University Press.

Laditka, J. N., Laditka, S. B., Olatosi, B., & Elder, K. T. (2007). The health trade-off of rural residence for impaired older adults: Longer life, more impairment. *Journal of Rural Health, 23,* 124–132.

Luloff, A. E., Bourke, L., Jacob, S., & Seshan, S. (1995). *Farm and non-farm interdependencies at the rural-urban interface.* Final Project Report for the Pennsylvania Department of Agriculture, The Pennsylvania State University, University Park, PA.

Luloff, A. E., Kassab, C. D., Bridger, J. C., Melbye, J., Liao, P., & Theodori, G. L. (2000). *Rural economic development and individual well-being.* Final Research Report prepared for the United States Department of Agriculture, Cooperative State Research, Education, and Extension Service. The Pennsylvania State University, University Park, PA.

Lutfey, K., & Freese, J. (2005). Toward some fundamentals of fundamental causality: Socioeconomic status and health in the routine clinic visit for diabetes. *American Journal of Sociology, 110,* 1326–1372.

MacKenzie, T. A., Wallace, A. E., & Weeks, W. B. (2010). Impact of rural residence on survival of male veterans affairs patients after age 65. *Journal of Rural Health, 26,* 318–324.

Mechanic, D. (2004). The rise and fall of managed care. *Journal of Health and Social Behavior, 45*(Extra Issue), 76–86.

Meng, H., Wamsley, B., Liebel, D., Dixon, D., Eggert, G., & Van Nostrand, J. (2009). Urban-rural differences in the effect of a medicare health promotion and disease self-management program on physical function and health care expenditures. *The Gerontologist, 49*(3), 407–417.

Miech, R. A., & Shanahan, M. J. (2000). Socioeconomic status and depression over the life cycle. *Journal of Health and Social Behavior, 41,* 162–176.

Mirowsky, J., & Ross, C. F. (2003). *Education, social status, and health.* New York, NY: Aldine de Gruyter.
Morton, L. W. (2004). Spatial patterns of rural mortality. In N. Glasgow, L. W. Morton & N. E. Johnson (Eds.), *Critical issues in rural health* (pp. 37–45). Ames, IA: Blackwell Publishing.
Phelan, J. C., Link, B. G., Diez-Roux, A., Kawachi, I., & Levin, B. (2004). Fundamental causes of social inequalities in mortality: A test of the theory. *Journal of Health and Social Behavior, 45,* 265–285.
Schieman, S., Van Gundy, K., & Taylor, J. (2001). Status, role, and resource explanation for age patterns in psychological distress. *Journal of Health and Social Behavior, 42,* 80–96.
Smith, M. H., Anderson, R. T., Bradham, D. D., & Longino, C. F. (1995). Urban and rural differences in mortality Americans 55 years and older: Analysis of the national longitudinal mortality study. *The Journal of Rural Health, 11,* 274–285.
Steele, J., Bourke, L., Luloff, A. E., Liao, P., Theodori, G. L., & Krannich, R. S. (2001). The drop-off/pick-up method for household survey research. *Journal of the Community Development Society, 32,* 238–250.
Stern, S., Merwin, E., Hauenstein, E., Hinton, I., Rovnyak, V., Wilson, M., … Mahone, I. (2010). The effects of rurality on mental and physical health. *Health Services and Outcomes Research Methodology, 10*(1), 33–66.
Szreter, S. (1997). Economic growth, deprivation, disease and death: On the importance of politics in public health for development. *Population and Development Review, 23,* 693–728.
Theodori, G. L. (1999). *The effects of community satisfaction and attachment on individual well-being.* PhD Dissertation, Department of Agricultural Economics and Rural Sociology, The Pennsylvania State University, University Park, PA.
Theodori, G. L. (2001). Examining the effects of community satisfaction and attachment on individual well-being. *Rural Sociology, 66,* 618–628.
Theodori, G. L., Luloff, A. E., & Willits, F. K. (1998). The association of outdoor recreation and environmental concern: Reexamining the dunlap-heffernan thesis. *Rural Sociology, 63,* 94–108.
Wallace, R. B., Grindeanu, L. A., & Cirillo, D. J. (2004). Rural/urban contrasts in population morbidity status. In N. Glasgow, L. W. Morton & N. E. Johnson (Eds.), *Critical issues in rural health* (pp. 15–26). Ames, IA: Blackwell Publishing.
Ware, J. E., & Sherbourne, C. D. (1992). The MOS 36-intem short form health survey (SF-36). I. Conceptual framework and item selection. *Medical Care, 30,* 473–483.
Warren, J. R. (2009). Socioeconomic status and health across the life course: A test of social causation and health selection hypotheses. *Social Forces, 87,* 2125–2154.
Yang, Y. (2007). Is old age depressing? Growth trajectories and cohort variations in late-life depression. *Journal of Health and Social Behavior, 48,* 16–32.
Young, F. W. (2004). Community structure and population health: The challenge of explanation. In N. Glasgow, L. W. Morton & N. E. Johnson (Eds.), *Critical issues in rural health* (pp. 261–270). Ames, IA: Blackwell Publishing.

PART 3
RACE/ETHNICITY AND SES FACTORS AND DISPARITIES

ETHNIC GROUP DIFFERENCES IN THE UTILIZATION OF PREVENTIVE MEDICAL CARE SERVICES AMONG FOREIGN-BORN ASIAN AND LATINO ADULTS IN THE UNITED STATES

Bridget K. Gorman and Cindy Dinh

ABSTRACT

Purpose – *To investigate ethnic group differences in the utilization of preventive medical care services among U.S. Asian and Latino immigrant adults.*

Methodology/approach – *Using data from the 2002–2003 National Latino and Asian American Study, we examined whether differences exist in the reporting of any preventive physical care or dental/optician visit during the last year across Asian and Latino immigrant groups. Following, we applied Andersen's (1995) Behavioral Model of Health Services Use to assess how ethnic disparities in preventive care use are a function of predisposing, enabling/impeding, and need-based factors.*

Social Determinants, Health Disparities and Linkages to Health and Health Care
Research in the Sociology of Health Care, Volume 31, 111–141
Copyright © 2013 by Emerald Group Publishing Limited
All rights of reproduction in any form reserved
ISSN: 0275-4959/doi:10.1108/S0275-4959(2013)0000031008

Findings – *Descriptive results showed that among Latinos, a much lower proportion of Mexican immigrants reported a preventive medical care visit during the last year than either Cuban or Puerto Rican immigrants. Asian immigrants show less variation in use, but significant differences still exist with Filipino immigrants reporting the highest level of use, followed by Vietnamese and then Chinese immigrants. Logistic regression models also indicated that predisposing characteristics, especially aspects of acculturation status, contribute strongly to ethnic group differences in preventive care use, while enabling/disabling and need-based characteristics are less important.*

Implications – *While studies of medical care use often treat Asians and Latinos as homogeneous groups, our findings illustrate the need for a more detailed view of the foreign-born population. Findings also highlight the role of acculturation status in shaping group differences in preventive medical care use – and as such, the importance of considering these differences when promoting the use of timely preventive care services among immigrant populations.*

Keywords: Medical Care; Asian; Latino; ethnicity; acculturation; immigrant

INTRODUCTION

While beneficial for their health, each year a substantial portion of U.S. adults do not receive preventive medical care services, thereby missing recommended screenings, timely diagnoses, and effective treatments that can promote management of acute and chronic health conditions. As such, delayed or no care may result in long-term problems that exacerbate illness and lead to health decline and/or premature death (Brown, Ojeda, Wyn, & Levan, 2000; U.S. Preventive Services Task Force, 1996). Research shows that a person's utilization of preventive health care is shaped by factors that go far beyond the nature of an illness and its related symptoms (McAlpine & Boyer, 2007). This includes nativity and racial/ethnic identity, as U.S. studies show that selected immigrant and racial/ethnic groups experience diminished access to and utilization of preventive medical care services (Blendon et al., 2007; Brown et al., 2000; Frisbie, Cho, & Hummer, 2001).

To date, research has focused on medical care use among pan-ethnic rather than specific ethnic groups (i.e., Asians rather than Vietnamese, Filipino, etc., and Latinos rather than Mexican, Cuban, etc.). This is problematic given that these are diverse groups (Saenz, 2010; Xie & Goyette, 2004), some of whom may have higher medical need than the native born but more limited knowledge and access to the health care system. Research shows that ethnic immigrants constitute underserved populations when it comes to health care access and utilization (Akresh, 2009; Derose, Bahney, & Lurie, 2009). To date, however, the manner in which preventive medical care use differs across ethnic immigrants groups is not well documented, thus serving as a barrier to the development of more targeted social and economic policy initiatives aimed at improving access and use of care across immigrant populations.

In this chapter, we investigate ethnic differences in the utilization of preventive medical care among immigrants using data from the National Latino and Asian American Study (NLAAS), a nationally representative study of health and health care use among U.S. Asian and Latino adults. We begin by exploring differences in use of preventive medical care services (specifically, whether any preventive physical and dental/optical health care visits occurred during the last year) among Asian (Vietnamese, Filipino, and Chinese) and Latino (Mexican, Cuban, and Puerto Rican) foreign-born adults. Following, we apply Andersen's (1995) Behavioral Model of Health Services Use to assess how ethnic disparities in preventive care use are a function of factors that (a) shape the predisposition to use care (e.g., age, acculturation, education), (b) enable or impede the use of care (e.g., income, medical insurance status), and (c) influence the perceived need for care (e.g., participation in unhealthy behaviors like smoking and heavy drinking). This focus is important, as knowledge of the predictors of use among disparate ethnic groups is understudied and remains inconclusive (see Zambrana & Carter-Pokras, 2010), and factors relating to access and utilization of health care are complex, multifaceted processes that are contingent upon illness status in addition to an array of individual and social factors (Andersen, 1995). As such, our analysis describes not only the pattern of preventive health care use across immigrant ethnic groups, it also establishes whether predisposing, enabling, and need-based factors mediate ethnic differences in use within Asian and Latino immigrant populations.

IMMIGRANTS, ETHNICITY, AND PREVENTIVE MEDICAL CARE USE

Latino and Asian ethnic groups are substantial and growing segments of the U.S. population. All together Latinos total 16.3% of the U.S. population, of whom one-third are foreign-born and hail from Spanish-speaking countries in Latin America, Spain, and the Caribbean (Terrazas & Batalova, 2009; U.S. Census Bureau, 2011b). While Mexicans are the largest segment of the U.S. Latino population (roughly two-thirds of all Latinos), Puerto Ricans are the second most prominent group, followed by Salvadoran, Cuban, and Dominicans (Saenz, 2010). Asian Americans are an even more diverse population whose origins trace to many national backgrounds, with members who speak a variety of languages and are characterized by diverse social and economic characteristics (Lee, 1998; Xie & Goyette, 2004). All together Asian Americans comprised 5.6% of the total U.S. population in 2010 with one-fifth classified as first-generation immigrants (U.S. Census Bureau, 2011a). Chinese Americans comprise the largest proportion (about 24%), followed by Filipino, Asian Indian, Vietnamese, and Korean Americans (Xie & Goyette, 2004).

While research demonstrates a clear gap in access and receipt of medical care across racial and ethnic groups (Blendon et al., 2007; Flores & Tomany-Korman, 2008; Kang-Kim et al., 2008), no published studies that we could identify examined ethnic group differences in medical care use among immigrants (e.g., Vietnamese immigrants, Cuban immigrants). Studies generally find that racial minorities, compared to whites, are more likely to have forgone a medical or dental visit last year (Flores & Tomany-Korman, 2008). Latinos in particular report less use than whites of preventive care, such as breast self-exams, mammography, and Pap testing, and higher outcomes of diabetes and being overweight or obese than non-Latinos (Kang-Kim et al., 2008; Rodriguez, Bustamante, & Ang, 2009; Tanningco, 2007). While Asians tend to do better than Latinos in terms of visits to the doctor or dentist, studies report diminished access and use in relation to whites. For example, Kim, Kronenfeld, and Rivers (2007) find that about half of Asians reported receiving any dental services last year, compared to 61% of whites.

Yet research on ethnic group differences is growing, with studies increasingly documenting significant diversity in medical care use within both pan-ethnic Asian and Latino groups. One recent study of medical care use compared 14 different ethnic groups, finding that while selected populations (i.e., Cubans, Mexicans, Vietnamese and Koreans) were the least likely to report receiving care from a health care professional last year, other groups (i.e., Japanese, Asian Indians) were actually *less* likely than whites to report receiving poor care (Blendon et al., 2007). In addition, while Solis and colleagues (1990) reported that Puerto Ricans are more likely than Cubans and Mexicans to use the hospital ER services as their usual source of care, this contradicts a newer study by Beal, Hernandez, and Doty (2009) which found that Puerto Ricans, because of their citizenship status, used preventive care services and reported having a regular source of care at a rate similar to whites.

Studies have shown that immigrant status, especially when combined with a lack of U.S. citizenship, is associated with diminished access to routine medical care services (Ku & Matani, 2001). For example, Goldman, Smith, and Sood (2006) in a study of Los Angeles County adults find that a large portion of foreign-born adults had no contact with the formal medical care system during the last year, with one-quarter of immigrants never receiving a routine medical checkup – a rate nearly double that of native-born adults. In addition, a recent analysis of the 2003–2005 National Health Interview Survey by Ye, Mack, Fry-Johnson, and Parker (2012) finds that foreign-born Asian American adults were less likely than native-born Asians to have seen or talked to a general doctor during the last year. While studies that systematically examine ethnic group differences in medical care use among immigrants are lacking, research does show that heterogeneity exists in the extent to which immigrants are vulnerable to inadequate health care (Derose, Escarce, & Lurie, 2007).

Explanations for Differences in Preventive Medical Care Use

To identify the factors that shape preventive care use across Asian and Latino ethnic immigrant groups, we apply the theoretical framework proposed by Andersen (1968, 1995). Specifically, in the Behavioral Model of Health Service Use, Andersen outlines how the use of health services is due to (a) the predisposition to use services, (b) factors which enable or impede use, and (c) the perceived need for care. Even though the behavioral model has been rarely examined among immigrants, this model is appropriate for our sample as Akresh (2009) finds that Anderson's behavioral model is well suited for predicting preventive medical care use among immigrant samples.

Predisposing characteristics include demographic and social structure components. Demographic traits like age and gender predispose health care utilization (Courtenay, Mccreary, & Merighi, 2002; Vaidya, Partha, & Karmakar, 2011), while aspects of an individual's social structure matter because they relate to status and the ability to cope and respond to health problems (Andersen, 1995). Notably for immigrants, factors related to acculturation status (or the process of adaption occurring through contact with a host culture; Salabarria-Pena et al., 2001) are important as behavioral choices are influenced by culturally based knowledge, attitudes, and beliefs

(Gor, 2010), and research shows that more acculturated adults use medical services more frequently than less acculturated adults (Lara, Gamboa, Kahramanian, Morales, & Bautista, 2005; Salant & Lauderdale, 2003). Compared to the native-born, immigrants often have different expectations of Western medicine, communication preferences, familiarity with navigating health systems, and facility with English – all of which may impede understanding of and access to benefits, services, and health information (Takeuchi, Alegria, Jackson, & Williams, 2007).

Following the works of Alegria, Sribney, Woo, Torres, and Guarnaccia (2007), Berry (2003), and Salant and Lauderdale (2003), we see acculturation as a multidimensional process, with adherence to a new host culture operating independently of how strongly ties are maintained to the culture of origin. While acculturation is a process of adaptation to a new culture, it is not necessarily a linear process, and thus may not lead to a loss of a person's ethnic identity and ties to their origin culture (Beck, Froman, & Bernal, 2005; Lara et al., 2005). Therefore, examining measures which gauge behaviors referenced against the country of origin and the United States, considering factors that represent both pre- and postmigration decisions and context, can allow for a more nuanced assessment of how acculturation influences medical care use (Arends-Tóth & van de Vijver, 2006; Berry, 2003). Indeed, while factors such as U.S. citizenship are relevant since it is an important determinant of access to health insurance (Derose et al., 2009; Ku & Matani, 2001), behaviors such as remitting and return visits may be pseudo-measures for less acculturation, as individuals are still closely tied financially and physically to their country of origin. Reasons for migration, and whether migration was a voluntary choice (or not), can also affect how the acculturation process operates for immigrants – including the likelihood that migration is accompanied by stressful circumstances (poverty, violence) and health conditions that shape the need for and ability to access medical care services (Salant & Lauderdale, 2003). In addition, while we examine differences in medical care use for persons who identify as members of various ethnic groups, the extent to which immigrants report feelings of belonging, commitment, and shared values with a group represents an important aspect of the acculturation process that goes beyond ethnic self-identification alone (Liebkind, 2006; Sam, 2006), and may therefore influence the extent to which health care is desired and accessed.

Research on acculturation and medical care use shows that patterns vary by ethnic group (Salant & Lauderdale, 2003), and may be influenced by language barriers (Facione, Giancarlo, & Chan, 2000). Indeed, language ability is especially relevant for health care use as over half of all U.S.

immigrants come from Latin America and Asia, the majority of whom do not speak English as their first language (Terrazas & Batalova, 2009). In particular, the Asian and Pacific Islander population represents over 50 racial/ethnic backgrounds and speaks over 100 different languages (Tseng et al., 2010). Furthermore, 40.7% of those who speak an Asian or Pacific Islander language and 35.6% of those who speak the Spanish language at home report speaking English less than very well in the latest Census (U.S. Census Bureau, 2010). Yet research shows that English fluency is an important resource for navigating and accessing health care services (DuBard & Gizlice, 2008), and Spanish-speaking Latinos have been shown to use less health care than English-speaking Latinos (Fiscella, Franks, Doescher, & Saver, 2002), with the lack of Spanish-speaking doctors a demonstrated barrier to health care for this group (Whitley, Samuels, Wright, & Everhart, 2005). In addition, Hu and Covell (1986) found that the frequency of general physical, vision, and dental checkups among Latino adults in San Diego was positively correlated with English use, compared to those who were bilingual or spoke primarily Spanish (Hu & Covell, 1986). Evidence also suggests that the relevance of English language use in medical care appears to differ by group, as Akresh (2009) found that English proficiency predicts dental visits among Latino but not Asian immigrants. Blendon et al. (2007) also found that nearly one in five Puerto Rican, Mexican and Vietnamese Americans reported receiving poor quality care because of how they spoke English. The few exceptions include Japanese, Asian Indian, Filipino, and Cuban Americans – groups who consistently report health care experiences similar to whites, which appears driven by their distinct historical context when immigrating, along with exposure to English in their countries of origin and to Western political systems and health beliefs (Akresh, 2009; Sakamoto, Goyette, & Kim, 2009).

Beyond acculturation, marriage and the composition of one's household can promote preventive medical care use through enhanced social and financial supports (Sandman, Simantov, & An, 2000), although little research to date has explored whether and how marital status shapes preventive medical care use (see review by Wood, Goesling, & Avellar, 2007). Other aspects of social structure are more established in their relevance for health care use, especially education. Research shows that educational attainment positively affects one's likelihood of using preventive health care and that employment is generally associated with better health (Ross & Wu, 1995). Studies show that immigrants who have on average higher educational and occupational levels tend to have smoother transitions to the United States, akin to older, European immigrant groups, a trend seen across racial groups (Frisbie et al., 2001; Lara et al., 2005). Studies show that Asian Americans, on average, tend to be well educated (Xie and Goyette, 2000), while Latinos report relatively low education levels, especially Mexican Americans (Brown et al., 2000). While Asians are often portrayed as model minorities and generally have high educational attainment (Frisbie et al., 2001; Sakamoto et al., 2009), these portrayals often mask documented health disparities and SES differences across subgroups, as recent immigrants face educational and linguistic barriers that in turn affect their economic and educational success, and social integration (Sakamoto et al., 2009; Tseng et al., 2010). Among Asians, educational attainment ranges from very high (Asian Indians and Japanese) to very low (Cambodians and Laotians), in part because completing secondary school was uncommon for the latter cohort of immigrants who arrived in the United States from mostly poor circumstances, including refugees from counties like Vietnam and Laos (Frisbie et al., 2001; Sakamoto et al., 2009).

Enabling resources must also be present to facilitate health care use (Andersen, 1995). Financial resources like health insurance and income are requirements for entry into the U.S. medical care system (Leclere, Jensen, & Biddlecom, 1994). Selected minority groups, including Latinos, tend to have lower incomes and lower rates of private health insurance coverage than whites and other groups, and insurance rates for Asians differ across ethnicities and generations (Ashton, Collins, Petersen, & Wray, 2003; Brown et al., 2000). Immigrant studies show substantial wage growth and insurance coverage with increasing time spent in the United States and acculturation more generally (Antecol, Kuhn, & Trejo, 2006; Rodriguez et al., 2009).

Enabling resources also include the quality of social relationships, both positive and negative. Social relationships are often seen as health-protective; they improve health through various routes, including the provision of supports (emotional, instrumental, and financial) that may facilitate the use of medical care (Berkman & Glass, 2000). At the same time, not all social relationships benefit health, as negative exchanges within social networks are associated with greater life stress and less supportive networks (Rook, 2003). Indeed, stressors related to immigration can influence one's need for and use of medical care services. For example, refugees from countries like Vietnam and Laos are more likely to enter the United States from poor circumstances with high levels of preexisting distress and posttraumatic stress from political and civil strife, adding to the typical stresses associated with immigration (Salant & Lauderdale, 2003). In addition, limited English proficiency often leads to communication difficulties between patients and health professionals, perceived discrimination, and problems associated with being poor and uninsured (Blendon et al., 2007). These problems are more pronounced for recent immigrants, who report higher racial and language discrimination. Yet at the same time, when compared to the U.S. dominant culture, Asian or Latino cultures are more likely to have strong familial and support networks that can help abate everyday stresses (Andersen, 1995; Foner, 1997). Such familism is embedded in most extended family structures but seems to rapidly deteriorate after U.S. arrival due to intergenerational conflict and tension from disconcerted values of individuality and independence (Alegria et al., 2007; Ying & Han, 2007).

Finally, Andersen's (1968, 1995) framework outlines the possibility that health care use is influenced by factors related to one's *perceived need for care*, represented by health behaviors and health status. Health statuses prompt people to seek medical care, and studies document elevated health problems among Latino immigrants compared to whites (Tanningco, 2007), and that more harmful health behaviors (e.g., less exercise) beset more acculturated Latinos than the less acculturated (Lara et al., 2005). While the health status of Asians also changes with acculturation and exposure to U.S. culture, strikingly, the burden of cancer and other morbidities are disproportionally distributed between Asian ethnic groups; in the United States, more than half of Hepatitis B carriers are of Asian descent, particularly among Vietnamese men (Gor, 2010).

Overall, studies exploring ethnic differences in immigrant health care use rarely test these three hypothesized pathways of use, and as such an important facet of our study is its ability to describe patterns in preventive care use among Latino and Asian adults who migrated from different sending nations, in addition to investigating the predisposing, enabling, and need-based factors that may drive these differences.

DATA, MEASURES, AND METHOD

We examine data on immigrant adults from the NLAAS. Collected in 2002–2003, the NLAAS is a nationally representative community household survey designed to examine mental health and health care among U.S. Latinos and Asians Americans aged 18 and older. A multistage, stratified national area probability sample was drawn from the noninstitutionalized U.S. population, with oversampling of areas with a moderate-to-high density of Latinos and Asian Americans. All interviewers were bilingual, and interviews were conducted in person and in English, Spanish, Vietnamese, Chinese (either Mandarin or Cantonese), or Tagalog. The overall response rate was 65.6% for Asian Americans and 75.5% for Latinos (see Heeringa et al., 2004 and Pennell et al., 2004 for detailed sampling descriptions). When weighted, the NLAAS includes a nationally representative sample of 4,649 adults, including 2,554 Latinos and 2,095 Asian Americans. We limit this sample to foreign-born adults and remove "other" Asian and Latino adults from the sample, given our interest in examining ethnic-group differences in medical care use – resulting in our final sample of 2,528 respondents. Rates of item nonresponse for our independent measures are nonexistent or small (under 5%), and are imputed using the ICE command in Stata 12.0. Missing values on dependent measures are not imputed. All analyses were run using the Stata 12.0 software package, and utilized Taylor-series-approximate methods with SVY commands (in conjunction with the MIM commands following multiple imputation of missing data) to adjust for the complex sample design of the NLAAS. All analyses are also weighted with the final sampling weight.

Measures

Measures of medical care use include (1) *any visits last year for a routine physical checkup*, and (2) *any visits last year to a dentist or optician for a routine checkup*. Following Andersen's model, we divide our predictors into three main categories: predisposing characteristics, enabling resources, and factors related to one's perceived need for care.

All models are stratified by Latino/Asian sample, and baseline models test the importance of predisposing characteristics, including *gender, age at interview*, and dummy variables for *ethnicity* (Vietnamese, Filipino, and Chinese [reference] for Asians, and Cuban, Puerto Rican, and Mexicans [reference] for Latinos). For both Latinos and Asians we select the largest ethnic group as the reference for comparison – Mexican immigrants for Latinos, and Chinese immigrants for Asians.

Previous health and health care studies typically measure acculturation status with a variety of proxy variables (Hunt, Schneider, & Comer, 2004; Lara et al., 2005), and we include measures that reference ties to both origin and U.S. culture. This includes two aspects of premigration context: whether *migration to the United States was voluntary* (1 = yes, 0 = no), and three yes–no dummy variables that gauge *reasons for migrating to the United*

States, including (1) to find a job, (2) to join other family members, and (3) to seek medical attention. We also include dichotomous measures of *age at U.S. migration* (1 = before age 18, 0 = age 18 +), whether they currently *remit money* to relatives in their country of origin (1 = yes, 0 = no), *how frequently they make return visits to their country of origin* (1 = never, 2 = rarely, 3 = sometimes, and 4 = often), and *citizenship status* (1 = U.S. citizen, 0 = other). We also examine a measure of strength of *co-ethnic ties*, based on the average response to four questions that ask respondents to rank how close they feel to others of the same racial/ethnic descent (e.g., "How closely do you identify with other people who are of the same racial and ethnic descent as yourself?," $\alpha = .66$).

We also include two measures of *language ability* that consider English language proficiency in tandem with native language proficiency. For English ability, respondents were asked to rate their ability to read, write, and speak English on a four-point scale (where 1 = poor and 4 = excellent), from which we calculated their average ability across these three domains of use ($\alpha = .97$). Similarly, respondents were asked to rate their ability to read, write, and speak their native language, and again we calculated their average ability ($\alpha = .89$). In our models, we also test the interaction between English proficiency and native language proficiency, since limited research finds different patterns of health care utilization for immigrants who are bilingual (Hu & Covell, 1986).

Additional predisposing characteristics in the baseline model include *marital status* (1 = married or cohabiting, 0 = otherwise), and the *number of adults and children living in the household*. We also include *years of completed schooling* and a dichotomous measure of *employment status* (1 = currently working, 0 = otherwise).

Building upon the baseline model that examines only predisposing characteristics, we next test a model that adds factors which may enable the use of health care services, including *poverty status* (1 = income below the 2001 federal poverty line, 0 = higher) and a continuous measure of the extent to which respondents report that they have *difficulty paying monthly bills* (1 = not at all difficult and 4 = very difficult). We gauge how easily adults can access care by considering *medical insurance status* (1 = no medical insurance, 0 = insured), and whether they report having a *regular doctor* for routine medical care (1 = yes, 0 = no).

For enabling resources we also include measures of the quality of social relationships, stress, and discrimination. *Positive social support* is constructed from six questions ($\alpha = .73$) that gauge the availability of support from friends and family (e.g., how much they can rely on relatives they don't live with if they have a serious problem), where $1 =$ less than once a month and $5 =$ almost every day, while *family cohesion* is constructed from 10 questions ($\alpha = .93$) that gauge family closeness and communication (e.g., family members like to spend free time with each other), where $1 =$ hardly ever or never, $2 =$ sometimes, and $3 =$ often. Measures of stress and discrimination include *acculturative stress*, which is a summed index ($\alpha = .71$) based on responses to nine yes–no questions about stress experienced since migrating to the United States (e.g., "Have you felt guilty about leaving family or friends in your country of origin?"). We also include the *frequency of day-to-day discriminatory treatment* on the basis of national origin/ancestry, race, or skin color (where $1 =$ never and $6 =$ almost everyday), constructed from the average of nine questions about routine experiences with racial discrimination (e.g., being treated with less respect than other people; $\alpha = .91$). *Negative social exchanges* is an averaged index based on four questions that ask how frequently friends and family argue with and make too many demands on the respondent (where $1 =$ less than once a month and $5 =$ almost every day; $\alpha = .68$), while *family cultural conflict* is an averaged index ($\alpha = .78$) based on five questions addressing issues of cultural and intergenerational conflict between respondents and families (e.g., arguments over different customs), where $1 =$ hardly ever or never, $2 =$ sometimes, and $3 =$ often (see Alegria et al., 2004).

Our final model includes factors related to one's perceived need for care. We control for three health behaviors, including dummy variables for *smoking status* (current smoker, former smoker, and never smoked), and *heavy drinking* (defined as two or more drinks per day for women, and three or more drinks per day for men; DHHS and Department of Agriculture, 2005). We also measure whether respondents are classified as *overweight or obese* ($1 =$ yes, $0 =$ no), based on their body mass index. For health status, we include two measures: *self-rated physical health* and *self-rated mental health* ($1 =$ poor and $5 =$ excellent).

RESULTS

Descriptive Statistics

Table 1 stratifies our sample by ethnic group, showing weighted means and percent values for all measures. Looking at utilization of preventive medical care in the first two rows, for Latino immigrants we see that as a group, Mexican immigrants report significantly lower use than either Cuban or

Table 1. NLASS Foreign-Born Adults: Sample Characteristics (Percentages and Means), by Latino and Asian Ethnic Group.

	Immigrant Asian Adults			Immigrant Latino Adults		
	Vietnamese	Filipino	Chinese	Mexican	Cuban	Puerto Rican
Any routine physical care visits last year	76.7***	81.3***	70.9	52.9	72.2***	80.4***
Any routine dental/optician visits	70.3***	75.2***	65.9	39.4	60.6***	65.9***
Predisposing characteristics						
Age at interview	44.4 (14.4)	46.7 (15.5)***	43.5 (13.3)	35.8 (11.9)	51.7 (16.3)***	47.0 (15.6)***
Female	54.0	57.0	54.6	45.2	48.2*	48.0
Voluntarily moved to the United States	82.5***	67.2	68.4	72.4	32.9***	71.8
Migrated to the United States in order to....						
Find a job	2.3 (0.9)*	2.7 (0.6)***	2.4 (0.8)	2.7 (0.7)	2.2 (0.9)***	2.5 (0.8)***
Join other family members	2.5 (0.9)***	2.4 (0.8)***	2.3 (0.8)	2.1 (0.9)	2.2 (0.9)***	2.2 (0.9)
Seek medical attention	1.7 (0.9)***	1.5 (0.8)	1.5 (0.7)	1.3 (0.6)	1.4 (0.8)***	1.5 (0.8)***
Migrated to United States before age 18	19.9	23.5	21.0	43.1	25.6***	52.3***
Remits money to relatives	63.5***	64.5***	35.7	43.0	40.6	16.9***
How often returns to country of origin	1.8 (0.9)***	2.4 (1.0)***	2.2 (0.9)	2.3 (1.0)	1.6 (0.8)***	2.8 (0.9)***
Strength of co-ethnic ties	3.5 (0.6)***	3.1 (0.5)***	3.0 (0.5)	3.1 (0.6)	3.3 (0.6)***	3.2 (0.5)**
Proficiency in country-of-origin language	3.2 (0.9)***	3.1 (1.0)**	3.0 (0.9)	3.0 (0.8)	3.3 (0.7)***	3.0 (0.9)
Proficiency in English	2.0 (0.9)***	3.2 (0.8)***	2.3 (1.0)	1.6 (0.9)	1.9 (1.1)***	2.4 (1.0)***
U.S. Citizen	71.6***	66.5***	59.3	20.5	54.6***	98.4***
Married or cohabiting	75.9	77.3*	74.0	76.1	65.2***	59.8***
Household size	3.5 (1.6)***	3.2 (1.7)***	2.7 (1.4)	3.5 (1.8)	2.5 (1.3)***	2.4 (1.4)***
Years of schooling	11.8 (3.8)***	13.6 (3.1)	13.4 (3.3)	8.9 (3.6)	11.8 (3.8)***	11.2 (3.6)***
Currently working	62.1*	66.1	65.6	64.7	57.5***	53.9***
Enabling/disabling characteristics						
Poor	37.6***	13.9***	27.0	52.1	34.5***	32.5***

Table 1. (Continued)

	Immigrant Asian Adults			Immigrant Latino Adults		
	Vietnamese	Filipino	Chinese	Mexican	Cuban	Puerto Rican
Extent of difficulty paying monthly bills	2.1 (1.0)***	1.9 (0.9)***	1.7 (0.8)	2.5 (0.9)	2.4 (1.1)	2.3 (1.0)***
No medical insurance	18.2	11.5***	15.8	56.0	25.0***	13.7***
Has a regular doctor	64.8	71.4*	67.5	40.4	69.7***	83.0***
Acculturative Stress	1.8 (1.5)***	1.2 (1.3)***	2.1 (1.6)	2.6 (1.8)	1.9 (1.5)***	1.5 (1.5)***
Frequency of discriminatory experiences	1.1 (0.8)	1.3 (1.0)***	1.1 (0.9)	1.2 (1.0)	1.0 (0.7)***	1.2 (1.0)
Negative social exchanges	1.5 (0.5)***	2.0 (0.5)***	1.7 (0.5)	1.7 (0.6)	1.6 (0.6)***	1.7 (0.6)
Family cultural conflict	1.2 (0.3)***	1.3 (0.4)*	1.3 (0.4)	1.3 (0.4)	1.2 (0.4)***	1.3 (0.4)**
Positive social support	2.0 (0.7)***	2.7 (0.7)***	2.4 (0.7)	2.5 (0.7)	2.9 (0.7)***	2.7 (0.7)***
Family cohesion	3.8 (0.4)***	3.8 (0.4)***	3.6 (0.5)	3.6 (0.5)	3.8 (0.4)***	3.6 (0.6)***
Need-based characteristics						
Smoking status						
Current smoker	17.4**	18.6***	13.8	21.8	20.3	26.0*
Former smoker	13.6**	21.6***	10.5	17.4	23.0***	28.9***
Never smoked	69.0***	59.9***	75.7	60.8	56.7**	45.1***
Current heavy drinker	3.6	12.2***	2.9	20.6	17.9*	21.5
Overweight or obese	17.7***	47.8***	22.3	70.5	69.1	69.6
Self-rated physical health	3.3 (1.2)***	3.6 (0.9)***	3.1 (0.9)	3.1 (1.1)	3.4 (1.2)***	3.1 (1.3)
Self-rated mental health	3.6 (1.1)**	4.0 (0.9)***	3.5 (1.0)	3.5 (1.1)	3.8 (1.1)***	3.7 (1.1)**
Sample size	501	349	473	487	501	217

Note: Standard deviations in (parentheses). *$p \leq .05$; **$p \leq .01$; ***$p \leq .001$ (two-tailed test, relative to Chinese for the Asian sample, and relative to Mexican adults for the Latino sample).

Puerto Rican immigrants. Just over half (52.9%) of Mexican immigrants had a preventive physical care visit last year, compared to 72.2% of Cuban and 80.4% of Puerto Rican migrants. While usage rates are lower for all groups, the pattern is similar for a routine dental or optical visit, with just over a third of Mexicans (39.4%) reporting any care last year, compared to 60.6% of Cubans and 65.9% of Puerto Ricans.

For the most part, Asian immigrants report greater use of preventive medical services than Latino immigrants, but rates differ by group even though we see less variation based on ethnicity. Filipinos do better on average than either Vietnamese or Chinese immigrants, but while significantly more Filipinos report a physical care visit than Chinese immigrants (81.3% vs. 70.9%), the difference with Vietnamese immigrants (76.7%) is not significant (additional test not shown). A similar pattern emerges for dental/optical use, with Filipino adults reporting the highest use rate (75.2%), which is significantly higher than Chinese (65.9%) but not Vietnamese immigrants (70.3%).

For predisposing measures, Table 1 shows that the Latino sample is slightly more male than female, with the Mexican sample containing the highest proportion of men (54.8%) and the youngest average age (35.8 years), compared to Puerto Ricans and Cubans who are substantially older (47.0 and 51.7 years, respectively). Mexican immigrants have the lowest education levels (average schooling: 8.9 years), while Cuban immigrants have the highest (11.8 years). Mexican immigrants also report the highest rate of employment and marriage/cohabitation, and they live in larger households than Cuban and Puerto Rican immigrants.

In certain respects, Mexican immigrants also report low acculturation levels; only one in five reports U.S. citizenship (compared to over half of Cubans and nearly all Puerto Ricans), and they report low-proficiency (in reading, writing, and speaking) English. However, Mexicans are less distinctive when other measures of acculturation are considered. While they report lower proficiency in Spanish than Cuban immigrants, their proficiency level is equivalent with Puerto Ricans. Mexican immigrants are also similar to Puerto Ricans in the frequency of visits to their home country, and both groups report more frequent visits than Cubans. Yet, Cubans also report the strongest co-ethnic ties of the three groups. Mexican immigrants do report the highest remittance rate (43.0%), but this number is very similar to Cubans (40.6%); only Puerto Ricans are substantially lower, at 16.9%. Perhaps this low remittance rate of Puerto Ricans reflects their longer-term ties to the United States, as over half report migrating to the United States as a child (followed by 43.1% of Mexicans and 25.6%

of Cubans), and over 70% report that migrating was a voluntary decision (a rate similar to Mexicans, but much higher than Cubans). And when we examine reasons for migrating, we see diversity across ethnic groups: Mexicans are most likely to agree that migration was motivated by the desire to find a job, compared to family reunification (which is a somewhat stronger motivation for Cuban and Puerto Rican immigrants), and seeking medical attention (which is mentioned most strongly by Puerto Rican immigrants).

For Asian immigrants, predisposing characteristics in Table 1 show that the Asian sample is more female than male, with Filipino immigrants reporting a slightly higher average age (46.7 years) than the other groups. Rates of marriage and cohabitation are also high for all Asian ethnic groups (about three out of four respondents), although Chinese immigrants report significantly smaller households (2.7 persons) than Filipino and Vietnamese immigrants (3.2 and 3.5 persons, respectively). And while Asian immigrants are more highly educated than Latino immigrants on average, we see that the Vietnamese stand out with significantly lower years of completed schooling (11.8) in comparison to Filipino (13.6) and Chinese adults (13.4). Vietnamese immigrants also report somewhat lower employment rates.

In terms of acculturation measures, Vietnamese immigrants also appear distinctive. Compared to Chinese and Filipino migrants, the Vietnamese report the highest rate of U.S. citizenship, the highest rate of voluntary movement to the United States, and the fewest visits to their country of origin. At the same time, however, Vietnamese immigrants also report the lowest proficiency in English but the highest proficiency in their native language, the highest remittance rate, and the strongest co-ethnic ties. The Vietnamese are also the least likely to agree that they migrated to the United States in search of a job, and more strongly agree that they migrated in order to join family members and to seek medical attention.

For enabling characteristics, within each sample Table 1 shows that Vietnamese and Mexican immigrants report the poorest socioeconomic standing while Filipinos and Puerto Ricans do the best. Indeed, Vietnamese and Mexicans report the highest level of poverty and difficulty paying bills, along with the lowest rate of insurance coverage and having a regular doctor. For measures of stress and support, however, we see different patterns of risk and support. Among Asians, while Chinese immigrants report the highest level of acculturative stress, Filipino immigrants stand out in reporting the most discrimination, family cultural conflict, and negative social exchanges – while simultaneously reporting high levels of positive social support and family cohesion. Among Latinos, Mexican immigrants report much higher levels of acculturative stress, and along with Puerto Ricans they report higher (and similar) levels of discrimination, family cultural conflict, and negative social exchanges; indeed, Cuban immigrants report the lower levels of stress overall, along with the highest levels of positive social support and family cohesion.

And finally, for need-based characteristics Table 1 shows that while smoking rates are slightly higher among Puerto Ricans, rates of heavy drinking are lowest among Cubans and rates of overweight/obesity are quite similar across groups. However, Cubans do report substantially higher self-rated physical and mental health when compared to Puerto Ricans and Mexicans. Among Asian immigrants, Chinese adults report the least smoking (13.8%) and heavy drinking (2.9%). In contrast, 12.2% of Filipinos are heavy drinkers and 47.8% are overweight or obese – more than double the Chinese (22.3%) and Vietnamese (17.7%) rate. Yet, for perceived health status Filipinos do best, reporting higher levels of self-rated mental and physical health than either Chinese or Vietnamese adults.

Logistic Regression Models: Any Preventive Medical Care Use Last Year

We start our multivariate analysis in Table 2 by examining unstandardized coefficients from logistic regression models predicting whether or not respondents received a doctor visit for a routine physical checkup last year. For Asian immigrants, adjusting for predisposing characteristics in Model 1 explains away the difference in having received a physical checkup between Filipino and Chinese immigrants, but as we saw in Table 1, Vietnamese adults remain significantly more likely to have had a visit last year than Chinese adults. Model 1 also shows that Asian immigrants are significantly more likely to have received a checkup when they are U.S. citizens, when migration for medical attention is a strong motivation for moving to the United States, and when they have completed more years of schooling; use decreases when Asian immigrants report that they are currently working.

In Model 2 we add enabling characteristics and see that the coefficients for ethnicity do not diminish, but actually increase in size, indicating that aspects of socioeconomic resources, stress, and support suppress some of the differences in physical care checkups across Asian ethnic immigrants. In particular, medical insurance and having a regular doctor are strongly associated with receiving a physical checkup, and those who report higher levels of day-to-day discrimination are also more likely to have received a routine physical care visit last year.

Table 2. Coefficients from Logistic Regression Models, Any Routine Physical Health Visits Last Year.

	Immigrant Asian Adults (n = 1,318)			Immigrant Latino Adults (n = 1,197)		
	Model 1	Model 2	Model 3	Model 1	Model 2	Model 3
Predisposing characteristics						
Age at interview	.01 (.01)	.01 (.01)	.01 (.01)	.03 (.01)**	.01 (.01)	.01 (.01)
Female	.91 (.20)***	.89 (.20)***	.92 (.23)***	1.02 (.20)***	.81 (.21)***	.65 (.26)*
Ethnicity (reference: Chinese or Mexican)						
Vietnamese	.54 (.22)*	.65 (.21)**	.65 (.21)**	–	–	–
Filipino	.27 (.19)	.30 (.24)	.23 (.24)	–	–	–
Cuban				.08 (.27)	–.21 (.26)	–.19 (.27)
Puerto Rican				.39 (.29)	.12 (.38)	.17 (.38)
Voluntarily moved to the United States	.02 (.17)	.06 (.16)	.07 (.16)	–.40 (.17)*	–.44 (.19)*	–.43 (.18)*
Migrated to the United States in order to....						
Find a job	.05 (.11)	.09 (.14)	.10 (.12)	.03 (.14)	–.11 (.13)	–.10 (.12)
Join other family members	.07 (.11)	.10 (.12)	.10 (.12)	–.32 (.07)***	–.29 (.08)***	–.29 (.09)**
Seek medical attention	.33 (.12)**	.35 (.11)**	.35 (.11)**	.48 (.14)***	.37 (.14)*	.40 (.15)**
Migrated to United States before age 18	–.25 (.27)	–.32 (.26)	–.35 (.27)	–.09 (.25)	–.07 (.31)	–.07 (.30)
Remits money to relatives in country of origin	–.07 (.17)	–.15 (.20)	–.13 (.20)	.14 (.20)	.37 (.21)	.34 (.20)
How often returns to country of origin	.16 (.11)	.08 (.12)	.08 (.12)	.18 (.11)	.12 (.15)	.12 (.15)
Strength of co-ethnic ties	.08 (.14)	.03 (.14)	.05 (.14)	–.05 (.15)	–.22 (.15)	–.23 (.16)
Language proficiency						
Country-of-origin language	–.21 (.23)	–.23 (.30)	–.25 (.29)	.50 (.27)	.58 (.34)	.54 (.36)
English language	.12 (.31)	–.22 (.35)	–.24 (.35)	.92 (.50)	.99 (.64)	.89 (.67)
Country-of-origin* English	.06 (.09)	.09 (.10)	.09 (.10)	–.19 (.14)	–.26 (.18)	–.24 (.18)

	1	2	3	4	5
U.S. Citizen	.40 (.18)*	.24 (.21)	.45 (.32)	.08 (.31)	.09 (.31)
Married or cohabiting	.48 (.26)	.28 (.28)	.35 (.24)	.34 (.26)	.31 (.26)
Household size	-.07 (.08)	-.02 (.09)	.05 (.05)	.06 (.05)	.06 (.05)
Years of schooling	.08 (.02)**	.08 (.03)**	.03 (.04)	.02 (.04)	.03 (.04)
Currently working	-.42 (.16)*	-.50 (.17)**	-.31 (.25)	-.30 (.29)	-.27 (.31)
Enabling/disabling characteristics					
Poor	.12 (.26)	.12 (.26)	.12 (.26)	.34 (.21)	.34 (.21)
Extent of difficulty paying monthly bills	-.01 (.12)	-.01 (.11)	-.01 (.11)	.15 (.13)	.14 (.13)
No medical insurance	-1.18 (.21)***	-1.16 (.21)***	-1.16 (.21)***	-1.10 (.21)***	-1.05 (.22)***
Has a regular doctor	1.41 (.21)***	1.42 (.22)***	1.42 (.22)***	1.66 (.18)***	1.66 (.18)***
Acculturative Stress	-.07 (.05)	-.07 (.05)	-.07 (.05)	-.04 (.08)	-.04 (.08)
Frequency of discriminatory experiences	.25 (.09)*	.24 (.09)*	.24 (.09)*	.07 (.13)	.05 (.13)
Negative social exchanges	.25 (.16)	.23 (.17)	.23 (.17)	-.09 (.15)	-.08 (.16)
Family cultural conflict	.16 (.27)	.17 (.27)	.17 (.27)	.47 (.23)*	.55 (.24)*
Positive social support	.16 (.12)	.17 (.12)	.17 (.12)	.11 (.16)	.09 (.16)
Family cohesion	.21 (.21)	.19 (.21)	.19 (.21)	.40 (.25)	.38 (.23)
Need-based characteristics					
Smoking status (reference: current smoker)					
Former smoker		.07 (.25)	.07 (.25)		.07 (.40)
Never smoked		.06 (.20)	.06 (.20)		.40 (.31)
Current heavy drinker		.09 (.45)	.09 (.45)		-.11 (.20)
Overweight or obese		.22 (.18)	.22 (.18)		.02 (.19)
Self-rated physical health		-.04 (.13)	-.04 (.13)		-.00 (.08)
Self-rated mental health		.07 (.13)	.07 (.13)		.07 (.10)

*p ≤ .05, **p ≤ .01, ***p ≤ .001.

Finally, Model 3 adds need-based characteristics, showing that adjusting for health behaviors and status mediates none of the difference in use between Vietnamese and Chinese adults. And indeed, none of these measures are direct predictors of having received a physical checkup during the last year.

For Latino immigrants, the story in Table 2 is somewhat different. Adjusting for predisposing characteristics in Model 1 explains away the lower rate of physical care checkups among Mexican immigrants relative to Cubans and Puerto Ricans, driven predominantly by the circumstances and motivations for migration. Specifically, Latino immigrants are less likely to report a physical checkup when they report that migration was voluntary and when they more strongly agree that they migrated to join other family members. At the same time, Latino immigrants are more likely to have had a physical care visit the more strongly they report migrating to the United States to seek medical attention.

For enabling characteristics, Model 2 shows that the likelihood of receiving a physical checkup increases when adults have medical insurance and a regular doctor, and as levels of family cultural conflict increase. For need-based characteristics, Model 3 shows no direct association between any measure of health status or behavior and receiving a physical care checkup among Latino immigrants.

Next, Table 3 shows unstandardized coefficients from logistic regression models predicting whether or not respondents received a routine optician or dental visit last year. For predisposing characteristics in Model 1, we see the same pattern as described for receiving a physical care checkup in Table 2; that is, ethnic group differences are no longer significant for Latino immigrants, and neither is the difference between Chinese and Filipino immigrants seen in the bivariate in Table 1. And again, Vietnamese immigrants remain significantly more likely to have received a routine checkup than Chinese immigrants. For Asian immigrants, the likelihood of a dental/optician visits is significantly higher among U.S. citizens, and declines with increasing proficiency in their native country language (in Model 2, however, once we adjust for enabling characteristics, the interaction between native and English language proficiency emerges as significant, indicating that the negative effect of native language proficiency is reduced with increasing proficiency in English). For Latino immigrants, the likelihood of a routine dental/optician is significantly higher among U.S. citizens and those who migrated to the United States in search of a job, and is lower among those who migrated to the United States voluntarily.

After adjusting for enabling characteristics in Model 2, we again see that the coefficients for ethnicity increase in size, indicating suppression based on

Table 3. Coefficients from Logistic Regression Models, Any Routine Dental/Optician Visits Last Year.

	Immigrant Asian Adults (n = 1,323)			Immigrant Latino Adults (n = 1,204)		
	Model 1	Model 2	Model 3	Model 1	Model 2	Model 3
Predisposing characteristics						
Age at interview	-.00 (.01)	-.01 (.01)	-.00 (.01)	.03 (.01)**	.01 (.01)	.01 (.01)
Female	.40 (.14)**	.24 (.13)	.20 (.16)	.47 (.19)*	.31 (.22)	.12 (.24)
Ethnicity (reference: Chinese or Mexican)						
Vietnamese	.52 (.25)*	.68 (.26)*	.64 (.26)*	—	—	—
Filipino	-.04 (.24)	-.09 (.24)	-.13 (.24)	—	—	—
Cuban	—	—	—	-.05 (.26)	-.18 (.26)	-.19 (.27)
Puerto Rican	—	—	—	-.03 (.22)	-.22 (.24)	-.15 (.25)
Voluntarily moved to the United States	-.14 (.22)	-.18 (.23)	-.19 (.22)	-.41 (.19)*	-.41 (.18)*	-.42 (.17)*
Migrated to the United States in order to....						
Find a job	.12 (.10)	.15 (.10)	.14 (.10)	.25 (.08)**	.24 (.10)*	.25 (.10)*
Join other family members	.01 (.11)	.03 (.12)	.03 (.12)	-.01 (.11)	.07 (.09)	.07 (.09)
Seek medical attention	-.15 (.11)	-.15 (.11)	-.13 (.11)	.17 (.10)	.08 (.12)	.10 (.13)
Migrated to United States before age 18	.14 (.27)	.09 (.25)	.06 (.26)	-.16 (.22)	-.28 (.23)	-.26 (.24)
Remits money to relatives in country of origin	.21 (.16)	.17 (.15)	.16 (.15)	.20 (.21)	.33 (.22)	.33 (.22)
How often returns to country of origin	.10 (.10)	.05 (.09)	.06 (.09)	.11 (08)	.02 (.09)	-.04 (.09)
Strength of co-ethnic ties	.04 (.19)	-.05 (.19)	-.04 (.19)	.15 (.15)	.15 (.16)	.10 (.17)
Language proficiency						
Country-of-origin language	-.44 (.18)*	-.51 (.19)**	-.53 (.17)**	.13 (.26)	.04 (.24)	-.03 (.26)
English language	.07 (.22)	-.20 (.21)	-.25 (.20)	.41 (.51)	.07 (.52)	-.11 (.56)
Country-of-origin * English	.11 (.06)	.14 (.06)*	.14 (.06)*	-.03 (.13)	.02 (.03)	.04 (.14)
U.S. Citizen	.30 (.14)*	.16 (.16)	.15 (.16)	.62 (.19)**	.36 (.23)	.40 (.24)
Married or cohabiting	.27 (.17)	.15 (.19)	.13 (.19)	-.39 (.20)	-.49 (.16)**	-.53 (.17)**

Table 3. (*Continued*)

	Immigrant Asian Adults (n = 1,323)			Immigrant Latino Adults (n = 1,204)		
	Model 1	Model 2	Model 3	Model 1	Model 2	Model 3
Household size	−.04 (.04)	−.01 (.04)	−.01 (.04)	.04 (.04)	.07 (.04)	.07 (.05)
Years of schooling	.05 (.03)	.04 (.03)	.04 (.02)	.06 (.05)	.05 (.05)	.05 (.05)
Currently working	.23 (.16)	.24 (.19)	.23 (.19)	.04 (.17)	−.02 (.18)	−.04 (.17)
Enabling/disabling characteristics						
Poor		.20 (.22)	.22 (.22)		−.34 (.25)	−.34 (.25)
Extent of difficulty paying monthly bills		−.13 (.11)	−.11 (.11)		−.19 (.09)*	−.20 (.09)*
No medical insurance		−.90 (.20)***	−.88 (.20)***		−.78 (.25)**	−.74 (.26)**
Has a regular doctor		.73 (.18)***	.75 (.18)***		1.08 (.20)***	1.12 (.19)***
Acculturative Stress		−.08 (.06)	−.07 (.06)		−.07 (.09)	−.08 (.07)
Frequency of discriminatory experiences		−.06 (.09)	−.07 (.09)		.02 (.08)	−.00 (.08)
Negative social exchanges		.41 (.20)*	.42 (.19)*		−.03 (.13)	.01 (.13)
Family cultural conflict		.10 (.27)	.08 (.26)		.79 (.24)**	.90 (.26)***
Positive social support		.17 (.16)	.15 (.16)		.05 (.14)	.02 (.13)
Family cohesion		.21 (.23)	.16 (.23)		−.15 (.20)	−.17 (.20)
Need-based characteristics						
Smoking status (reference: current smoker)						
Former smoker			.02 (.35)			.06 (.29)
Never smoked			.21 (.23)			.35 (.20)
Current heavy drinker			.50 (.49)			−.29 (.23)
Overweight or obese			.00 (.19)			−.26 (.19)
Self-rated physical health			.11 (.09)			.07 (.06)
Self-rated mental health			.11 (.10)			.17 (.08)*

*p ≤ .05, **p ≤ .01, ***p ≤ .001.

socioeconomic resources, stress, and support. Medical insurance and having a regular doctor are strongly associated with receiving a physical checkup for both Latino and Asian immigrants. And while the financial stress of reporting difficulty in paying monthly bills depresses the likelihood of a dental/optician visit among Latino immigrants, interpersonal aspects of stress (negative social exchanges among Asian immigrants, and family cultural conflict among Latino immigrants) is positively associated with receiving a dental/optician checkup last year.

Finally, need-based factors relating to health behaviors and status continue to show little explanatory power in terms of ethnic group differences, and little direct effect overall, on preventive medical care use among immigrants in our sample. No measures significantly predict a dental/optician visit among Asian immigrants, while only one measure – self-rated mental health – shows a positive relationship to use among Latino immigrants.

CONCLUSION

This chapter had two broad objectives. First, we sought to establish whether ethnic group variation exists in the utilization of preventive medical care services across Latino and Asian immigrant groups – and as expected, we find substantial differences. Other work has documented low rates of medical care use among Mexican-origin adults (Beal et al., 2009; Lara et al., 2005), and our study finds a much lower rate of preventive care service use among Mexican relative to Cuban and Puerto Rican immigrant adults. Indeed, for both types of care a significantly higher proportion of Cuban (approximately 20% higher) and Puerto Rican immigrants (just over 25% higher) report a visit during the last year. However, in contrast to Latinos where Mexican immigrants stand-out due to their very low rate of use, among Asians immigrants we found that ethnic group divisions are less pronounced, but still significant. For both types of preventive services, Filipino immigrants secure care at the highest rate, followed by Vietnamese and then Chinese immigrants. These findings indicate that those who use broad, pan-ethnic categories to describe medical care use among immigrant populations will mask substantial variation that exists across specific ethnic groups.

Our analyses then explored factors related to use, organized around Andersen's (1995) Behavioral Model of Health Services Use framework. Specifically, we investigated whether group differences in predisposing, enabling/disabling, and need-based characteristics accounted for ethnic gaps in the proportion using medical care services over the last year. In the aggregate, we found that Asian and Latino immigrants display important similarities and differences in the characteristics that relate to their use of preventive medical care services. Most prominently, we found substantial evidence that *predisposing characteristics* contribute strongly to ethnic group differences in having had a routine care visit during the last year for both Latino and Asian immigrants. Indeed, logistic regression models (for both outcomes) showed that adjusting for predisposing characteristics explained away the lower rate of use among Chinese relative to Filipino (but not Vietnamese) immigrants, and it explained away the lower rate of use among Mexican relative to both Cuban and Puerto Rican immigrants. More specifically, these models illustrated the strong role that group differences in acculturation status plays in shaping variation in preventive care use among both Asian and Latino immigrants.

For the Filipino–Chinese difference, additional models (not shown) indicated that the coefficient for having had a physical care visit was reduced to nonsignificance by adjusting for acculturation status measures, while for dental/optician visits adjusting for language use alone caused the coefficient for Filipino to lose significance. Other research has shown that English fluency is a primary contributor to ethnic disparities in access to health care (Fiscella et al., 2002; Solis et al., 1990), and that it may be a more potent factor shaping doctor visits for Asians than Latinos (Akresh, 2009). This complements other studies linking language barriers with fewer physician visits and reduced receipt of preventive services, even with adjustment for literacy, health status, health insurance, source of care, and economic indicators (Management Sciences for Health, 2011).

In-line with a multidimensional perspective on acculturation (Alegria et al., 2007; Berry, 2003; Salant & Lauderdale, 2003), Filipinos in our sample show characteristics indicative of adaption to U.S. culture (i.e., higher rates of U.S. citizenship and especially English language proficiency when compared to Chinese adults) in addition to the maintenance of significant ties with Filipino culture (e.g., more frequent return trips and remittances to family in the Philippines). This pattern of dual connection has been shown to predict positive psychosocial outcomes among immigrants (Schwartz, Unger, Zamboanga, & Szapocznik, 2010), and our findings indicate that, for Filipino immigrants, the benefits extends to the utilization of preventive medical care services as well.

For Vietnamese immigrants, however, adjusting for acculturation status and other predisposing characteristics does not explain their heightened use of preventive care services in relation to Chinese adults. While in some respects Vietnamese immigrants in our sample show stronger ties to the United States and their native homeland when compared to the Chinese (e.g., higher U.S. citizenship rates, more remittances to relatives), in other respects they display more risk on factors related to diminished use of medical care services (e.g., lower English proficiency). Altogether, our findings indicate that the acculturation profile of Vietnamese immigrants is not what drives their elevated use of preventive medical care relative to Chinese immigrants.

Among Latinos, differences on both outcome measures between Mexican and Puerto Rican immigrants were reduced to nonsignificance by adjusting for acculturation status measures as a whole (but especially citizenship status when predicting a dental/optician visit; additional models not shown). Overall, our sample of Puerto Rican migrants show stronger ties to U.S. culture than Mexican migrants (i.e., near universal U.S. citizenship, a higher proportion who migrated during childhood, better English proficiency) in addition to retaining strong ties to some aspects of Puerto Rican culture (e.g., more frequent return visits and stronger co-ethnic ties) while also reporting more agreement that they migrated to the U.S. mainland to seek medical attention. Together, these characteristics combine to shape their higher rate of preventive care use when contrasted against Mexican immigrant adults, and again provide evidence of the health benefits associated with ties to both United States and country of origin culture.

Acculturation status is also relevant for the contrast between Cuban and Mexican immigrants, in that the heightened use of dental/optician visits among Cubans was explained with adjustment for all acculturation measures (but especially for whether the decision to migrate was voluntary). Only one-third of Cubans in our sample report voluntary migration to the United States (compared to almost two-thirds of Mexican and Puerto Rican migrants), which is negatively associated with reporting a routine care checkup during the last year. For physical care visits, however, our models showed the relevance of gender, as the Cuban sample is significantly more female than the Mexican sample. Since previous research has shown that women use more preventive medical services than men (e.g., Courtenay et al., 2002), once we adjust for the gender imbalance across samples the difference between Cuban and Mexican migrants in reporting a routine physical care checkup is reduced to nonsignificance.

Beyond predisposing characteristics, our models also explored the role of *enabling and disabling characteristics* – and here we see no evidence that adjusting for these measures explains group differences in preventive care use, for either Asian or Latino immigrants. Indeed, accounting for these characteristics actually caused an amplification of ethnic group differences for nearly all contrasts (although not to the extent that any nonsignificant contrasts reemerged as significant). As expected, however, we do find that having medical insurance and a regular doctor are positively associated with both forms of preventive care, for both Asian and Latino immigrants.

Furthermore, it is worth noting the significance of stressful experiences in these models, as we found that higher levels of family cultural conflict is positively associated with both forms of care for Latino immigrants, and that discriminatory experiences and negative social exchanges are positively associated with care among Asian immigrants. While studies document how social support influences physical and mental health statuses, less is known about why stressful family exchanges bring a greater use of health care services (Berkman & Glass, 2000). Regardless of the positive or negative role family plays, we posit that family members may point out and stress the severity of the individual's health problems and prompt them to seek care. Within their social network, experienced immigrants may pass along local knowledge and shared norms around health behaviors, which thereby improves access to resources and material goods that can facilitate use of high-quality health care (Berkman & Glass, 2000; Falicov, 2007). Research shows that Latinos and other immigrant groups develop health benefits through family networks who help pool financial resources and help them feel connected (Documét & Sharma, 2004; Mulvaney-Day, Alergria, & Sribney, 2007); however, families are also a potential source of conflict. Although cultural conflict is present, it could be that a sense of obligation to the family and deference to elders serves as an underlying behavioral referent for immigrants, influencing them to seek care (Alegria et al., 2007; Ying & Han, 2007). In addition, research has repeatedly shown that stressors are damaging to physical health (Thoits, 2010), and as such immigrants who report exposure to stress may require more medical care services than those who do not.

Finally, our models showed that *need-based characteristics* played little-to-no role in shaping preventive care use among immigrants – directly, or in mediating ethnic group differences in the use of care during the previous year, for either Asians or Latinos. Yet, despite the potential value of our findings, it is important to keep in mind that the NLAAS is a cross-sectional survey, prohibiting more rigorous assessment of the causal dynamics of how ethnicity shapes preventive medical care use among immigrants. Replication of our study with panel data, and across a wider range of measures related to medical care use, is needed.

In conclusion, while studies of medical care use often treat Asians and Latinos as homogeneous groups, our findings illustrate the need for a more detailed view of the foreign-born population. It is important to note ethnic differences in medical care utilization when working to achieve the *Healthy People 2010* principles, as health disparities are likely to grow if not addressed in a manner most efficacious to the needs of the target population. While it may be more feasible to bring change through enabling factors than through predisposing characteristics (Andersen & Newman, 1973), our findings highlight the role of acculturation status in shaping group differences in preventive medical care use – and as such, the importance of considering these differences when promoting the use of timely preventive care services among immigrant populations.

REFERENCES

Akresh, I. R. (2009). Health service utilization among immigrants to the United States. *Population Research and Policy Review, 28*, 795–815.

Alegria, M., Sribney, W., Woo, M., Torres, M., & Guarnaccia, P. (2007). Looking beyond nativity: The relation of age of immigration, length of residence, and birth cohorts to the risk of onset of psychiatric disorders for latinos. *Research in Human Development, 4*(1), 19–47.

Alegria, M., Vila, D., Woo, M., Canino, G., Takeuchi, D., Vera, M., ... Shrout, P. (2004). Relevance and equivalence in the NLAAS instrument: Integrating etic and emic in the development of cross-cultural measures for a psychiatric epidemiology and services study of latinos. *International Journal of Methods in Psychiatric Research, 13*(4), 270–288.

Andersen, R., & Newman, J. F. (1973). Societal and individuals determinants of medical care utilization in the United States. *The Milbank Memorial Fund Quarterly, 51*(1), 95–124.

Andersen, R. M. (1968). *Behavioral model of families' use of health services.* Research Series No. 25. Chicago, IL: Center for Health Administration Studies, University of Chicago.

Andersen, R. M. (1995). Revisiting the behavioral model and access to medical care: Does it matter? *Journal of Health and Social Behavior, 36*(March), 1–10.

Antecol, H., Kuhn, P., & Trejo, S. J. (2006). Assimilation via prices or quantities? Sources of immigrant earnings growth in Australia, Canada, and the United States. *The Journal of Human Resources, 41*(4), 821–840.

Arends-Tóth, J., & van de Vijver, F. J. R. (2006). Acculturation: A conceptual overview. In M. H. Bornstein & L. R. Cote (Eds.), *Acculturation and parent-child relationships: Measurement and development* (pp. 13–30). New York, NY: Lawrence Erlbaum Associates, Inc.

Ashton, C. M., Collins, T. C., Petersen, L. A., & Wray, N. P. (2003). Racial and ethnic disparities in the use of health services. *Journal of General Internal Medicine, 18*, 146–152.

Beal, A., Hernandez, S., & Doty, M. (2009). Latino access to the patient-centered medical home. *Journal of General Internal Medicine, 24*(Suppl. 3), 514–520.

Beck, C. T., Froman, R., & Bernal, H. (2005). Acculturation and postpartum depression in hispanic mothers. *The American Journal of Maternal Child Nursing, 30*(5), 299–304.

Berkman, L., & Glass, T. (2000). Social integration, social networks, social support, and health. In L. Berkman & I. Kawachi (Eds.), *Social epidemiology* (pp. 137–173). Oxford: Oxford University Press.

Berry, J. W. (2003). Conceptual approaches to acculturation. In K. M. Chun, P. B. Organista & G. Marín (Eds.), *Acculturation: Advances in theory, measurement, and applied research* (pp. 17–37). Washington, DC: American Psychological Association.

Blendon, R., Buhr, T., Cassidy, E., Perez, D., Hunt, K., Fleischfresser, C., ... Herrmann, M. (2007). Disparities in health: Perspectives of a multi-ethnic, multi-racial America. *Health Affairs, 26*(5), 1437–1447.

Brown, E. R., Ojeda, V. D., Wyn, R., & Levan, R. (2000). *Racial and ethnic disparities in access to health insurance and health care*. Los Angeles, CA: UCLA Center for Health Policy Research.

Courtenay, W. H., Mccreary, D. R., & Merighi, J. R. (2002). Gender and ethnic differences in health beliefs and behaviors. *Journal of Health Psychology, 7*(3), 219–231.

Derose, K. P., Bahney, B. W., & Lurie, N. (2009). Immigrants and health care access, quality, and cost. *Medical Care Research and Review, 66*(4), 355–408.

Derose, K. P., Escarce, J. J., & Lurie, N. (2007). Immigrants and health care: Sources of vulnerability. *Health Affairs, 26*(5), 1258–1268.

Documét, P. I., & Sharma, R. K. (2004). Latinos' health care access: Financial and cultural barriers. *Journal of Immigrant Health, 6*(1), 5–13.

DuBard, A. C., & Gizlice, Z. (2008). Language spoken and differences in health status, access to care, and receipt of preventive services among US hispanics. *American Journal of Public Health, 98*(11), 2021–2027.

Facione, N., Giancarlo, C., & Chan, L. (2000). Perceived risk and help-seeking behavior for breast cancer: A Chinese-American perspective. *Cancer Nursing, 23*(4), 258–267.

Falicov, C. (2007). Working with transnational immigrants: Expanding meanings of family, community, and culture. *Family Process, 46*(2), 157–171.

Fiscella, K., Franks, P., Doescher, M. P., & Saver, B. G. (2002). Disparities in health care by race, ethnicity, and language among the insured. *Medical Care, 40*(1), 52–59.

Flores, G., & Tomany-Korman, S. (2008). The language spoken at home and disparities in medical and dental health, access to care, and use of services in US children. *Pediatrics, 121*(6), e1703–e1714.

Foner, N. (1997). The immigrant family: Cultural legacies and cultural changes. *International Migration Review, 31*(4), 961–974.

Frisbie, P. W., Cho, Y., & Hummer, R. (2001). Immigration and the health of asian and pacific islander adults in the United States. *American Journal of Epidemiology, 153*, 372–380.

Goldman, D. P., Smith, J. P., & Sood, N. (2006). Immigrants and the cost of medical care. *Health Affairs, 25*(6), 1700–1711.

Gor, B. (2010). *Health needs of Asian & Pacific islander Americans: Stories from the model minority*. [PowerPoint Slides]. Retrieved with permission of the author from Rice University Health Disparities in the U.S. Blackboard.

Heeringa, S. G., Wagner, J., Torres, M., Duan, N., Adams, T., & Berglund, P. (2004). Sample designs and sampling methods for the collaborative psychiatric epidemiology studies (CPES). *International Journal of Methods in Psychiatric Research, 13*(4), 221–240.

Hu, D., & Covell, R. (1986). Health care usage by hispanic outpatients as function of primary language. *Western Journal of Medicine, 144*(4), 490–493.

Hunt, L., Schneider, S., & Comer, B. (2004). Should "acculturation" be a variable in health research? A critical review of research on US hispanics. *Social Science & Medicine, 59*, 973–986.

Kang-Kim, M., Betancourt, J., Ayanian, J., Zaslavsky, A., Yucel, R., & Weissman, J. (2008). Access to care and use of preventive services by hispanics. *Medical Care, 46*(5), 507–515.

Kim, S., Kronenfeld, J., & River, P. (2007). Racial and socioeconomic differences in predictors of dental care use. Access quality and satisfaction with care: Concerns of patients, providers and insurers. *Research in the Sociology of Health Care, 24*, 61–79.

Ku, L., & Matani, S. (2001). Left out: Immigrants' access to health care and insurance. *Health Affairs, 20*(1), 247–256.

Lara, M., Gamboa, C., Kahramanian, M. I., Morales, L., & Bautista, D. H. (2005). Acculturation and latino health in the United States: A review of the literature and its sociopolitical context. *Annual Review of Public Health, 26*, 367–397.

Leclere, F. B., Jensen, L., & Biddlecom, A. E. (1994). Health care utilization, family context, and adaptation among immigrants to the United States. *Journal of Health and Social Behavior, 35*(4), 370–384.

Lee, S. M. (1998). Asian Americans: Diverse and growing. *Population Bulletin, 53*(2). Washington, DC: Population Reference Bureau.

Liebkind, K. (2006). Ethnic identity and acculturation. In D. L. Sam & J. W. Berry (Eds.), *The Cambridge handbook of acculturation psychology* (pp. 78–96). New York, NY: Cambridge University Press.

Management Sciences for Health. (2011). *The provider's guide to quality and culture: Understanding minority, immigrant and refugee populations, Asians.* Retrieved from http://erc.msh.org/mainpage.cfm?file = 5.1.0f.htm&module = provider&language = english. Accessed on January 9, 2011.

McAlpine, D. D., & Boyer, C. A. (2007). Sociological traditions in the study of mental health services utilization. In W. R. Avison, J. D. McLeod & B. A. Pescosolido (Eds.), *Mental health, social mirror* (pp. 355–378). New York, NY: Plenum.

Mulvaney-Day, N., Alergria, M., & Sribney, W. (2007). Social cohesion, social support, and health among latinos in the United States. *Social Science & Medicine, 64*, 477–495.

Pennell, B.-E., Bowers, A., Carr, D., Chardoul, S., Cheung, G.-Q., Dinkelmann, K., … Torres, M. (2004). The development and implementation of the national comorbidity survey replication, the national survey of American life, and the national latino and Asian American survey. *International Journal of Methods in Psychiatric Research, 13*(4), 241–269.

Rodriguez, M., Bustamante, A., & Ang, A. (2009). Perceived quality of care, receipt of preventive care, and usual source of health care among undocumented and other latinos. *Journal of General Internal Medicine, 24*(3), 508–513.

Rook, K. S. (2003). Exposure and reactivity to negative social exchanges: A preliminary investigation using daily diary data. *Journal of Gerontology: Psychological Sciences, 58B*(2), 100–p111.

Ross, C. E., & Wu, C.-L. (1995). The links between education and health. *American Sociological Review*, *60*(5), 719–745.

Saenz, R. (2010). *Latinos in America 2010 population bulletin update*. Washington, DC: Population Reference Bureau.

Sakamoto, A., Goyette, K., & Kim, C. H. (2009). Socioeconomic attainments of Asian Americans. *Annual Review of Sociology*, *35*, 255–276.

Salabarria-Pena, Y., Trout, P. T., Gill, J., Morisk, D., Muralles, A., & Ebin, V. (2001). Effects of acculturation and psychosocial factors in latino adolescents' TB-related behaviors. *Ethnicity and Disease*, *11*(4), 661–675.

Salant, T., & Lauderdale, D. S. (2003). Measuring culture: A critical review of acculturation and health in Asian immigrant populations. *Social Science & Medicine*, *57*(1), 71–90.

Sam, D. L. (2006). Acculturation: Conceptual background and core components. In D. L. Sam & J. W. Berry (Eds.), *The Cambridge handbook of acculturation psychology* (pp. 11–26). Cambridge: Cambridge University Press.

Sandman, D., Simantov, E., & An, C. (2000). *Out of touch: American men and the health care system*. Retrieved from http://www.commonwealthfund.org/Publications/Fund-Reports/2000/Mar/Out-of-Touch–American-Men-and-the-Health-Care-System.aspx. Accessed on January 14, 2012.

Schwartz, S. J., Unger, J. B., Zamboanga, B. L., & Szapocznik, J. (2010). Rethinking the concept of acculturation. *American Psychologist*, *65*(4), 237–251.

Solis, J., Marks, G., Garcia, M., & Shelton, D. (1990). Acculturation, access to care, and use of preventive services by hispanics: Findings from HHANES 1982-1984. *American Journal of Public Health*, *80*(Suppl), 11–19.

Takeuchi, D., Alegria, M., Jackson, J., & Williams, D. (2007). Immigration and mental health: Diverse findings in Asian, black, and latino populations. *American Journal of Public Health*, *97*(1), 11–12.

Tanningco, M. (2007). *Revisiting the latino health paradox the Thomas Rivera policy institute*. Retrieved from http://www.trpi.org/PDFs/Latino%20Paradox%20Aug%202007%20 PDF.pdf. Accessed on December 13, 2010.

Terrazas, A., & Batalova, J. (2009). *Frequently requested statistics on immigrants and immigration in the United States*. Migration Policy Institute. Retrieved from http://www.migrationinformation.org/USfocus/display.cfm?ID=747#2. Accessed on November 10, 2010.

Thoits, P. A. (2010). Stress and health: Major findings and policy implications. *Journal of Health and Social Behavior*, *51*(extra issue), S41–S53.

Tseng, W., McDonnell, D., Takahashi, L., Ho, W., Lee, C., & Wong, S. (2010). *Ethnic health assessment for Asian Americans, native hawaiians and pacific islanders in California*. Berkeley, CA: School of Public Health. California Program on Access to Care.

U.S. Census Bureau. (2010). *Language spoken at home by ability to speak english for the population 5 years and over*. [Data file B16001]. Retrieved from http://factfinder2.census. gov/faces/tableservices/jsf/pages/productview.xhtml?src=bkmk. Accessed on August 23, 2012.

U.S. Census Bureau. (2011a). *Asian/Pacific American Heritage Month: May 2011*. Retrieved from http://www.census.gov/newsroom/releases/archives/facts_for_features_special_ editions/cb11-ff06.html. Accessed on August 23, 2012.

U.S. Census Bureau. (2011b). *Overview of race and hispanic origin: 2010*. Retrieved from http:// www.census.gov/prod/cen2010/briefs/c2010br-02.pdf. Accessed on August 23, 2012.

U.S. Department of Health and Human Services and U.S. Department of Agriculture. (2005). *Dietary guidelines for Americans, 2005* (6th ed.). Washington, DC: U.S. Government Printing Office.

U.S. Preventive Services Task Force. (1996). *Guide to clinical preventive services* (2nd ed.). Baltimore, MD: Williams & Wilkins.

Vaidya, V., Partha, G., & Karmakar, M. (2011). Gender differences in utilization of preventive care services in the United States. *Journal of Women's Health, 21*(2).

Whitley, E. M., Samuels, B. A., Wright, R. A., & Everhart, R. M. (2005). Identification of barriers to healthcare access for underserved men in denver. *The Journal of Men's Health & Gender, 2*(4), 421–428.

Wood, R. G., Goesling, B., & Avellar, S. (2007). *The effect of marriage on health: A synthesis of recent research evidence.* Washington, DC: U.S. Department of Health and Human Services.

Xie, Y., & Goyette, K. A. 2004. *A demographic portrait of Asian Americans.* Retrieved from http://www.prb.org/Articles/2004/DemographicPortraitofAsianAmericans.aspx. Accessed on July 14, 2012.

Ye, J., Mack, D., Fry-Johnson, Y., & Parker, K. (2012). Health care access and utilization among US-born and foreign-born Asian Americans. *Journal of Immigrant and Minority Health, 14*(5), 731–737.

Ying, W.-W., & Han, M. (2007). The longitudinal effect of intergenerational gap in acculturation on conflict and mental health in southeast Asian American adolescents. *American Journal of Orthopsychiatry, 77*(1), 61–66.

Zambrana, R. E., & Carter-Pokras, O. (2010). Role of acculturation research in advancing science and practice in reducing health care disparities among latinos. *American Journal of Public Health, 100*(1), 18–23.

BIRTH OUTCOMES OF PATIENTS ENROLLED IN "FAMILIAS SANAS" RESEARCH PROJECT

Kathryn Connors, Dean V. Coonrod, Patricia Habak, Stephanie Ayers and Flavio Marsiglia

ABSTRACT

Purpose – *This chapter examines birth outcomes of patients enrolled in* Familias Sanas *(Healthy Families), an educational intervention designed to reduce health disadvantages of low-income, immigrant Latina mothers by providing social support during and after pregnancy.*

Methodology/approach – *Using a randomized control-group design, the project recruited 440 pregnant Latina women, 88% of whom were first generation. Birth outcomes were collected through medical charts and analyzed using regression analysis to evaluate if there were any differences between patients enrolled in* Familias Sanas *compared to those patients who followed a typical prenatal course.*

Findings – *Control and intervention groups were found to be similar with regard to demographic characteristics. In addition, we did not observe a decrease in rate of a number of common pregnancy-related complications. Likewise, rates of operative delivery were similar between the two groups as were fetal weight at delivery and use of regional anesthesia at delivery.*

Social Determinants, Health Disparities and Linkages to Health and Health Care
Research in the Sociology of Health Care, Volume 31, 143–159
ISSN: 0275-4959/doi:10.1108/S0275-4959(2013)0000031009

Research limitations/implications – *The lack of improvements in birth outcomes for this study was perhaps because this social support intervention was not significant enough to override long-standing stressors such as socioeconomic status, poor nutrition, genetics, and other environmental stressors.*

Originality/value of chapter – *This study was set in an inner-city, urban hospital with a large percentage of patients being of Hispanic descent. The study itself is a randomized controlled clinical trial, and data were collected directly from electronic medical records by physicians.*

Keywords: Birth outcomes; social support; intervention; pregnant Latina women

BACKGROUND

Hispanics/Latinos are the largest ethnic/racial minority group with more than 50 million people (U.S. Census Bureau, 2011). Since 2000, Latinos accounted for half or more of the population growth in the nation (US Census Bureau, 2011) with a fertility rate of 2.4 compared to 1.8 for non-Hispanic whites (Passel, Livingston, & Cohn, 2012). Latinos are also disproportionately represented among the nation's poor; more than 30% of Latinos aged 18 years or younger are living in poverty (Martin, Hamilton, & Ventura, 2011). Thus, Latino individuals, particularly those of Mexican heritage, bear a disproportionate burden of economic disadvantage among Latinos and consequently, carry a disproportional vulnerability to disease, disability, and death associated with preventable health conditions (CDC, 2011). Birth outcomes can impact not only Latinos more disparately than non-Hispanic Whites, but within Hispanic sub-groups, differences in birth outcomes emerge as well. For example, while Cuban women have low infant mortality and preterm birth (Hummer, Eberstein, & Nam, 1992), Mexican women have a higher risk of delivering a preterm and low-weight baby (Singh & Yu, 1996; Zambrana, Scrimshawe, Collins, & Dunkel-Schetter, 1997) and a higher risk of receiving inadequate prenatal care (Frisbie & Song, 2003).

One way to reduce these disparities is through culturally grounded health promotional activities which can influence knowledge, attitudes, and behaviors (Novilla et al., 2006; Padilla & Villalobos, 2006). For Mexican/Mexican American women, offering choices and counseling in health care decisions need to resonate culturally and draw on the strength of culture rather than view culture as a barrier to receiving healthcare (Padilla & Villalobos, 2006). One aspect of Mexican culture that has been shown to significantly influence health outcomes is social support, which embraces the values of familism, respect, and collectiveness (Padilla & Villalobos, 2006). Social support in general has been shown to be a "major factor predicting their excellent birth weight outcomes in spite of very low SES levels" (McDuffie, Beck, Bischoff, Cross, & Orleans, 1996, p. 3).

Given that the importance of prenatal care for maternal and child health is well established (Alexander & Kotelchuck, 2001) and the promotion of medical care can improve pregnancy-related outcomes and potentially reduce societal cost (Cefalo & Moos, 1995), understanding disparities faced by Mexican/Mexican American women is not only an examination of health care access, quality, and utilization, but also a consideration of programs that can encourage, promote, and support better health outcomes for Mexican/Mexican American women.

BARRIERS TO UTILIZATION AND RECEIPT OF CARE

The unique stressors often faced by Mexican women, particularly for immigrant women, through limited financial resources, cultural beliefs regarding health and illness, lack of social support, and inadequate English language mastery, have been associated with poorer birth outcomes (Harley & Eskenazi, 2006). Utilization of prenatal care is lower for Hispanic women compared to non-Hispanic women, and among Hispanic women, Mexican/ Mexican American women utilize less prenatal care than other Hispanic subgroups (Collins & Shay, 1994; Guendelman & English, 1995; Singh & Yu, 1996). The long-term benefits of receiving prenatal care expand past the mother's health to the child's health as well. Hispanic mothers who receive prenatal care not only have better overall health outcomes for the baby (Singh & Yu, 1996; Zambrana et al., 1997) but are also more likely to utilize well-child services including immunizations and well-child visits (Kogan, Alexander, Jack, & Allen, 1998; Moore & Hepworth, 1994; Wiecha & Gann, 1994).

Limited financial resources, living in poverty, and lacking health insurance are key barriers which create disparities in access to and utilization of health care for Mexican/Mexican Americans (Pérez-Escamilla, Garcia, & Song, 2010).

Studies consistently report that immigrants, both citizen and noncitizen, are less likely to have and maintain consistent health insurance compared to U.S.-born individuals (Carrasquillo, Carasquillo, & Shea, 2000; Thamer, Richard, Casebeer, & Ray, 1997; Trevino, Moyer, Valdez, & Stroup-Benham, 1991), and even when an immigrant transitions from being undocumented to documented, having health insurance remains significantly less than the general U.S. adult population (Brown, Ojeda, Lara, & Valenzuela, 1999) – 33% in the Latino population compared to 16% in the general US population (McDonald & Hertz, 2008). Lack of health care access is also influenced by limited English proficiency, being foreign-born, and being a noncitizen (DuBard & Gizlice, 2008). Spanish-speaking individuals are less likely to have health insurance, a regular source of care, and utilize preventive medicine compared to English-speaking individuals (DuBard & Gizlice, 2008). While immigrants, in general, are less likely to utilize health care, if insured, immigrants have similar utilization rates as U.S.-born individuals (Siddiqi, Zuberi, & Nguyen, 2009). Latinos are more likely to have multiple risk factors for the receipt of health insurance and health care utilization, including work status (i.e., having an employer offering health insurance) and residency status (i.e., having access to government-funded health insurance) (Marcelli, 2004). Even when health insurance is present, living in poverty presents the challenge of paying for office visits, prescriptions, and health insurance premiums (Amirehsani, 2010).

Cultural norms and beliefs can influence the perceptions of the importance to seek medical care during and after pregnancy, and the provider–patient relationship can be shaped by cultural assumptions and expectations (Carrillo, Green, & Betancourt, 1999). Cultural beliefs shape the interpretation of the origins of the illness (etiology) and the best methods of healing. These cultural beliefs, if not addressed, can often act as barriers to care (Eshiett & Parry, 2003). Hispanic women receiving prenatal care report concerns about receiving "humanistic care" from providers and other health care professions. Having the personal processes of healthcare (respect, caring, understanding, patience, and dignity), the availability of Spanish-speaking healthcare providers and the inclusion of family members in healthcare decisions were of utmost importance to the women (Berry, 1999; Warda, 2000). Having not only ethnic concordance, but language and gender concordance, can impact the quality of care. Spanish-speaking patients have been found to be at a double disadvantage in encounters with English-speaking monolingual physicians. For example, Hispanic women are more likely to feel embarrassed during medical procedures, particularly if the medical provider is a male (Byrd, Mullen, Selwyn, & Lorimor, 1996). Feeling embarrassed or being ignored can result in less treatment adherence and poorer medical outcomes (Rivadeneyra, Elderkin-Thompson, Silver, & Waitzkin, 2000). Lack of culturally similar social support networks may also act as a barrier to utilization, particularly for immigrants who have lived in the United States for a longer period of time or for those who are U.S. born. Immigrant women, who have lived in the United States longer, tend to become more socially integrated into the host culture and create new social networks to take the place of those in Mexico (Harley & Eskenazi, 2006). As social networks are replaced and acculturation occurs, women of Mexican heritage adopt poorer health behaviors, particularly during pregnancy (Harley & Eskenazi, 2006). These "Americanized" health behaviors include using substances during pregnancy like cigarettes, alcohol, or illicit drugs (Vega, Kolody, Hwang, Noble, & Porter 1997; Wolff & Portis, 1996) and eating a diet poor in nutrition (Harley, Eskenazi, & Block, 2005). These "Americanized" health behaviors have been linked to poorer health outcomes, such as low birth weight and preterm babies, for U.S.-born Mexican American women (Singh & Yu, 1996; Zambrana et al., 1997).

CULTURALLY GROUNDED HEALTH PROMOTIONAL ACTIVITIES

During the past three decades, social support has been cited as having a positive impact on a wide array of health outcomes and behaviors during pregnancy (Harley & Eskenazi, 2006), including increased birth weight (Feldman, Dunkel-Schetter, Sandman, & Wadhwa, 2000), reduced rates of complications during pregnancy (Norbeck & Anderson, 1989), earlier initiation of prenatal care (Zambrana et al., 1997), higher use of prenatal vitamins (Harley & Eskenazi, 2006), and lower rates of smoking (Schaffer & Lia-Hoagberg, 1997).

Engaging community members in the provision of health education has been identified as an effective strategy to provide social support and bridge the cultural gap between providers and patients. These community members, often called *promotoras de salud* (health promoters), live in the communities they serve, distribute health information, encourage utilization of health care services, and reinforce Mexican cultural practices and beliefs (Larkey, 2006; McGlade, Saha, & Dahlstrom, 2004; Ramos, May, & Ramos, 2001). This approach has been successfully used in the Latino community through the engagement of paraprofessional women from the community (Hunter et al., 2004; Larkey, 2006) to have a positive impact on utilization, access, and overall health outcomes (Hunter et al., 2004; Larkey, 2006).

The focus of this study is to examine birth outcomes of patients enrolled in *Familias Sanas* (Healthy Families), an educational intervention designed to reduce health disadvantages of low-income, immigrant Latina mothers by providing social support during and after pregnancy. The original study sought to determine if participants enrolled in the intervention utilized the postpartum visit at rates higher than those seen in the control group (Marsiglia, Bermudez-Parsai, & Coonrod, 2010). This secondary study seeks to evaluate birth outcomes in the intervention and control groups with the intent to determine if improved outcomes were seen in the group receiving social support.

Familias Sanas sought to empower women to take an active part in the management of their health by encouraging them to advocate for themselves. In partnership with Women's Care Clinic at Maricopa Integrated Health Systems, the overall aim of *Familias Sanas* was to increase Latina mothers' access to and utilization of interconception care as a means of enhancing the overall well-being of the mothers and their children. In addition to visiting with a health care professional, the patient met with a prenatal partner during each clinic visit of the pregnancy at the Women's Care Clinic at Maricopa Integrated Health Systems, a prenatal clinic located at a major urban hospital in the Southwest United States. Prenatal partners used this opportunity to establish rapport with the patient. In the following meetings the prenatal partner provided education on prenatal care, discussed the patient's concerns, and developed a plan for regular prenatal and postpartum visits. Participants in the intervention group met with prenatal partners from 1 to 20 times, from the time of recruitment to the time they delivered their babies.

Familias Sanas took a one-on-one approach connecting Latino patients to Latino female professional health educators that served as prenatal partners. Prenatal partners were Master Level students, bilingual and bicultural, and highly experienced and committed to work with the Latino population. These partners provided basic health education, translating (culturally as well as linguistically) and reinforcing the medical advice provided to pregnant women by the health care professionals. They also worked with the patient to identify barriers to care and possible solutions, building on existing cultural assets and empowering patients to utilize those assets. Prenatal partners helped women navigate the health care system and empower them to advocate for themselves. The education component of *Familias Sanas* was based on a book that the clinic distributed among all pregnant women that sought medical services at the Clinic: "Hola Bebe." This book is divided in chapters that contribute easy-to-read information about each month of a woman's pregnancy and including things they could do to increase the likelihood of experiencing a healthy pregnancy (e.g., taking folic acid, attending medical appointments), and how to get ready for the birth of the baby. The book is beautifully illustrated and appealing, even to mothers with low literacy levels. The *Familias Sanas* team prepared five minute summaries of each chapter, and utilized the book illustrations to put together a short curriculum that was used as the educational piece. In addition, the *Familias Sanas* team focused on support and empowerment. During the educational sessions, prenatal partners encouraged women to discuss/share any issues related to their pregnancies and to medical care. When women shared concerns or had questions, prenatal partners helped them brainstorm ways to ask those questions from their health care providers. Patients were empowered to go back to the health care provider for clarifications and/or answers to their questions.

Methods

Using a randomized control-group design, the project recruited 440 pregnant Latina women attending the Women's Care Clinic at Maricopa Integrated Health Systems, a hospital providing services to a low-income, prisoner, or immigration-detainee populations who are mostly receiving Medicaid/Medicare insurance. In order to participate, women needed to (1) self-identify as Latina/Hispanic, (2) be 18 years of age or older, and (3) be less than 35-weeks pregnant. Patients meeting the inclusion criteria were recruited for the study during their first clinic visit between December 1, 2007 and April 30, 2009. The 440 participants were near evenly distributed between the two conditions (intervention $N = 221$; control $N = 219$). Sealed envelopes with the group assignment (treatment or control) and with accompanying baseline assessment instruments were maintained at the clinic. Each patient in the treatment condition received the intervention from her first clinic visit (i.e., recruitment into the study) until birth and was followed for two months after birth with prenatal partners (as described above). Each patient in the control condition received care as usual. Control group participants were recruited into the study during their first clinic visit and were followed until two months after birth.

Sample
The vast majority of women were of Mexican origin (81%) and first generation (88%) with a mean age of 27 (SD = 5.95). The average annual income was $15,792, with 78% of women reporting annual incomes of less than $20,000. While 68% of women reported less than a high school degree, one quarter (25%) had completed less than six years of schooling.

Data Collection
Upon enrollment, participants completed a baseline survey which asked questions about acculturation, social support, stress, and demographics. To obtain medical outcomes for the participants and babies, electronic medical charts were reviewed to collect information about the following variables: age, gravity and parity, length of hospital stay, gestational age at delivery, birth weight, maternal medical complication of diabetes, hypertension, preeclampsia, post-partum fever, hemorrhage, route of delivery, induction of labor, use of epidural, and whether or not the patient planned to breastfeed after delivery. The chart review was approved by the Institutional Review Board at Maricopa Medical Center prior to data extraction. This information was found in the scanned archives of the medical record, including the standard history forms, the delivery note, the admission history and physical examination, the discharge summary, and nursing delivery notes. Data were collected by healthcare providers familiar with the delivering facility and the record-keeping system. In total, out of the 440 patients enrolled in the study, we were able to collect complete data on 356 of the participants with 169 in the control group and 187 in the intervention group. Outcome data were not available on 84 of the initially enrolled patients for a variety of reasons including transfer of care, delivery outside of our hospital system, and loss of pregnancy prior to term. We did not collect delivery information on patients that did not deliver at Maricopa Medical Center.

Measures
Medical outcome measures were collected on both the baby and the mother. *Gestational age* is measured as the age of the fetus at the time of birth with a full-term gestational age equal to 40 weeks, though average gestational age ranges between 38 and 42 weeks. *Birth weight* of the baby is measured in grams, with an average full-term baby weighing between 2700 and 4000 grams. *Length of stay* in the hospital measured, in days, the total days from admission to discharge. *Anesthesia* was measured by use of an epidural during delivery. *Induction* refers to if the labor was induced. *Delivery route*

refers to delivery of the baby through a vaginal delivery, a cesarean section (C Section), or an operative vaginal delivery (vaginal delivery through use of forceps or vacuum). Numerous *maternal complication* data were collected including the presence of gestational hypertension (GHNT), chronic hypertension (CHNT), preeclampsia (PreEcc), gestational diabetes (GDM), diabetes prior to pregnancy (PreDM), postpartum hemorrhage (PPH), and maternal postpartum fever (Fever). Data were reviewed using regression analysis to evaluate if there was any difference in birth or delivery outcomes of the patients who had a prenatal partner compared to those patients who followed a typical prenatal course.

Results

Control and intervention groups were found to be similar with regard to demographic characteristics. The mean age of the participants was 26 in the control and 27 in the intervention group. Mean gravidity and parity were the same with mean gravidity of 3 and mean parity of 2. The mean gestational age at delivery was 38.5 weeks for the control group and 38.6 weeks for the intervention and intervention group (Fig. 1). Mean birth weights were 3,267 grams and 3,229 grams for the control and the intervention group, respectively (Fig. 2). Length of the hospital stay postdelivery was an average of 3.3 days for the control group and 3.6 for the intervention patients (Fig. 3). When investigating the mode of anesthesia, 44% of control

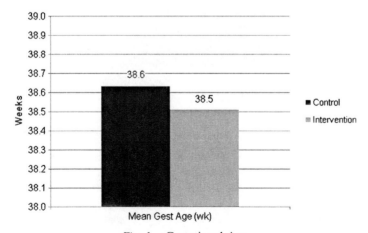

Fig. 1. Gestational Age.

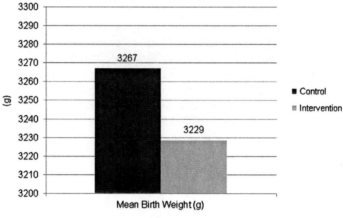

Fig. 2. Birth Weight.

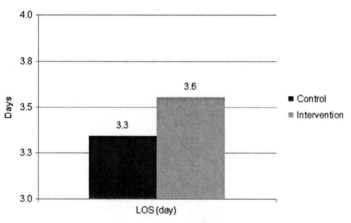

Fig. 3. Length of Stay.

participants utilized epidural compared to 49% of the intervention group. The percentage of patients who used no anesthesia was 37% and 32%, respectively; a spinal (typically used with cesarean section) was utilized 17% in the control and 18% in the intervention and general anesthesia which is used in an emergency setting was 2% and 1%, respectively (Fig. 4). None of these findings were found to be statistically significant.

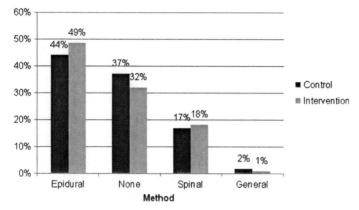

Fig. 4. Anesthesia.

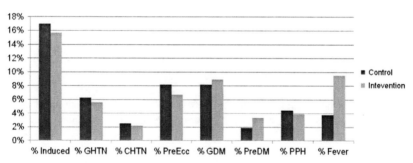

Fig. 5. Induction and Maternal Complication Data.

Maternal medical complications occurred with similar frequency in the control and intervention groups. There was no statistically significant difference in outcomes of hypertensive diseases of pregnancy, pre-gestational diabetes, gestational diabetes, postpartum hemorrhage, and maternal fever (Fig. 5). Likewise, induction rates were similar between the intervention and control groups at 15.5% and 17%, respectively.

Delivery route was also investigated. The number of patients with spontaneous vaginal delivery was 75% in the control compared to 68% in the intervention group. Operative vaginal delivery, comprising both forceps and vacuum deliveries occurred 5% and 7%, respectively. A cesarean section totaled 20% of the patients in the control group and 25% in the intervention group (Fig. 6).

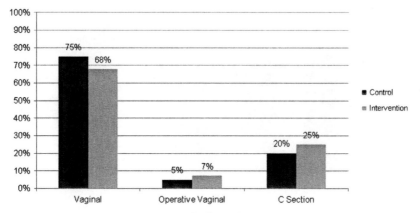

Fig. 6.   Delivery Route.

Conclusions

Familias Sanas was originally designed to evaluate if pairing prenatal care patients with a Prenatal Partner/*Promotora* would increase compliance with the postpartum visit. In the primary study, patients in the intervention group did have a higher rate of postpartum follow up than a control group of patients who did not have contact with the prenatal partner during the course of prenatal care (Marsiglia et al., 2010). This study was a secondary analysis of the aforementioned study which aimed to determine if patients in the intervention group experienced improved birth outcomes compared to patients who did not have contact with a prenatal partner. We did not observe a decrease in rate of a number of common pregnancy-related complications. Likewise, rates of operative delivery were similar between the two groups as were fetal weight at delivery and use of regional anesthesia at delivery.

One of the greatest strengths of this study is that it was a randomized controlled clinical trial. The control and intervention groups were found to be similar in terms of demographic and clinical characteristics. Further-more, the outcome information was obtained directly from electronic medical records by physicians familiar with collecting the clinical data assessed. Therefore the outcome data are felt to be detailed and accurate. The study was performed at an inner-city, urban hospital with a large percentage of patients being of Hispanic descent. This allowed for relatively easy recruitment of patients from this often under-studied population.

However, significant differences were not seen in birth outcomes between the women intervention and control groups. This could be explained by the fact that there were a large number of patients for whom delivery information was not available. Although there was a large number initially recruited, nearly one quarter of enrolled patients did not have data available to collect – meaning they either delivered elsewhere or had a miscarriage. Additionally, this is a secondary analysis of a prior study. The original study was designed to investigate compliance with postpartum follow-up visit; improvement in birth outcomes was not a goal targeted in the study design. It could be that there was more emphasis on the postpartum follow-up and less on prenatal care, or that the study was not tailored to the goal of altering delivery outcomes. Since there was a statistical difference in the number of patients returning for postpartum follow up in the original study, one could postulate those same patients will be more likely to continue to receive well-woman visits for themselves in the future. As noted previously, Hispanic mothers who receive prenatal care have better health outcomes for baby and are more likely to utilize well-child visits and have their children immunized (Kogan et al., 1998; Moore & Hepworth, 1994; Singh & Yu, 1996; Wiecha & Gann, 1994; Zambrana et al., 1997). It may be that women who were encouraged to present for the postpartum visit will be more likely to continue to access healthcare services for their children although this outcome was unfortunately not assessed in this secondary outcome study. Women enrolled in the intervention were better able to deal with complications, have improved mental health or exhibit a decrease in postpartum depression, although again this secondary analysis did not examine these outcomes. Decreased postpartum depression has been seen in low-income women with improved quality of social support (Collins, Dunkel-Schetter, Lobel & Scrimshaw, 1993).

One final explanation for the lack of improvement in birth outcomes for this study may be that this social support intervention was not significant enough to override long-standing stressors such as socioeconomic status, poor nutrition, genetics, and other environmental stressors (Harley & Eskenazi, 2006; Pérez-Escamilla, Garcia, & Song, 2010). In the initial study patients were eligible to participate if they presented for prenatal care at less than 34 weeks gestation – relatively late in pregnancy. Some of the documented benefits of culturally grounded health promotional activities include increased birth weight (Feldman et al., 2000), earlier initiation of prenatal care (Zambrana et al., 1997), higher use of prenatal vitamins (Harley & Eskenazi, 2006), and lower rates of smoking (Schaffer & Lia-Hoagberg, 1997). It is likely that many of the patients assessed in this study were admitted to the intervention too late in pregnancy to see measurable health benefits by the time of delivery. Many of the obstetric complications which were evaluated in the secondary analysis, in particular preeclampsia and gestational diabetes, are felt to be established early in the pregnancy or even prior to pregnancy, making it less likely that an intervention begun at entry into prenatal care would have a measurable clinical benefit.

There are many factors that affect the health of a pregnancy including preconception health of the patient, genetics, socioeconomics, and prior birth history. While it is has been demonstrated that Mexican women have a higher risk of delivering a preterm and low-weight baby (Singh & Yu, 1996; Zambrana et al., 1997), the exact mechanisms at play are still unknown. For Mexican women, when compared to other Mexican women, the role of social support may not have as significant of a role as these other factors. Social support is an important part of women's lives; however, it is unclear if it has any role in improving birth outcomes in pregnancy.

ACKNOWLEDGMENTS

This study was supported by the Hispanic Health Services Grant Program/ Centers for Medicare and Medicaid Services, award 1H0CMS03207. It was hosted by the Southwest Interdisciplinary Research Center, an exploratory center of excellence on minority health and health disparities research funded by award P20MD002316 of the National Center on Minority Health and Health Disparities (NCMHD) of the National Institutes of Health (NIH). The content is solely the responsibility of the authors and does not necessarily represent the official views of the Centers for Medicare and Medicaid Services, the National Center on Minority Health and Health Disparities, or the National Institutes of Health.

REFERENCES

Alexander, G. R., & Kotelchuck, M. (2001). Assessing the role and effectiveness of prenatal care: History, challenges, and directions for future research. *Public Health Report*, *116*(4), 306–316.

Amirehsani, K. A. (2010). Mexican Americans with type 2 diabetes in an emerging latino community: Evaluation of health disparity factors and interventions. *Home Health Care Management Practice*, *22*, 470–478.

Berry, A. B. (1999). Mexican American women's expressions of the meaning of culturally congruent prenatal care. *Journal of Transcultural Nursing, 10*(3), 203–212.

Brown, E. R., Ojeda, V. D., Lara, L. M., & Valenzuela, A. (1999). *Undocumented immigrants: Changes in health insurance coverage with legalized immigration status.* Los Angeles, CA: UCLA Center for Health Policy Research.

Byrd, T. L., Mullen, P. D., Selwyn, B. J., & Lorimor, R. (1996). Initiation of prenatal care by low-income Hispanic women in Houston. *Public Health Reports, 111*(6), 536.

Carrasquillo, O., Carasquillo, A., & Shea, S. (2000). Health insurance coverage of immigrants living in the United States: Differences by citizenship status and country of origin. *American Journal of Public Health, 90*, 917–923.

Carrillo, J. E., Green, A. R., & Betancourt, J. R. (1999). Cross-cultural primary care: A patient-based approach. *Annals of Internal Medicine, 130*, 829–834.

Cefalo, R. C., & Moos, M. K. (1995). *Preconceptional health care: A practical guide.* St. Louis, MO: Mosby.

Centers for Disease Control. (2011). *Health disparities and inequalities report – United States, 2011. Morbidity and mortality weekly report, supplement, Vol. 60.* Atlanta, GA: Center for Disease Control.

Collins, J., & Shay, D. (1994). Prevalence of low birth weight among Hispanic infants with United States-born and foreign-born mothers: the effect of urban poverty. *American Journal of Epidemiology, 139*(2), 184–192.

Collins, N. L., Dunkel-Schetter, C., Lobel, M., & Scrimshaw, S. C. (1993). Social support in pregnancy: Psychosocial correlates of birth outcomes and postpartum depression. *Journal of Personality and Social Psychology, 65*, 1243–1258.

DuBard, C. A., & Gizlice, Z. (2008). Language spoken and differences in health status, access to care, and receipt of preventive services among US Hispanics. *American Journal of Public Health, 98*(11), 2021–2028.

Eshiett, M. U., & Parry, E. H. (2003). Migrants and health: A cultural dilemma. *Clinical Medicine, Journal of the Royal College of Physicians, 3*(3), 229–231.

Feldman, P. J., Dunkel-Schetter, C., Sandman, C. A., & Wadhwa, P. D. (2000). Maternal social support predicts birth weight and fetal growth in human pregnancy. *Psychosomatic Medicine, 62*(5), 715–725.

Frisbie, W. P., & Song, S. E. (2003). Hispanic pregnancy outcomes: Differentials over time and current risk factor effects. *Policy Studies Journal, 31*(2), 237–252.

Guendelman, S., & English, P. (1995). Effect of United States residence on birth outcomes among Mexican immigrants: an exploratory study. *American Journal of Epidemiology, 142*(9), S30–S38.

Harley, K., & Eskenazi, B. (2006). Time in the United States, social support and health behaviors during pregnancy among women of Mexican descent. *Social Science & Medicine, 62*(2006), 3048–3061.

Harley, K., Eskenazi, B., & Block, G. (2005). The association of time in the US and diet during pregnancy in low-income women of Mexican descent. *Pediatric and Perinatal Epidemiology, 19*(2), 125–134.

Hummer, R. A., Eberstein, I. W., & Nam, C. (1992). Infant mortality differentials among hispanic groups in Florida. *Social Forces, 70*, 1055–1075.

Hunter, J. B., de Zapien, J. G., Papenfuss, M., Fernandez, M. L., Meister, J., & Giuliano, A. R. (2004). The impact of a promotora on increasing routine chronic disease prevention among women aged 40 and older at the US-Mexico border. *Health Education & Behavior, 31*(4 suppl), 18S–28S.

158 KATHRYN CONNORS ET AL.

Kogan, M., Alexander, G., Jack, B., & Allen, M. (1998). The association between adequacy of prenatal care utilization and subsequent pediatric care utilization in the United States. *Pediatrics*, *102*(1), 25–30.

Larkey, L. (2006). Las mujeres saludables: Reaching Latinas for breast, cervical and colorectal cancer prevention and screening. *Journal of community health*, *31*(1), 69–77.

Marcelli, E. A. (2004). The unauthorized residency status myth: Health insurance coverage and medical care use among Mexican immigrants in California. *Migraciones Internacionales*, *2*(4), 5–35.

Marsiglia, F. F., Bermudez-Parsai, M., & Coonrod, D. (2010). Familias sanas: An intervention designed to increase rates of postpartum visits among Latinas. *Journal of Health Care for the Poor and Underserved*, *21*, 119–131.

Martin, J. A., Hamilton, B. E., Ventura, S. J., et al. (2011). *Births: Final data for 2009. National vital statistics reports (Vol. 60, no. 1)*. Hyattsville, MD: National Center for Health Statistics.

McDuffie, R., Beck, A., Bischoff, K., Cross, J., & Orleans, M. (1996). Effect of frequency of prenatal care visits on perinatal outcome among low-risk women. *JAMA*, *275*, 847–851.

McDonald, M., & Hertz, R. P. (2008). *A profile of uninsured persons in the United States*. Pfizer Facts. Retrieved from http://www.pfizer.com/files/products/Profile_of_uninsured_persons_in_the_United_States.pdf

McGlade, M. S., Saha, S., & Dahlstrom, M. E. (2004). The Latina paradox: An opportunity for restructuring prenatal care delivery. *Journal Information*, *94*(12).

Moore, P., & Hepworth, J. (1994). Use of perinatal and infant health services by Mexican-American medicaid enrollees. *JAMA*, *272*(4), 297–304.

Norbeck, J. S., & Anderson, N. J. (1989). Psychosocial predictors of pregnancy outcomes in low-income Black, Hispanic, and White women. *Nursing Research*, *38*(4), 204–209.

Novilla, M., Lelinneth, B., Barnes, M. D., De La Cruz, N. G., Williams, P. N., & Rogers, J. (2006). Public health perspectives on the family. *Family & Community Health*, *29*(1), 28–42.

Padilla, Y. C., & Villalobos, G. (2006). Cultural responses to health among Mexican American women and their families. *Family & Community Health*, *30*(1S), S24–S33.

Passel, J., Livingston, G., & Cohn, D. (2012). *Explaining why minority births now outnumber White births*. Pew Research Social & Demographic Trends. Retrieved from http://www.pewsocialtrends.org/2012/05/17/explaining-why-minority-births-now-outnumber-white-births/. Accessed on January 20, 2012.

Pèrez-Escamilla, R., Garcia, J., & Song, D. (2010). Health care access among Hispanic immigrants: ¿Alguien está escuchando? [Is anybody listening?]. *NAPA Bulletin*, *34*(1), 47–67.

Ramos, I. N., May, M., & Ramos, K. S. (2001). Field action report. Environmental health training of promotoras in colonias along the Texas-Mexico border. *American Journal of Public Health*, *4*(91), 4.

Rivadeneyra, R., Elderkin-Thompson, V., Silver, R. C., & Waitzkin, H. (2000). Patient centeredness in medical encounters requiring an interpreter. *The American Journal of Medicine*, *108*(6), 470–474.

Schaffer, M. A., & Lia-Hoagberg, B. (1997). Effects of social support on prenatal care and health behaviors of low-income women. *Journal of Obstetric, Gynecologic, and Neonatal Nursing*, *26*(4), 433–440.

Siddiqi, A., Zuberi, D., & Nguyen, Q. C. (2009). The role of health insurance in explaining immigrant versus non-immigrant disparities in access to health care: Comparing the United States to Canada. *Social Science & Medicine, 69*(10), 1452–1459.

Singh, G., & Yu, S. (1996). Adverse pregnancy outcomes: Differences between US and foreign-born women in major US racial and ethnic groups. *American Journal of Public Health, 86*(6), 837–843.

Thamer, M., Richard, C., Casebeer, A. W., & Ray, N. F. (1997). Health insurance coverage among foreign-born US residents: The impact of race, ethnicity, and length of residence. *American Journal of Public Health, 87*, 96–102.

Trevino, F. M., Moyer, M. E., Valdez, R. B., & Stroup-Benham, C. A. (1991). Health insurance coverage and utilization of services by Mexican Americans, mainland Puerto Ricans and Cuban Americans. *JAMA, 265*, 233–237.

U.S. Census Bureau. (2011). Statistical abstract of the United States: 2012 (131st ed.). Washington, DC. Retrieved from http://www.census.gov/compendia/statab/

Vega, W. A., Kolody, B., Hwang, J., Noble, A., & Porter, P. A. (1997). Perinatal drug use among immigrant and native-born Latinas. *Substance Use & Misuse, 32*(1), 43–62.

Warda, M. R. (2000). Mexican Americans' perceptions of culturally competent care. *Western Journal of Nursing Research, 22*(2), 203–224.

Wiecha, J., & Gann, P. (1994). Does maternal prenatal care use predict infant immunization delay? *Family Medicine, 26*(3), 172–178.

Wolff, C. B., & Portis, M. (1996). Smoking, acculturation, and pregnancy outcome among Mexican Americans. *Health Care for Women International, 17*(6), 563–573.

Zambrana, R. E., Scrimshawe, S. C., Collins, N., & Dunkel-Schetter, C. (1997). Prenatal health behaviors and psychological risk factors in pregnant women of Mexican origin: The role of acculturation. *American Journal of Public Health, 87*(6), 1022–1026.

VARIATIONS IN PARENTS' PERCEPTIONS OF THEIR CHILDREN'S MEDICAL TREATMENT: THE EFFECT OF DISSATISFACTION ON PREVENTIVE CARE AND UNMET NEED

Hanna Jokinen-Gordon and Jill Quadagno

ABSTRACT

Purpose – *This chapter examines social variations in parent dissatisfaction with children's medical care and tests whether greater dissatisfaction is associated with less preventive care and unmet medical need.*

Methodology/approach – *The 2007 National Survey of Children's Health (NSCH) is a nationally representative cross-sectional sample of parents of U.S. children age 0–17 years (N = 78,523). We use a combination of ordinary least squares (OLS) and binary logistic regression to analyze parent dissatisfaction, preventive care, and unmet medical need.*

Social Determinants, Health Disparities and Linkages to Health and Health Care
Research in the Sociology of Health Care, Volume 31, 161–185
Copyright © 2013 by Emerald Group Publishing Limited
All rights of reproduction in any form reserved
ISSN: 0275-4959/doi:10.1108/S0275-4959(2013)0000031010

Findings – *Our results indicate that parents' dissatisfaction scores are significantly higher for racial/ethnic minorities, non-English speakers, lower socioeconomic status (SES) respondents, and the uninsured. Furthermore, parent dissatisfaction has a significant and robust association with lack of preventive care and reports of unmet medical need.*

Research limitations/implications – *Due to the cross-sectional research design, we were unable to determine whether dissatisfaction caused parents to delay children's medical care, thus resulting in a lack of annual preventive care and greater unmet needs.*

Originality/value of chapter – *Although there is extensive research on adult perceptions of their own medical care, few sociological studies have examined parents' perceptions about their children's care. Yet, there is substantial evidence that parents transmit health-related attitudes, beliefs, and behaviors to their children. As with adult patients, parent satisfaction with their child's medical care is stratified by social characteristics; however, we also find a strong association between dissatisfaction and use of other important health services. It may be the case that when parents feel that they did not receive satisfactory care, they are more likely to delay, or to forgo, preventive and other health services.*

Keywords: Health care satisfaction; children/youth; unmet medical need

A fundamental precept of life course research is that the foundation of future life chances is grounded in the early conditions of childhood (Graham 2002; Wadsworth 1997). During childhood, important socialization processes occur that shape subsequent health and well-being (Singh-Manoux & Marmot, 2005). Because children are perceptive about how the adults in their lives deal with adversity, they learn from them important health-related behaviors and attitudes (Lau, Quadrel, & Hartman, 1990; Roche, Ahmed, & Blum, 2008; Wickrama, Conger, Wallace, & Elder, 1999). This means that parents' interactions with the health care system have the potential to influence their children's health, not only in early life, but well into adulthood.

Although there is extensive research on adult perceptions of their own care, few studies have examined parents' perceptions of their children's care from a sociological standpoint (Becker & Newsom, 2003; Cooper-Patrick et al., 1999; Lillie-Blanton, Brodie, Rowland, Altman, & McIntosh, 2000). Yet a number of studies have shown that children learn to mirror their parents' health-related behaviors (Lau et al., 1990), including smoking (Ennett et al., 2010), alcohol consumption (Latendresse et al., 2008), dietary behaviors, and physical exercise (Burgess-Champoux et al., 2008; Rimal, 2003). Children also learn from the adults in their lives important health-related attitudes (Lau et al., 1990; Roche et al., 2008; Wickrama et al., 1999). If parents feel distrustful about the medical care they receive, their children may grow up holding similar views (Rimal, 2003). For example, Lau et al. (1990) found that as children approach adulthood, their health beliefs and attitudes converged with those of their parents. Similarly, in a small sample, Byczkowski, Kollar, and Britto (2010) found concordance between parents and their adolescent children's perceptions of care.

Research on adult perceptions of their own medical care finds that feelings of trust and satisfaction with care affect both adherence to prescribed treatment and also health in general (Roche et al., 2008; Street, Makoul, Arora, & Epstein, 2009). Patients who feel that their doctor is acting in their best interests are more likely to comply with treatment and to have better self-rated health and clinical outcomes (Franks et al., 2006; Lee & Lin, 2009). By contrast, patients who view the doctor–patient interaction in negative terms tend to be less trusting and more dissatisfied with the quality of care and experience greater stress and frustration (Armstrong, Ravenell, McMurphy, & Putt, 2007; Dovidio et al., 2008). Thus, patients' satisfaction with their interaction with the medical system has significant implications for health outcomes (Boyer & Lutfey, 2010; Street et al., 2009).

Parental attitudes may also affect their children's medical care. Some studies suggest that parents who have confidence in those who provide care to their children are more likely to schedule regular physician visits and comply with instructions, while parents who are dissatisfied are less likely to do so (DiMatteo, 2004). Thus, positive parental attitudes may ensure that children receive preventive care and adequate treatment and transmit the message that regular care is necessary and important.

Research suggests that there is significant variation in the ability to navigate the clinical setting based on such factors as race and ethnicity, social class, and insurance coverage. Although many studies have examined how social disparities affect adult satisfaction, fewer studies have considered whether parents' perceptions of their child's medical care vary on the same dimensions. In this chapter we examine the effect of race/ethnicity, socioeconomic status (SES), insurance coverage, and language on parents' satisfaction with their children's medical care and assess whether dissatisfaction is associated with fewer preventive visits and greater unmet medical need.

FACTORS ASSOCIATED WITH ADULTS' PERCEPTIONS OF HEALTH CARE

Race and Ethnicity

Many studies have found that racial and ethnic minorities perceive their treatment and interactions in the clinical setting in more negative terms. Compared to white patients, racial and ethnic minorities are more likely to rate their experience negatively, less likely to view their medical care as satisfactory, and more likely to believe that they receive lower quality care (Armstrong et al., 2007; Cooper-Patrick et al., 1999; Lillie-Blanton et al., 2000). Studies of parents' experiences with their children's medical care providers suggest that race/ethnicity is an important correlate of both physician–family engagement and overall parent satisfaction (Berdahl et al., 2010; Bethell et al., 2011; Cox et al., 2012; Wilkins, Elliott, Richardson, Lozano, & Mangione-Smith, 2011). Berdahl et al. (2010) examined both receipt and quality of children's medical care and found that minority youth were less likely to report receiving particular services and less likely to report patient-centered care. When the authors examined racial disparities by income group, racial disparities were present even in higher SES groups. These findings point to an independent influence of race/ethnicity on parent assessments of children's medical care.

The effect of race/ethnicity on parents' evaluations of care may be explained by differences in both the way that physicians interact with minority families and/or by differences in the way that families engage in, and value, aspects of the care exchange (Wilkins et al., 2011). For example, when Cox et al. (2012) examined racial/ethnic variations in family–physician engagement, they found that when physicians visited Asian families, they were less likely to engage in communications that facilitated relationship building. Further, compared to white families, African American families were less likely to be engaged in decision-making while Latino families were less likely to gather information. They also found, however, that these differences were a function of SES. Among adult patients, physicians are more likely to perceive minority patients in negative terms compared to white patients (van Ryn & Burke, 2008). Such attitudes may be transmitted to patients in both direct and subtle ways that influence how patients experience the interaction. These attitudes, in turn, have significant consequences for compliance, for minority patients who believe they are being discriminated against may react by being more skeptical of providers and less accommodating of treatment (Schnittker, Pescosolido, & Croghan, 2005).

Although there is extensive evidence suggesting racial disparities in patient trust and satisfaction, there is also some contradictory evidence. One survey found that race or ethnicity had no effect on adults' trust of physicians (Hall, Camacho, Dugan, & Balkrishnan, 2002). Another study found that when patients were asked to directly indicate their level of trust in a physician, race effects were not significant, but when trust was measured using indirect statements rooted in personal experiences with providers, minority patients reported significantly lower trust (Stepanikova, Mollborn, Cook, Thom, & Kramer, 2006). Thus, the wording of the question may affect the response received.

Socioeconomic Status

As noted, above, SES is another factor that influences patient perceptions of medical care. Compared to middle or high SES individuals, lower SES parents and individuals tend to report less satisfaction with their primary care provider (Berdahl et al. 2010; Campbell, Ramsay, & Green, 2001; Stevens & Shi, 2003) and have lower scores on multiple measures of satisfaction (Haviland, Morales, Dial, & Pincus, 2005). Individuals living in poverty are significantly more likely than others to report negative perceptions of care, and among the very poor negative attitudes toward health care are even greater (Haviland et al., 2005).

There are several reasons why SES influences attitudes toward medical care. Low SES parents bring less cultural health capital in the form of "knowledge of medical topics and vocabulary" and in "the ability to communicate social privilege and resources" (Shim, 2010, p. 3). As a result, they are more likely to be perceived by physicians as unintelligent and less likely to comply with treatment recommendations (van Ryn & Burke, 2000). These beliefs can spill over into the doctor–patient interaction in negative ways that influence patient's perceptions of care. Further, because families with low SES are limited in their ability to choose health care providers, they are more likely to utilize overburdened public health services and also lack in a regular source of care. As a result, doctors may be forced by the volume of patients they see to limit their interactions with these patients (Lutfey & Freese, 2005). Not having a usual source of care also undermines the development of a trusting relationship.

Insurance Coverage

Health insurance is a key resource that patients bring to the clinical interaction. In 2012 55 percent of children under age 18 were insured through either an employer or other private insurance and about 34 percent were covered through public programs such as the State Children's Health Insurance Program (SCHIP) or Medicaid (Kaiser Family Foundation 2012). Yet because states vary widely in the coverage provided and requirements for participation, approximately 10 percent of children are uninsured.

Several studies have found that patients believe they receive differential treatment based on their insurance coverage. One study found that when patients were asked why they felt discriminated against, the most common response involved type of insurance. Their perceptions may have been correct, because those who perceived discrimination were less likely to receive preventive testing (Trivediand Ayanian, 2006). Another study found that trust in physicians was higher among fee-for-service patients compared to patients in capitated or managed care plans (Kao, Green, Zallavsky, Koplan, & Cleary, 1998). These perceptions are anchored in real experiences, because physicians do appear to discriminate against patients based on type of insurance coverage. A study of internists in California found that 77 percent would be willing to accept new patients with private insurance, while only 31 percent would accept new Medicaid patients and 43 percent new uninsured patients (Komaromy, Lurie, & Bindman, 1995). In this study, physicians' attitudes were most negative toward publicly insured patients, which might influence how such patients are treated and thus how they perceive their care. However, there is also evidence of bias against uninsured patients (Hadley, 2003), so one would expect both groups to have more negative perceptions of the health care experience and less trust in their physicians.

Language Barriers

Health literacy is derived from linguistic facility and is central to the full exchange of information between patients and providers (Shim, 2010).

Evidence suggests that when physicians do not speak the patient's language, communication barriers can lead to frustration and confusion and reduce patient satisfaction (Gonzalez, Vega, & Tarraf, 2010). For example, Hispanic patients who only speak Spanish experience lower patient satisfaction than those who are bilingual. Further, patients with limited English proficiency have difficulty finding bilingual physicians and have less access to care and poorer adherence to treatment regimens (Flores, 2006; Regenstein, Mead, Muessig, & Huang, 2009). This is especially problematic for immigrant children who face considerable barriers in accessing health care (Flores, 2006). Language barriers may inhibit a family's ability to navigate publicly funded children's health insurance programs and negatively affect their experiences with the health care system (Chung, Lee, Morrison, & Schuster, 2006; Flores & Tomany-Korman, 2008a). However, when patients receive "linguistically competent" primary care, language barriers can be overcome (O'Brien & Shea, 2011).

Although many studies have examined adult patients' perceptions, what is less known is whether the same factors that shape adults perception of their own medical care also influence how they perceive their children's medical care and whether or not dissatisfaction decreases the likelihood of receiving needed medical care. In our analysis, we critically examine the relationship between social factors and parents' perceptions of their child's medical care and then consider whether dissatisfaction is associated with receipt of preventive care and with unmet need. Based on the literature cited above, we test the following hypotheses:

Hypotheses

1. Parents of minority children will have more negative assessments of their children's medical care.
2. Parents with language barriers will have more negative assessments of their children's medical care.
3. Parents with lower SES will have more negative assessments of their children's medical care.
4. Parents of publicly insured and uninsured children will have more negative assessments of their children's medical care than parents of privately insured children.
5. Children whose parents have higher dissatisfaction scores will be less likely to have received preventive care and more likely to have unmet medical needs.

Data and Methods

To test these hypotheses, we use data from the 2007 National Survey of Children's Health (NSCH). The 2007 NSCH is a nationally representative, random digit dial survey of the health of children age 0–17 years conducted by the Center for Disease Control and the National Center for Health Statistics. Households were selected from each of the 50 states and the District of Columbia. One child from the household was selected at random. Respondents were the parent or guardian who knew the most about the selected child, most often the mother. For the study sample 74 percent of respondents were the child's biological, step or adoptive mother. The weighted response rate was 51.2 percent. Additional details regarding the methodology and survey design have been published and can be found online (Blumberg, Foster, & Frasier, 2009).

The full final sample size of the 2007 NSCH was 91,642 youth age 0–17 years. For this analysis, we limited the sample to children who were living with at least one parent, including both biological parents, a two-parent stepfamily, an adoptive parent family or a single parent household ($n = 85,893$). Because SES is both a household and a parent-specific measure, we exclude children living in other family arrangements. The sample was further limited to those children without missing values on the dependent and independent variables. If the selected child (S.C.) did not receive medical care in the past year or if the parent refused or responded that they did not know, the dissatisfaction measure was set as missing ($n = 4,951$). The independent variable with the most missing values was race, approximately six percent of respondents. The final sample size was $n = 78,523$.

Dependent Variables

Parent Dissatisfaction with Care
The dependent variable for the analysis was a mean item index of parent dissatisfaction with medical care. The measure was generated using five questions meant to assess parent satisfaction with their child's medical care visit. Respondents were asked to think about their child's most recent experience in the past 12 months and answer questions regarding their satisfaction using a Likert-type scale. Questions included: (1) when [the S.C.] is seen by a doctor or other health providers, how often are they sensitive to your families values and customs, and (2–5) during the past twelve months, or since [S.C.'s] birth, how often did doctors or other health providers

(2) spend enough time with [him/her], (3) listen carefully to you, (4) give you the specific information you needed, and (5) make you feel like a partner in your child's health care. We reverse coded the response so that a higher score on the index indicated greater dissatisfaction. Responses ranged from always ("0"), usually ("1"), sometimes ("2"), but never ("3"). The index measured the respondents mean dissatisfaction score. Scores ranged from 0 to 3. The index was reliable with a Cronbach's alpha of 0.83. Because the responses in the index were positively skewed, subsequence multivariate analyses employed a square root transformation. After the transformation, skewness and kurtosis estimates were reduced from 1.59 and 5.42 to 0.42 and 2.01, respectively. Respondents whose child did not receive any medical care in the past year were coded as missing responses.

Medical Care
Two measures were used to assess children's medical care. First, a dichotomous measure was used to indicate those children who did not receive at least one preventive visit in the past 12 months ("1"). A second dichotomous measure was used to indicate whether the child had any unmet medical care needs. The original question asked parents if, at any point in the past 12 months, the child needed health care that was delayed or not received. Parents were then asked to indicate whether the care that was delayed or not received was a medical, dental, mental health, or other health care need. For this analysis we focused only on parents who reported that their child had an unmet medical care need ("1").

Key Independent Variables

Race and Ethnicity
Race and ethnicity were measured using a set of dichotomous variables. Respondents were asked about their race using the following categories: White, Black/African American, American Indian or Alaska Native, Asian, Native Hawaiian or Pacific Islander. Respondents who reported more than one category were coded as multiracial. Verbatim responses were also included and later back coded into the listed categories. Responses which could not be back coded were set as missing. To protect respondent anonymity, the responses were further collapsed into: white, black, multirace, and other. For the analysis, race was measured using three mutually exclusive categories. We generated two dummy indicators of race, black ("1"), multirace/other ("1"), and we used non-Hispanic white as

the referent. Ethnicity was a dichotomous indicator of whether the parent identified the child as Hispanic ("1") or not ("0").

Language
To measure the respondent's language, we used a dummy variable to indicate whether the preferred language used at home was something other than English ("1").

Socioeconomic Status
SES was measured using two variables. First, we included the family's income as a percentage of the federal poverty limit. This measure was useful because it was adjusted for household size and was directly related to public insurance eligibility. The family's poverty status was measured using a categorical variable coded as follows: "3" for 0–99 percent of the federal poverty limit, "2" for 100–199 percent, "1" for 200–399 percent , and "0" for 400 percent and higher. We also included a second measure of SES, parent's educational attainment. Respondents were asked to list the highest level of education received by the selected child's father and mother. If the father's highest level of education was missing (17.8 percent), we used the mother's highest level of education. In this sample, those respondents living in single mother households (16.7 percent) were most likely to have a missing value on father's education. Responses included less than high school, high school, some college or more. We collapsed the categories so that parents with a high school diploma or less were coded as "1" and all others were set to '0."

Insurance Status
The child's insurance status was measured using a set of dummy variables. Respondents were asked to indicate whether the S.C. was privately insured, publicly insured, or without insurance coverage. Children with public insurance were asked specifically whether the child was enrolled in the respondent's home state SCHIP or Medicaid program, using the name of the program. However, to ensure confidentiality, all children enrolled in either Medicaid or SCHIP were coded as having public insurance. We use two dichotomous indicators of insurance status, publicly insured children ("1") and uninsured children ("2"), with privately insured children as the reference category.

Other Covariates
In addition to the key independent variables, we included other covariates that may influence satisfaction with medical care. The sex of the S.C. was

measured using a dichotomous indictor for which male is coded as "1." The child's age in years was measured with a continuous variable ranging from 0 to 17. The parent's assessment of the selected child's physical health was measured with a categorical variable ranging from excellent ("3"), very good ("2"), good ("1"), and fair/poor ("0"). Finally, we included whether the S.C. has a usual source of medical care or a medical home, that is, a regular physician. Respondents whose child did not have a usual source of care or medical home were coded "1."

Analytic Strategy

To assess the relationship between social characteristics and dissatisfaction with medical care, we proceed in three steps. First, we present unweighted descriptive statistics for the study sample. Next we assess the multivariate relationship between social factors and parent dissatisfaction scores. Finally, we examine whether parent dissatisfaction scores are associated with children's receipt of medical care and unmet medical need.

Using a set of nested ordinary least squares regression models, our analytic strategy for the prediction of parent dissatisfaction involves four steps. In Model 1, we test the effects of race/ethnicity and language, while controlling for age and sex. Model 2 includes the measures of SES, household poverty status and parent's highest level of education. Model 3 adds the measures of insurance status and the control for no medical home. Finally, Model 4 controls for the parent rated measure of child health. The decision to use ordinary least squares (OLS) was based on multiple sensitivity analyses. We tested multiple versions of the dependent variable using both OLS and other generalized linear regression models. The results were consistent across multiple models.

The final stage of our analysis tests whether parent dissatisfaction scores are related to the children's receipt of preventive and needed medical treatment. For this phase, we employ two binary logistic regression models (Table 3). The first regresses the full model covariates, as well as parent dissatisfaction, on the odds that the child did not receive preventive medical treatment in the past 12 months. The second model repeats this analysis for a measure of unmet or delayed medical care need. However, in this model we include an additional covariate for no preventive care. In analyses not shown here, for both binary outcomes we tested nested models like those for the dissatisfaction index. Since the inclusion of the dissatisfaction measure did not alter the direction or relationship between lack of preventive care or

unmet medical need, only the findings from the full models are displayed in
Table 3.

Because the NSCH 2007 used a complex sampling design, appropriate
weighting procedures were applied using STATA 11.0. Additional analyses
were performed to test for multicollinearity with the "collin" command used
to examine the variance inflation factors for each regression coefficient. For
all variables the VIF statistics were well below two, indicating that the
standard errors are not biased due to multicollinearity.

RESULTS

Descriptive Analysis

Table 1 provides unweighted descriptive statistics for the study sample. In
general, the children in this sample live above the federal poverty limit. Only
10 percent of the children in the sample reside in households below 100
percent of the federal poverty line (FPL). Most parents have completed
more than a high school education; 69.9 percent report more than
high school as their highest level of education. In terms of the racial and
ethnic composition of the sample, the majority of children are non-Hispanic
white; slightly more than 10 percent are black, 10 percent are in the
multiracial/other category, and 8.4 percent are Hispanic. Most of the
children are privately insured with 19.2 percent publicly insured and 6.1
percent uninsured. Most children live in predominately English-speaking
households with 2.7 percent residing in primarily non-English-speaking
households.

According to the descriptive statistics, the average respondent scored very
low on the dissatisfaction index. Most children were likely to receive
preventive care and unlikely to have a delayed or unmet medical care need.
In a bivariate analysis not presented here, we found significant associations
between model predictors and dependent variables in the hypothesized
directions.

Multivariate Analyses

Table 2 presents the results from the OLS regression models predicting
dissatisfaction with care. First, we estimate the effects of race/ethnicity and
language while controlling for age and sex. Second, we include the measures

Table 1. Sample Summary Statistics and Percentages.

		Score	Sq. Rt. Score
Dependent Variables			
Dissatisfaction Index			
	Min.-Max.	0–3	0–1.73
	Mean	0.47	0.50
	Std. Deviation	0.60	0.47
	Alpha	0.83	
Preventative Care			
	No (= 1)	9.76	
	Yes	90.24	
Unmet or Delayed Medical Need			
	Yes (= 1)	3.91	
	No	96.09	
Covariates			
SES			
Federal Poverty Status			
	0–99 percent	9.74	
	100–199	15.64	
	200–399	34.59	
	400 or more	40.03	
Parent Education			
	High School or Less	30.04	
	More than High School	69.96	
Race			
Black		10.12	
Multirace/Other		10.36	
White		79.53	
Ethnicity			
Hispanic		8.41	
Non-Hispanic		91.59	
Type Insurance			
Privately Insured		74.71	
Publicly Insured		19.22	
Uninsured		6.07	
Language			
Non-English Household		2.74	
Controls			
Male		51.89	
Parent-Rated Health			
	Excellent	67.05	
	Very Good	22.64	
	Good	8.38	
	Fair/Poor	1.93	
Age		9.10(5.32)	
No Medical Home		3.48	
		N = 78,5233	

Table 2. OLS Regression Coefficients of Sq. Root of Dissatisfaction Index Scores on Social Characteristics.

	Model 1		Model 2		Model 3		Model 4	
	b	SE	b	SE	b	SE	b	SE
Race (white)								
Black	0.150***	0.012	0.114***	0.012	0.105***	0.012	0.094***	0.012
Multirace/Other	0.135***	0.016	0.131***	0.015	0.126***	0.016	0.118***	0.016
Ethnicity (non-Hispanic)								
Hispanic	0.080**	0.023	0.068**	0.023	0.064**	0.023	0.058*	0.023
Language (English)								
Non-English	0.251***	0.035	0.195***	0.035	0.158***	0.035	0.118**	0.035
SES								
Federal Poverty Status			0.038***	0.005	0.034***	0.005	0.024***	0.024
High School or Less (more than high school)			0.033**	0.009	0.028***	0.028	0.021*	0.021
Insurance Status (privately insured)								
Publicly Insured					-0.001	0.014	-0.013	0.014
Uninsured					0.170***	0.017	0.129***	0.017
Controls								
Male (female)	0.002	0.008	0.002	0.008	0.001	0.008	-0.002	0.008
Age	0.010***	0.001	0.010***	0.007	0.010***	0.001	0.009***	0.001
No Medical Home					0.169***	0.025	0.159***	0.025
Parent-Rated Health							-0.092***	0.007
Constant	0.352	0.009	0.302		0.299		0.654	
Model Statistics								
Model F	81.25***		69.72***		62.33***		67.24***	
R-squared	0.053		0.067		0.085		0.103	
N = 78,523								

Note: OLS = ordinary least squares. Reference categories are identified in parentheses within stub columns. *$p < .05$, **$p < .01$, ***$p < .001$.

of SES to test whether they mediate any of the race effect. Then we include insurance status while controlling for whether the child has a usual source of medical care. Finally, we add the control for the parent-rated child health measure. Table 3 presents the results of two binary logistic regression models used to assess the relationship between parent dissatisfaction scores and lack of preventive care and unmet medical need.

Model 1 of Table 2 shows that both race/ethnicity and speaking a language other than English at home are significantly related to parents' dissatisfaction with their child's medical care. Controlling for age and sex,

Table 3. Logistic Regression of the Odds of Reporting No Preventive Care and Unmet or Delayed Medical Care Need.

	No Preventive Care		Unmet Health Care Need	
	OR's	95% C.I.	OR's	95% C.I.
Parent Dissatisfaction Index	1.754***	1.593–1931	2.318***	2.048–2.624
Race (white)				
Black	0.466***	0.361–0.613	0.921	0.705–1.203
Multirace/Other	0.959	0.754–1.220	0.901	0.645–1.257
Ethnicity (non-Hispanic)				
Hispanic	1.024	0.729–1.437	1.155	0.774–1.722
Language (English)				
Non-English	0.556*	0.340–.909	0.224***	0.119–0.421
SES				
Federal Poverty Status	1.110**	1.103–1.92	1.195**	1.070–1.334
High School or Less (more than high school)	1.051	0.918–1.203	0.713**	0.573–0.888
Insurance Status (privately insured)				
Publicly Insured	0.684***	0.572–0.818	1.514**	1.153–1.987
Uninsured	1.480***	1.199–1.819	2.653***	1.903–3.698
Controls				
Male (female)	0.094	0.832–1.057	0.975	0.803–1.184
Age	1.113***	1.102–1.125	0.984	0.965–1.003
No Medical Home	1.609**	1.196–2.164	0.895	0.656–1.221
Parent-Rated Health	1.138**	1.048–1.236	0.619***	0.549–0.696
No Preventive Care			0.951	0.717–1.260
N = 78,523				

*$p < .05$, **$p < .01$, ***$p < .001$.

the results of the regression of dissatisfaction scores on race/ethnicity and language are consistent with our first and second hypotheses. They suggest that parents of minority children and those in non-English-speaking households are far more likely to have negative perceptions of their medical care interaction.

The addition of SES in Model 2 mediates a considerable portion of the effect of being black and residing in a non-English-speaking household. However, SES has less effect on the dissatisfaction scores of multirace/other and Hispanic respondents. This suggests that there may be something unique about multirace/other and Hispanic parent's perceptions of the health care interaction independent of SES. In the full cumulative model, race/ethnicity continues to exert a significant effect on dissatisfaction scores. The inclusion of the other covariates such as insurance status, usual source of care, and parent-rated health considerably reduce the magnitude of the effect of being black and living in a non-English-speaking household, but the coefficients for being multirace/other and Hispanic remain relatively consistent. Given that parents of multirace/other children are persistently more dissatisfied, it may be that these parents perceive a unique type of discrimination that is tied less to the covariates that partially mediate other race and language effects. When age and sex are controlled, race/ethnicity and language explain approximately five percent of the variation in the square root of parent dissatisfaction scores.

Household poverty status and parents' education are added in Model 2 of Table 2. As in the descriptive analyses, results from the multivariate analyses reveal a consistent association between income and parent dissatisfaction with care. In Model 2, those living closer to the federal poverty limit have a significantly higher likelihood than more affluent respondents of reporting a negative experience. As respondents move closer to 0–99 percent of the FPL, their scores on the dissatisfaction index increase. When insurance status and having a usual source of care are included in Model 3, the magnitude of the effect of poverty status is reduced slightly. The effect of poverty remains significant even in the final cumulative model. Parents in households living closer to the FPL consistently score higher on the dissatisfaction index.

We also consider whether parents' education levels influence their perception of care and find that parents with less education are more likely to be dissatisfied. As shown in Model 2, parents with a high school-level education or less have significantly higher dissatisfaction scores than parents who have more than a high school education. The inclusion of education in Model 2 increases the explained variation in parent dissatisfaction by slightly more than one percent. When the other covariates are included, the effect of parent education is reduced but not fully mediated. In the full model, parents with a high school-level education or less are significantly more likely to report being more dissatisfied.

Insurance status is added in Model 3 of Table 2. Contrary to our hypothesis, we do not find a significant difference between publicly and privately insured children. However, being uninsured significantly increases negative assessments of medical care. Parents whose child is uninsured have higher ratings of dissatisfaction with their child's most recent care interaction. In the final model, being uninsured continues to influence parent's perceptions of care. Parents of uninsured children consistently report higher dissatisfaction. While modest, the *R*-squared in the final model with all covariates demonstrates the importance of social characteristics in shaping parent dissatisfaction. Together the model covariates explain 10.3 percent of the variation in parent dissatisfaction scores.

Table 3 displays the odds ratios from two binary logistic models. The first column in Table 3 presents the odds ratios from a binary logistic model predicting the odds of the child not receiving a preventive health care visit in the past 12 months. As hypothesized, parents who have higher scores on the dissatisfaction index have significantly higher odds of reporting that their child did not receive any preventive care in the past year. As a parent's score on the dissatisfaction index increases, the odds of the child not receiving preventive care increases by 75 percent ($p < .001$). One interpretation of this finding is that parents who feel dissatisfied with their child's medical care interaction are less likely to schedule routine check-ups with their child's health care provider. Alternatively, these parents may be more dissatisfied because their child does not have a regular physician and their most recent medical visit was in an emergency room or walk-in clinic. Somewhat surprisingly, black children ($p < .001$) and those living in non-English-speaking households ($p < .05$) have significantly lower odds of receiving no preventive care. More impoverished parents ($p < .01$) and the uninsured ($p < .001$) have higher odds of reporting no preventive care. Parents whose child is covered by public insurance are far less likely to report no preventive care. Finally, older children, those with no usual source of care or medical home, and those in better health have greater odds of not receiving preventive medical care.

The third column of Table 3 shows the multivariate results predicting that a child has a delayed or unmet medical care need. Similar to the results regarding preventive care, parents with higher dissatisfaction score have significantly higher odds of reporting that their child has an unmet medical care need. Greater dissatisfaction is associated with a 2.3 times higher odds of reporting that their child has a delayed or unmet need ($p < .001$). On the one hand, it may be that parents who feel greater dissatisfaction are more likely to delay needed medical care. On the other hand, it might be that parents who perceive that their child has medical care needs that are delayed or unmet are more dissatisfied with their child's treatment. Again, parents residing in non-English-speaking households have significantly lower odds of reporting unmet medical need, perhaps due to cultural differences in perceptions of what constitutes needs. Parents with a high school education or less ($p < .01$) also have lower odds of reporting unmet or delayed medical need. Not surprisingly, families living closer to the federal poverty limit ($p < .01$), those with uninsured children ($p < .001$), and those who report their child is in worse health ($p < .001$) have greater odds of reporting a delayed or unmet medical care need.

DISCUSSION

This study employed data from the 2007 NSCH to examine the social patterning of parent dissatisfaction with their children's medical care. Our findings support our hypotheses that members of racial/ethnic minority groups, non-English speakers, those with lower income and less education, and the uninsured are significantly more likely than their counterparts to rate their medical interactions poorly. We also examined whether parent dissatisfaction with care was associated with the lack of preventive care and delayed or unmet medical care need. Our results support our hypotheses that greater dissatisfaction is related to higher odds of reporting no preventive care and higher odds of reporting delayed or unmet medical need.

As is true of research on adult patients, we found that the parents of racial/ethnic minorities were more likely than white respondents to report dissatisfaction. Black, multiracial/other, and Hispanic respondents consistently reported lower satisfaction with their child's medical treatment. Racial variations in perceptions of care may be affected by an individual's past experiences with discrimination, both in and outside of the health care system (Street, Gordon, & Haidet, 2007). Studies show that patients who have had previous experiences with discrimination are more likely to report differential treatment by health care providers (Malat & Hamilton, 2006). Variation in the way that physicians communicate with minority patients also likely contribute to our findings of greater dissatisfaction among the parents of racial and ethnic minority children.

While SES and insurance coverage mediated a considerable portion of the race effect for black respondents, this was not necessarily the case for other minority groups, particularly for parents of multiracial children. As the trend toward interracial unions continues to rise (Fryer, 2007), medical sociologists should note that the experience of multiracial patients may differ in distinct and substantial ways from other racial minorities. This may be particularly true when the parent and child are not racially concordant. These parents may experience the physician–patient interaction in a qualitatively different way.

Parents who speak a language other than English at home also were consistently more likely to be dissatisfied. In part, this finding reflects the communication challenges and lack of cultural health capital faced by non-native speakers in medical care interactions. If linguistic barriers prevent parents from successfully navigating the physician–patient interaction, this may further exacerbate existing inequalities in both care and overall well-being of their children.

Several studies have found that among adult patients, individuals with lower SES are less likely than others to be satisfied with their medical care (Campbell, Ramsay, & Green, 2001; Haviland et al., 2005). Our analyses revealed a similar pattern for parent satisfaction. Respondents living in poverty and those with only a high school education or less were far more likely to be dissatisfied with their child's care. Poor families have limited resources and often face constrained choices about medical care. The lack of autonomy regarding a choice of providers may produce feelings of frustration with the health care system. If parents with lower SES feel that their child is receiving unsatisfactory treatment, they are less able to seek alternative providers and may instead choose to discontinue treatment.

Although having health insurance coverage is closely tied to SES and race, being uninsured exerts an independent effect on parents' perceptions of their children's medical treatment. When children are uninsured, they are less likely to have a regular physician and more likely to seek medical care only in extreme circumstances from emergency rooms, public health clinics, and walk-in clinics. Thus, it is not surprising that respondents whose child is uninsured are far less likely than parents of insured children to report satisfaction. Contrary to our expectations, however, we did not find greater dissatisfaction among parents of publicly insured children. Given the wide variation in the requirements and type coverage provided by SCHIP and Medicaid across states, it is difficult to determine how public coverage affects the patient–doctor interaction.

While negative assessments of the medical care interaction have been shown to exert an independent effect on compliance with treatment and health outcomes in adults, few studies have considered whether children whose parents are dissatisfied also are less likely to receive preventive services or have unmet medical needs. Our results indicate that greater parent dissatisfaction is associated with a greater likelihood of children not receiving important medical treatment. Due to data limitations, however, we were unable to test the direction of this association. In future research, it would be helpful to examine these questions longitudinally to determine whether parents who feel displeased with their child's care are more likely to forgo future routine medical check-ups.

Our findings help explain the social and structural factors that influence parental attitudes toward their children's medical care. One caveat is that the dependent variable in this analysis asks the parent to think only about the child's most recent healthcare visit and does not address general beliefs and attitudes about medical care. It may be that some parents are not generally displeased with the quality of their child's care but recently have had a bad experience. Yet the consistency of the findings across groups suggests that this is not the case.

CONCLUSION

Despite efforts to improve health providers cultural competence (Betancourt, Green, Carrillo, & Anach-Firempon, 2003) and encourage patient-centered communication (Audet, 2006), disparities based on SES and race/ethnicity persist. These disparities may be the result of "aversive racism" and inadvertent discrimination in the way providers interact with patients who bring less cultural health capital to the clinical setting. As with adult patients, physicians may see parents of minority and low-income children as less likely to comply with treatment and information and thus communicate less effectively with them. A less participatory communication style may translate into lower satisfaction with medical care. When parents have lower satisfaction with medical care, they may communicate feelings of distrust to their children. Thus, a vicious cycle is created that can contribute to lifelong inequalities in health.

Patient satisfaction is not solely a product of micro-level interactions, however, but also is influenced by broader trends in the health care system. With the dramatic rise in the cost of medical care over the past few decades, the United States has entered what medical sociologists term the "era of managerial control and market mechanisms" (Wright & Perry, 2010). This shift has prompted significant changes in the role of both patient and physician (Boyer & Lutfey, 2010). Patients no longer are passive recipients of treatment but instead have become active consumers of health services who are empowered to make choices. Yet the shift toward the "patient as consumer paradigm" has highlighted the importance of education, financial resources, and the ability to pay for services, at times overshadowing the concern with quality care. When health becomes a commodity that can be bought and sold, social inequalities are amplified, and individuals with fewer resources and from socially marginalized groups have less autonomy and choice regarding their health care.

Physicians and care providers also are torn between competing interests (Timmermans & Oh, 2010). In addition to responding to the needs of patients and their own desire to provide quality care, physicians have a financially vested interest in complying with organizational and managerial requirements. Constraints imposed by insurance company regulations can limit physicians' ability to act in the patient's best interest and make it challenging to provide equitable care. As Shim (2010, p. 6) notes, such constraints "are likely to curb providers' ability to work with patients to maximize the cultural health capital available in the clinical encounter." Instead patients may be viewed as commodities and treatments as liabilities. Although patient-advocacy organizations coupled with a growing emphasis on patient-centered communication have ameliorated the strain for some, market and structural forces remain impediments for those with the fewest resources to bring to the doctor–patient interaction. On a more positive note, the passage of the Patient Protection and Affordable Care Act of 2010 expands Medicaid, includes a mandate that individuals purchase health insurance, and provides subsidies to help low-income people afford coverage. The new law should significantly improve access to health care and reduce the number of uninsured children (Quadagno, 2011).

ACKNOWLEDGMENT

We thank Terrence Hill and Don Lloyd for helpful comments on a previous draft of this manuscript.

REFERENCES

Armstrong, K., Ravenell, K. L., McMurphy, S., & Putt, M. (2007). Racial/ethnic differences in physician distrust in the United States. *American Journal of Public Health, 97*(7), 1283–1289.

Audet, A. D. K. (2006). Adoption of patient-centered care practices by physicians: Results from a national survey. *Archives of Internal Medicine, 166*(7), 754–759.

Becker, G., & Newsom, E. (2003). Socioeconomic status and dissatisfaction with health care among chronically ill African Americans. *American Journal of Public Health, 93*(5), 742–748.

Berdahl, T., Owens, P. L., Dougherty, D., McCormick, M. C., Pylypchuk, Y., & Simpson, L. A. (2010). Annual report on health care for children and youth in the United States: Racial/ ethnic and socioeconomic disparities in children's health care quality. *Academic Pediatrics, 10*(2), 95–118.

Betancourt, J. R., Green, A. R., Carrillo, J. E., & Ananeh-Firempong, O. (2003). Defining cultural competence: A practical framework for addressing racial/ethnic disparities in health and health care. *Public Health Reports, 118*(4), 293–302.

Bethell, C. D., Kogan, M. D., Strickland, B. B., Schor, E. L., Robertson, J., & Newacheck, P. W. (2011). A national and state profile of leading health problems and health care quality for US children: Key insurance disparities and across-state variations. *Academic Pediatrics, 11*(3, Supplement), S22–S33.

Blumberg, S. J., Foster, E. B., & Frasier, A. M. et al. (2009, May). *Design and operation of the National Survey of Children's Health, 2007.* Vital Health Stat, Series 1: Program and Collection Procedures.National Center for Health Statistics.. Retrieved from http:// ftp.cdc.gov/pub/health_Statistics/NCHS/slaits/nsch07/2_Methodology_Report/NSCH_ Design_and_Operations_052109.pdf

Boyer, C. A., & Lutfey, K. E. (2010). Examining critical health policy issues within and beyond the clinical encounter. *Journal of Health and Social Behavior, 51*(Suppl. 1), S80–S93.

Burgess-Champoux, T. L., Larson, N., Neumark-Sztainer, D., Hannan, P. J., & Story, M. (2008). Are family meal patterns associated with overall diet quality during the transition from early to middle adolescence? *Journal of Nutrition Education and Behavior, 41*(2), 79–86.

Byczkowski, T. L., Kollar, L. M., & Britto, M. T. (2010). Family experiences with outpatient care: Do adolescents and parents have the same perceptions? *Journal of Adolescent Health, 47*(1), 92–98.

Campbell, J. L., Ramsay, J., & Green, J. (2001). Age, gender, socioeconomic, and ethnic differences in patients' assessments of primary health care. *Quality in Health Care, 10*(2), 90–95.

Chung, P. J., Lee, T. C., Morrison, J. L., & Schuster, M. A. (2006). Preventive care for children in the United States: Quality and barriers. *Annual Review of Public Health, 27*, 491–515.

Cooper-Patrick, L., et al. (1999). Race, gender, and partnership in the patient-physician relationship. *JAMA: The Journal of the American Medical Association, 282*(6), 583–589.

Cox, E. D., Nackers, K. A., Young, H. N., Moreno, M. A., Levy, J. F., & Mangione-Smith, R. M. (2012). Influence of race and socioeconomic status on engagement in pediatric primary care. *Patient Education and Counseling, 87*(3), 319–326.

DiMatteo, M. R. (2004). The role of effective communication with children and their families in fostering adherence to pediatric regimens. *Patient Education and Counseling, 55*(3), 339–344.

Dovidio, J. F., Penner, L. A., Albrecht, T. L., Norton, W. E., Gaetner, S. L., & Nicole Shelton, J. (2008). Disparities and distrust: The implications of psychological processes for understanding racial disparities in health and health care. *Social Science and Medicine, 67*, 478–486.

Ennett, S. T., et al. (2010). A social contextual analysis of youth cigarette smoking development. *Nicotine & Tobacco Research, 12*(9), 950–962.

Flores, G. (2006). Language barriers to health care in the United States. *New England Journal of Medicine, 355*, 229–231.

Flores, G., & Tomany-Korman, S. C. (2008a). Racial and ethnic disparities in medical and dental health, access to care, and use of services in U.S. children. *Pediatrics, 121*(2), e286–e298.

Franks, P., Jerant, A. F., Fiscella, K., Shields, C. C., Tancredi, D. J., & Epstein, R. M. (2006). Studying physician effects on patient outcomes: Physicians interactional style and performance on quality of care indicators. *Social Science and Medicine, 62*, 422–432.

Fryer, R. G., Jr. (2007). Guess who's been coming to dinner? Trends in interracial marriage over the 20th century. *The Journal of Economic Perspectives, 21*(2), 71–90.

Gonzalez, H. M., Vega, W. A., & Tarraf, W. (2010). Health care quality perceptions among foreign-born latinos and the importance of speaking the same language. *Journal of American Board of Family Medicine, 23*(6), 745–752.

Graham, H. (2002). Building an inter-disciplinary science of health inequalities: The example of lifecourse research. *Social Science & Medicine, 55*(11), 2005–2016.

Hadley, J. (2003). Sicker and poorer – The consequences of being uninsured: A review of the research on the relationship between health insurance, medical care use, health, work, and income. *Medical Care Research and Review, 60*(2 suppl), 3S–75S.

Hall, M., Camacho, F., Dugan, E., & Balkrishnan, R. (2002). Trust in the medical profession: Conceptual and measurement issues. *Health Services Research, 37*(5), 1419–1439.

Haviland, M. G., Morales, L. S., Dial, T. H., & Pincus, H. A. (2005). Race/ethnicity, socioeconomic status, and satisfaction with health care. *American Journal of Medical Quality, 20*(4), 195–203.

Kaiser Family Foundation. (n.d.). Health policy research, analysis, polling, facts, data and journalism. Retrieved from http://kff.org/. Accessed on July 15, 2013.

Kao, A., Green, D., Zallavsky, A., Koplan, J., & Cleary, P. (1998). The relationship between method of physician payment and patient trust. *JAMA, 290*(19), 1708–1714.

Komaromy, M., Lurie, N., & Bindman, A. (1995). California physicians' willingness to care for the poor. *Western Journal of Medicine, 162*(2), 127–132.

Latendresse, S. J., et al. (2008). Parenting mechanisms in links between parents' and adolescents' alcohol use behaviors. *Alcoholism: Clinical and Experimental Research, 32*(2), 322–330.

Lau, R. R., Quadrel, M. J., & Hartman, K. A. (1990). Development and change of young adults' preventive health beliefs and behavior: Influence from parents and peers. *Journal of Health and Social Behavior, 31*(3), 240–259.

Lee, Y.-Y., & Lin, J. L. (2009). The effect of trust in a physician on self-efficacy, adherence and diabetes outcomes. *Social Science and Medicine, 68*, 1060–1068.

Lillie-Blanton, M., Brodie, M., Rowland, D., Altman, D., & McIntosh, M. (2000). Race, ethnicity, and the health care system: Public perceptions and experiences. *Medical Care Research and Review, 57*(4 Suppl.), 218–235.

Lutfey, K., & Freese, J. (2005). Toward some fundamentals of fundamental causality: Socioeconomic status and health in the routine clinic visit for diabetes. *American Journal of Sociology, 110*, 1136–1172.

Malat, J., & Hamilton, M. A. (2006). Preference for same-race health care providers and perceptions of interpersonal discrimination in health care. *Journal of Health and Social Behavior, 47*, 173–187.

O'Brien, M., & Shea, J. (2011). Disparities in patient satisfaction among Hispanics: The role of language preference. *Journal of Immigrant and Minority Health, 13*(2), 408–412.

Quadagno, J. (2011). Interest group influence on the patient protection and affordability act of 2010: Winners and losers in the health care reform debate. *Journal of Health Politics, Policy and Law, 36*(3), 449–454.

Regenstein, M., Mead, H., Muessig, K., & Huang, J. (2009). Challenges in language services: Identifying and responding to patients' needs. *Journal of Immigrant and Minority Health, 11*, 476–481.

Rimal, R. N. (2003). Intergenerational transmission of health: The role of intrapersonal, interpersonal, and communicative factors. *Health Education & Behavior, 30*(1), 10–28.

Roche, K. M., Ahmed, S., & Blum, R. W. (2008). Enduring consequences of parenting for risk behaviors from adolescence into early adulthood. *Social Science & Medicine, 66*(9), 2023–2034.

Schnittker, J., Pescosolido, B., & Croghan, T. (2005). Are African Americans really less willing to use health care? *Social Problems, 52*, 255–271.

Shim, J. (2010). Cultural health capital: A theoretical approach to understanding health care interactions and the dynamics of unequal treatment. *Journal of Health and Social Behavior, 51*(1), 1–12.

Singh-Manoux, A., & Marmot, M. (2005). Role of socialization in explaining social inequalities in health. *Social Science & Medicine, 60*(9), 2129–2133.

Stepanikova, I., Mollborn, S., Cook, K. S., Thom, D. H., & Kramer, R. M. (2006). Patients' race, ethnicity, language and trust in a physician. *Journal of Health and Social Behavior, 47*, 390–405.

Stevens, G. D., & Shi, L. (2003). Racial and ethnic disparities in the primary care experiences of children: A review of the literature. *Medical Care Research and Review, 60*(1), 3–30.

Street, R., Makoul, G., Arora, N., & Epstein, R. (2009). How does communication heal? Pathways linking clinician-patient communication to health outcomes. *Patient Education and Counseling, 74*(3), 295–301.

Street, R. G., Jr., Gordon, H., & Haidet, P. (2007). Physicians' communication and perceptions of patients: Is it how they look, how they talk, or is it just the doctor? *Social Science and Medicine, 65*, 586–598.

Timmermans, S., & Oh, H. (2010). The continued transformation of the medical profession. *Journal of Health and Social Behavior, 51*, S94–S106.

Trivedi, A. N, & Ayanian, J. Z (2006). Perceived discrimination and use of preventive health services. *Journal of General Internal Medicine, 21*(6), 553–558.

van Ryn, M., & Burke, J. (2008). The effect of patient race and socio-economic status on physicians' perceptions of patients. *Social Science and Medicine, 50*, 813–828.

Wadsworth, M. E. J. (1997). Health inequalities in the life course perspective. *Social Science & Medicine, 44*(6), 859–869.

Wilkins, V., Elliott, M. N., Richardson, A., Lozano, P., & Mangione-Smith, R. (2011). The association between care experiences and parent ratings of care for different racial, ethnic, and language groups in a medicaid population. *Health Services Research, 46*(3), 821–839.

Wickrama, K. A. S., Conger, R. D., Wallace, L. E., & Elder, G. H. (1999). The intergenerational transmission of health-risk behaviors: Adolescent lifestyles and gender moderating effects. *Journal of Health and Social Behavior, 40*(3), 258–272.

Wright, E. R., & Perry, B. L. (2010). Medical sociology and health services research: Past accomplishments and future policy challenges. *Journal of Health and Social Behavior, 51*(S), S107–S119.

AN APPLICATION OF THE ANDERSEN MODEL OF HEALTH UTILIZATION TO THE UNDERSTANDING OF THE ROLE OF RACE-CONCORDANT DOCTOR–PATIENT RELATIONSHIPS IN REDUCING HEALTH DISPARITIES

Galen H. Smith, III and Teresa L. Scheid

ABSTRACT

Purpose – *The race concordance hypothesis suggests that matching patients and health providers on the basis of race improves communication and patients' perceptions of health care, and by extension, encourages patients to seek and utilize health care, which may reduce health disparities. However, relatively few studies have examined the impact of race concordance on the utilization of health services. This chapter is*

Social Determinants, Health Disparities and Linkages to Health and Health Care
Research in the Sociology of Health Care, Volume 31, 187–214
Copyright © 2013 by Emerald Group Publishing Limited
All rights of reproduction in any form reserved
ISSN: 0275-4959/doi:10.1108/S0275-4959(2013)0000031011

grounded on Andersen's Emerging Model of Health Services Utilization (Phase 4) and extends that model to include race concordance.

Methodology/approach – *The data were collected from a stratified random sample of adult beneficiaries enrolled in North Carolina Medicaid's primary care case management delivery system in 2006– 2007. Propensity score matching techniques were used to sort respondents on their propensity for race concordance and indices were constructed to generate key control variables. Poisson regression was used to examine the impact of race concordance on the utilization of primary care and emergency room care, under the assumption that race concordance would increase the use of primary care and decrease the use of emergency care for minority patients.*

Findings – *While blacks (compared to whites) used less primary care and had more emergency care visits, race concordance was not a statistically significant predictor of either primary care or emergency room use. However, patients' satisfaction with their primary care providers was associated with significantly fewer primary care and emergency care visits while trust in one's provider was associated with more primary care visits.*

Research implications – *The study findings suggest that the central premises of the race concordance hypothesis require further study to confirm the assumption that better patient – primary care provider relationships result in less utilization of more costly and resource-intensive forms of health care.*

Value of chapter – *The study makes a valuable contribution by expanding the relatively small body of literature dedicated to exploring the impact of race concordance on health services utilization. Additionally, by virtue of researching the experience of Medicaid enrollees, the study controls for health insurance status.*

Keywords: Race concordance; utilization; satisfaction; trust; Medicaid

INTRODUCTION

The Institute of Medicine's report *Unequal Treatment: Confronting Racial and Ethnic Disparities in Health Care* (2003) suggests that racial and ethnic disparities in the U.S. health care system may be at least partially attributable to aspects of the patient–physician relationship. Cooper and Powe (2004) assert that "race-discordant" relationships, which are defined as patients seeking care from health providers with different racial or ethnic backgrounds compared to their own and which may result from the under-representation of minorities in the various health professions, adversely influence health care quality in terms of less involvement in decision-making (Kaplan, Gandek, Greenfield, Rogers, & Ware, 1995), less partnership with physicians (Cooper-Patrick et al., 1999), lower levels of trust in physicians (Boulware, Cooper, Ratner, LaVeist, & Powe, 2003; Doescher, Saver, Franks, & Fiscella, 2000), and lower levels of satisfaction with care (Saha, Komaromy, Koepsell, & Bindman, 1999). Conversely, Cooper and Powe (2004) examined the link between patient–physician race concordance (i.e., the patient's race is aligned with physician's race) and patient satisfaction and health outcomes and argue that racial and ethnic concordance is associated with higher levels of patient satisfaction and better health care processes.

The governmental entity tasked with evaluating the rationale for diversity in the medical professions provides a clear explanation of the *concordance hypothesis* – a specific aspect of the patient–practitioner relationship that is relevant to reducing race-based disparities (U.S. Department of Health and Human Services, 2006). Concordance theory suggests that minority patients who see a practitioner from their own racial or ethnic group or who speak their primary language will experience better health outcomes, including increased use of appropriate health care. In this context, Cooper and Powe (2004) and LaVeist, Nuru-Jeter, and Jones (2003) suggest increasing the number of minority health care providers as a means of creating more patient–physician race-concordant relationships toward the end of reducing disparities in health care. Others (Atkinson, 1983; Sue, 1988) argue that moral, ethical, and political principles should drive any increases in the number of female, ethnic, or racial minority providers. However, very few studies to date have directly examined the impact of race concordance on the utilization of health services, a key component in the link between race concordance and the narrowing of health disparities (Cooper & Powe, 2004). Demonstrating that racial concordance actually increases the utilization of appropriate health services (i.e., primary and preventative care as opposed to emergency room care) supports the notion that achieving more race-concordant relationships may eventually reduce health disparities. Fig. 1 summarizes the race concordance hypothesis and its relationship to health disparities.

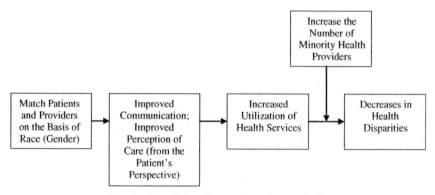

Fig. 1. The Race Concordance Hypothesis.

In this chapter we provide a modification of the Andersen's Emerging Model (Phase 4) to not only include race concordance as a component of what Andersen (1995) referred to as predisposing characteristics, but to also focus on the role of aspects of consumer satisfaction as important outcomes to race-concordant relationships which themselves have an independent effect on the utilization of health services.

BACKGROUND AND SIGNIFICANCE

A substantial body of literature linking racial concordance with patient satisfaction has been established. Saha et al. (1999) used data obtained in the Commonwealth Fund 1994 National Comparative Survey of Minority Health Care to analyze the responses of the 2,201 respondents who indicated that they had a regular physician and discovered that black respondents with black physicians were more likely to rate their physician as excellent, more likely to report receiving preventive care, and more likely to report receiving all needed care compared to black respondents with nonblack physicians. The same study revealed that Hispanics who had Hispanic physicians were inclined to report that they were very satisfied with their overall health care compared to Hispanics with non-Hispanic physicians. LaVeist and Nuru-Jeter (2002) used the same data set and discovered that physician satisfaction was greater for respondents in race-concordant relationships among each racial or ethnic group compared to respondents who were not race concordant. LaVeist and Carroll (2002) used

Commonwealth Fund Minority Health Survey data and reported that physician satisfaction was higher among the 745 African-American respondents with race-concordant physicians compared to those with race-discordant physicians. Cooper-Patrick et al. (1999) researched participatory decision-making, an important component of patients' satisfaction with their physicians, and reported that patients in race-concordant relationships with their physicians rated their physicians' decision-making style as more participatory compared to patients in race-discordant relationships. Cooper et al. (2003) found that race-concordant visits were longer and had higher ratings of patient positive affect, a composite variable that summarizes engagement, interest, friendliness, and responsiveness. The authors suggest that factors such as patient and physician attitudes may mediate the relationship between race concordance and higher patient ratings of care.

There is also a considerable volume of research that reveals patients' preferences for physicians of their own race or ethnicity. LaVeist and Carroll (2002) studied 745 African-American respondents in the Commonwealth Fund Minority Health Survey and reported that having a choice in the selection of a physician was a significant predictor of race concordance. Saha, Taggart, Komaromy, and Bindman (2000) analyzed data obtained in the Commonwealth Fund 1994 National Comparative Survey of Minority Health Care and reported that black and Hispanic Americans sought care from physicians of their own race based primarily on personal preference and language proficiency compared to geographic accessibility. Gray and Stoddard (1997) analyzed 1987 National Medical Expenditure Survey data and found that after controlling for a number of socioeconomic variables, minority patients were five times more likely than nonminority patients to report that their primary physician was a member of a racial or ethnic minority. Moy and Bartman (1995) studied a representative sample of 15,081 U.S. adults using 1987 National Medical Expenditure Survey data and indicated that individuals receiving care from minority physicians were more likely to be ethnic minorities. Specifically, they found that minority patients were more than four times more likely to receive care from nonwhite physicians compared to non-Hispanic white patients and that nonwhite physicians were more likely to care for medically indigent and sicker patients. Murray-Garcia, Garcia, Schembri, and Guerra (2001) examined the impact of language on the patient–provider relationship in a cross-sectional study of billing data from 13,681 patient visits at a Northern California pediatric medical center and found that African-American, Asian, and Latino pediatric residents were more likely to serve patients of their own ethnicity, regardless of language proficiency. The authors contend that "a (medical) resident's race or ethnicity may reflect a unique set of skills that is highly valued by patients or health care systems" (p. 1232). Other researchers have drawn similar conclusions (Brotherton, Stoddard, & Tang, 2000; Cohen, Cantor, Barker, & Hughes, 1990; Keith, Bell, Swanson, & Williams, 1985; Rabinowitz, Diamond, Veloski, & Gayle, 2000; Xu et al., 1997).

Despite the relatively abundant literature examining the relationship of race concordance with communication, satisfaction, trust, and empowered decision-making, there has been less research that has linked race concordance with health utilization (Cooper & Powe, 2004). A notable exception is LaVeist et al. (2003), who examined the utilization of health services in the context of race concordance and reported that white, black, Asian, and Hispanic patients in racially concordant relationships with their physicians were more likely to use needed health services and less likely to postpone seeking health care. King, Wong, Shapiro, Landon, and Cunningham (2004) analyzed data from a prospective, cohort study of a national probability sample of 1,241 adults receiving HIV care with linked data from 287 providers and found that African-American patients with white providers received protease inhibitors significantly later (in relation to the U.S. Food and Drug Administration (FDA) approval date of the first protease inhibitor) than the African-American patients with African-American providers. Additionally, Traylor, Schmittdiel, Uratsu, Mangione, and Subramanian (2010) examined the relationship between patient race/ethnicity and patient language and patient–physician race/ethnicity and language concordance on adherence of cardiovascular disease medications in patients with diabetes and concluded that race and language concordance may improve medication adherence for African-Americans and Spanish-speaking patients. A recent chapter by the first author (Smith, 2013) examines the impact of race concordance on prescription drug use in white and black subpopulations of North Carolina Medicaid enrollees and reveals no statistical differences in the probability for using prescription drugs among concordant and discordant whites. However, race-concordant blacks had a lower probability for using prescription drugs compared to race-discordant blacks.

In summary, there is considerable research linking race concordance to patient preferences, physician preferences, and satisfaction with care but relatively little that specifically examines the impact of racial concordance on the utilization of health services. This study seeks to fill that void and expand the knowledge base in this area by examining the effect of race concordance on the utilization of primary care and emergency room visits.

The study utilizes data collected from North Carolina Medicaid beneficiaries enrolled in a primary care case management delivery system.

THEORETICAL FRAMEWORK AND RESEARCH OBJECTIVES

The Andersen's Emerging Model (Phase 4) (1995) identifies numerous
components (the impact of the health care system, specific measures of
health services use, consumer satisfaction, health status outcomes, and the
impact of the external environment on health services' use), which have an
impact on health utilization and outcomes and are compatible with the data
used in this research. LaVeist et al. (2003) applied the Andersen model in
their analysis of the association between doctor–patient race concordance
and the utilization of health services. They broadly categorized the
independent variables in their study as predisposing variables, enabling
factors, and need variables. The dependent variable, health care utilization,
was measured in three different ways: failure to use needed care, delay in
seeking needed care, and entry into care. The authors included doctor–
patient race concordance as a predisposing independent variable and
"hypothesize[d] that patients who are race-concordant with their doctor
have a greater predisposition to utilize health services after controlling for
need, enabling, and other predisposing factors" (p. 314). We build upon the
work done by LaVeist et al. (2003). In addition to addressing the primary
question about the impact of race concordance on the utilization of primary
care and emergency care, this research also modifies the Andersen model to
examine those factors that can explain differences between blacks and
whites in health care utilization.

Fig. 2 presents the modified conceptual model that guides this research,
and includes the major variables examined in the data analysis. In this
chapter, health utilization serves as the dependent variable with two different forms of health care utilization – primary care and emergency care –
under the assumption that race concordance between patients and their
primary care providers would increase the use of primary care and decrease
the use of emergency care. Andersen identifies consumer satisfaction as an
important outcome that affects health care utilization and influences the
predisposing characteristics and enabling resources. We include *evaluated*
need, which is determined by enrollment in a disease management program.
Self-reported health status is also included, but we consider it as an indicator

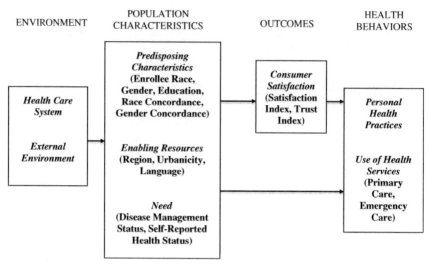

Fig. 2. Adaptation of the Andersen Model. (Adapted from Andersen, 1995.)

of the *perceived* need for health care, and include it under *population characteristics*. We control for the environment in that the study includes only patients enrolled in Medicaid managed care networks, and hence all also have access to the same health care benefits. Race and gender concordance are included as predisposing characteristics, consistent with LaVeist's previous use of the Andersen model to study race concordance. We focus on race concordance, but include gender concordance as an important control. We also include race, gender, and age as predisposing characteristics and enrollee urbanicity, region of residence, and language as enabling characteristics.

The data were collected at a single point in time and contain an obvious selection bias in that there is no way to control for respondent's self-selection into race-concordant or race-discordant relationships with their providers. We used propensity scoring to transform the study design into a posttest only comparison group design. Propensity scoring ensures concordant and discordant groups are matched in terms of critical background variables, which would influence respondents' self-selection into concordant or discordant groups. While the number of included respondents may be slightly reduced, depending on the specific type of propensity score matching employed, we feel this methodological technique adds to the significance of our findings.

In this chapter, we address the following research questions:

1. Do race-concordant doctor–patient relationships lead to increased use of primary care and reduce the use of emergency room services?
2. What impact do other variables in the Andersen model have on health utilization, and consequently, how can we reframe the Andersen model to better account for those variables that have the greatest impact on reducing health disparities?

RESEARCH DESIGN AND METHODS

Data and Methods

The data used in this study were collected from October 2006 through March 2007 from adult beneficiaries enrolled in North Carolina's Medicaid program who had landline telephones and had been continuously enrolled for six months in the network programs of the state's Medicaid Community Care of North Carolina (CCNC) primary care case management program. The research protocol was approved by the University of North Carolina at Charlotte's Institutional Review Board and conformed to the standards associated with research involving human subjects. The data collection instrument was derived from the Consumer Assessment of Health Plans and Systems (CAHPS) 3.0 Health Plan Survey, which was designed to evaluate beneficiary satisfaction, access, utilization, and health status and administered by the UNC Charlotte Urban Institute using computer assisted telephone interview (CATI) methods. Certain categories of Medicaid enrollee eligibility, including dual eligibles and institutionalized long-term care recipients, were specifically excluded from the study. The sampling frame consisted of 100,014 adults and was subsequently stratified into 14 groups based upon an enrollee's care network. The rationale for using the care network as the stratification variable was to facilitate cross-network comparisons in contexts where these comparisons would be particularly useful or valuable. A random sample of approximately 2,200 beneficiaries was subsequently drawn from each of the 14 care networks ($n = 29,122$) in order to compile a list of potential survey respondents. A total of 2,815 surveys were completed representing approximately 200 from each of the 14 networks. This number was chosen to satisfy statistical power requirements and to detect small effect sizes when comparing (health plans) networks (U.S. Department of Health and Human Services, 2008). The response rate to the survey was calculated at 27.1 percent using the standards and definitions determined by the American Association for Public Opinion Research (2006). Possible explanations for this observation include the well-documented difficulties locating Medicaid respondents to telephone surveys, lower than average literacy levels, high mobility, and high rates of inaccurate or unavailable telephone numbers among Medicaid recipients (Brown, Nederend, Hays, Short, & Farley, 1999).

The study data were collected at a single point in time (a cross-sectional observation research design) and, compared to classic experimental designs, contain a selection bias in that there is no way to control for respondents' self-selection into race-concordant or race-discordant relationships with their providers. Propensity score matching was invoked in order to neutralize these shortcomings and, in effect, to create a posttest only comparison group design where individuals were assigned to either a treatment group (the race-concordant group) or a comparison group (the race-discordant group) based upon their propensity scores. Briefly, propensity scoring creates two groups where individuals have been randomly assigned to either a treatment group (race concordant) or comparison group (race discordant) based upon their propensity score, which is defined as the "conditional probability of being assigned to a treatment group, given a set of pre-treatment characteristics" (Weitzen, Lapane, Toledano, Hume, & Mor, 2004, p. 841). In accordance with best practices associated with propensity score matching procedures, the outcome variables (primary care visits and emergency room visits) were set aside and an initial list of covariates with the potential to predict race concordance was evaluated in terms of balance and bias before and after matching. The list of covariates was modified in accordance with the results of the balance and bias before and after matching tests.

The data were subsequently truncated to include only those respondents who were white or black, in part because some respondents could not be accurately categorized as concordant or discordant due to ambiguities associated with reporting of either their race or the race of their providers. Thus, the data consisted of survey respondents who were white and stated that their primary care provider was either white or black and survey respondents who were black and stated that their primary care provider was either white or black. After listwise deletion of cases to account for missing values on any variable, the data set subject to analysis of primary care visits consisted of 1,912 cases and the data set subject to analysis of emergency care visits consisted of 1,964 cases.

Operationalization of Variables

The variables are organized according to the Andersen framework, beginning with the dependent variables and moving backward eventually to the predisposing characteristics and the enabling resources (see Fig. 2). The Environment section of the Andersen framework was not modeled due to limitations in the data set. However, a key feature of the Health Care System – health insurance status – is controlled to some degree by virtue of the fact that all subjects have access to health services, albeit to varying degrees, via their Medicaid enrollment.

There are two primary outcome variables – the *number of primary care visits* and the *number of emergency care visits*. In the case of both variables, the survey instrument accurately depicted instances of "zero," "one," "two," "three," or "four" visits in the preceding six months, but responses of "five" or more visits were upper- or right-censored (see Meyer, 2006 and Jöreskog, 2002 for a more comprehensive discussion of upper-censored variables). Specifically, the instrument was structured for respondents to choose "five-to-nine" visits and "ten-or-more" visits. Additionally, both variables are characterized by a relatively large number of "zero" values. As a result, specialized regression techniques are necessary to analyze this unique situation. Table 1 contains the frequency distribution for the dependent variables, and compares race-concordant and race-discordant groups.

Table 1. Frequency Distributions of Health Services Visits Among Individuals Matched on Propensity for Race Concordance.

Number of Visits	Primary Care				Emergency Room			
	Concordant		Discordant		Concordant		Discordant	
0	168	13.4%	115	17.4%	810	62.7%	395	58.8%
1	157	12.5%	96	14.6%	221	17.1%	118	17.6%
2	227	18.1%	118	17.9%	128	9.9%	69	10.3%
3	166	13.3%	85	12.9%	66	5.1%	33	4.9%
4	105	8.4%	58	8.8%	30	2.3%	31	4.6%
5–9	240	19.2%	116	17.6%	27	2.1%	18	2.7%
10 or more	189	15.1%	72	10.9%	10	0.8%	8	1.2%
	1,252		660		1,292		672	
Pearson Chi-square (6) and *p*-value	$\chi^2 = 12.2822$ $p = 0.056$				$\chi^2 = 10.2249$ $p = 0.115$			

Andersen's Emerging Model (Phase 4) describes consumer satisfaction as an outcome of health services in a bidirectional relationship with health services utilization. In this study, however, we reconceptualize consumer satisfaction as a predictor of primary care and emergency room visits. The concept of consumer satisfaction is operationalized by two variables – "satisfaction" and "trust" – that were created as indices from several items that appeared in the survey questionnaire, with high scores representing high levels of enrollee satisfaction and trust with their providers. In terms of consumer satisfaction, we have measures of both satisfaction and trust. Satisfaction was assessed by three questions, with a Cronbach's alpha score of 0.556 for emergency care visits and 0.563 for primary care visits.

• In the last six months, not counting times you needed health care right away, how often did you get an appointment for health care as soon as you wanted?
• In the last six months, when you called during regular office hours, how often did you get the help or advice you needed?
• In the last six months, how much of a problem, if any, was it to get the care, tests, or treatments you or a doctor believed necessary?

Trust was derived from the five survey questions appearing below and had a Cronbach's alpha score of 0.634 for emergency care visits and 0.684 for primary care visits.

• I think my doctor or nurse may not refer me to a specialist when needed.
• I sometimes think that my doctor or nurse might perform unnecessary tests or procedures.
• My doctor's or nurse's medical skills are not as good as they should be.
• I trust my doctor or nurse to put my medical needs above all other considerations when treating my medical problems.
• My doctor or nurse always pays full attention to what I am trying to tell him or her.

The Andersen framework also conceptualizes two types of need – *perceived* need and *evaluated* need. Perceived need considers how people experience their symptoms of illness and how they view their own health and functional state. On the other hand, evaluated need refers to a more formal situation where an individual's health status and the need for medical care are established by the professional judgment of a health care practitioner. A health status index, where high scores represent higher levels of self-reported health status, was created from five survey items to operationalize perceived need and had a Cronbach's alpha of 0.772 for emergency care visits and 0.782 for primary care visits.

- In general, how would you rate your overall health now? (This item carried the greatest proportional weight in the creation of the health status index at 0.6 compared to a proportional weight of 0.1 for each of the remaining health status index items.)
- Do you have a physical or medical condition that seriously interferes with your independence, participation in the community, or quality of life?
- Do you now have any physical or medical conditions that have lasted for at least three months? (Women: Do not include pregnancy.)
- In the last six months, have you seen a doctor or health provider more than twice for any of these conditions?
- Have you been taking prescription medicine for at least three months for any of these conditions?

Evaluated need is operationalized by the enrollee's disease management program enrollment status. This data was obtained from enrollment files provided by N.C. Medicaid administrators and is based on claims or provider recommendations as opposed to the recall ability of respondent's memory. Three formal disease management programs – asthma, diabetes, and asthma with diabetes – existed at the time that the sampling was conducted. The variable was created as a binary variable by collapsing the various program categories into a single "enrolled" category with the "no program enrollment" category representing the comparison group in the regression analyses. Table 2 contains the frequency distribution for disease management enrollment status.

The enabling resources in this study are conceptualized by three variables: enrollee language, region, and urbanicity. The language variable consists of three values: English, Spanish, and Other languages. English was the predominant language spoken in the home amongst these individuals and

Table 2. Frequency Distribution of Disease Management Enrollment Status Among Individuals Matched on Propensity for Race Concordance.

Program Enrollment Status	Primary Care Visits				Emergency Room Visits			
	Concordant		Discordant		Concordant		Discordant	
Not enrolled	1,031	82.4%	542	82.1%	1,062	82.2%	553	82.3%
Enrolled	221	17.6%	118	17.9%	230	17.8%	119	17.7%
	1,252		660		1,292		672	
Fisher's Exact Test, two-tailed (*p*-value)	0.900				1.000			

serves as the reference category in this analysis. However, the predominance of English as the primary spoken language among respondents and the lack of variation among values of the variable potentially lead to elimination of the variable in some of the regression analyses. Region is a nominal-level variable that categorizes the four different land regions that typify North Carolina – the Mountains, Piedmont, Coastal Plain, and Tidewater regions (Diemer & Bobyarchick, 2000). The Piedmont region represents the comparison category for this variable. Urbanicity classifies the enrollee's residential status as either urban, rural, or a mixed state between the two extremes and was derived from the 2003 Rural–Urban Continuum Codes employed by the Economic Research Services of the U.S. Department of Agriculture (U.S. Department of Agriculture, 2004). The urban category was selected as the comparison category for the purposes of statistical analysis. Table 3 contains the frequency distributions of the enabling characteristics.

Variables included among the predisposing characteristics are the respondent's race (white or black, with white assigned as the reference category), gender (male designated as the comparison category), education

Table 3. Profile of Enabling Resources Among Individuals Matched on Propensity for Race Concordance.

	Primary Care Visits				Emergency Room Visits			
	Concordant		Discordant		Concordant		Discordant	
Region								
Mountains	254	20.3%	23	3.5%	282	21.8%	24	3.6%
Piedmont	717	57.3%	414	62.7%	720	55.7%	421	62.7%
Coastal Plain	214	17.1%	193	29.2%	216	16.7%	197	29.3%
Tidal	67	5.4%	30	4.6%	74	5.7%	30	4.5%
	1252		660		1292		672	
Urbanicity								
Urban	756	60.4%	424	64.2%	759	58.8%	429	63.8%
Mixed	323	25.8%	148	22.4%	335	25.9%	154	22.9%
Rural	173	13.8%	88	13.3%	198	15.3%	89	13.2%
	1,252		660		1,292		672	
Language								
English	1,247	99.6%	658	99.7%	1,287	99.6%	670	99.7%
Spanish	*	<1%	*	<1%	*	<1%	*	<1%
Other	*	<1%	*	<1%	*	<1%	*	<1%
	1,252		660		1,292		672	

Note: Asterisks in the table replace actual numbers as a mechanism to attempt to protect the confidentiality and anonymity of research subjects who are categorized in cells of exceptionally small cell size.

level, age, gender concordance, and race concordance status. Six binary variables – 8th grade or less, some high school education without graduation, high school graduate or GED certificate, some college attendance without four-year degree, four-year college degree, and college attendance beyond the four-year degree – represent the different values of the education variable, with the 8th grade or less category as the comparison group. The enrollee's age is a continuous variable and was determined by calculating the number of years (expressed in thousandths of a year) that had elapsed between the enrollee's date of birth and March 31, 2006, the date that the sampling frame was established. Table 4 contains the frequency distributions for the predisposing characteristics.

Table 4. Profile of Predisposing Characteristics Among Individuals Matched on Propensity for Race Concordance.

	Primary Care Visits				Emergency Room Visits			
	Concordant		Discordant		Concordant		Discordant	
Race								
White	992	79.2%	140	21.2%	1,031	79.8%	144	21.4%
Black	260	20.8%	520	78.8%	261	20.2%	528	78.6%
	1,252		660		1, 292		672	
Gender								
Male	310	24.8%	152	23.0%	319	24.7%	152	22.6%
Female	942	75.2%	508	77.0%	973	75.3%	520	77.4%
	1,252		660		1,292		672	
Age								
18–25 yrs	241	19.3%	127	19.2%	248	19.2%	130	19.4%
25–34 yrs	275	22.0%	139	21.1%	286	22.1%	142	21.1%
35–44 yrs	256	20.5%	139	21.1%	265	20.5%	141	21.0%
45–54 yrs	270	21.6%	137	20.8%	274	21.2%	137	20.4%
55+ yrs	210	16.8%	118	17.9%	219	17.0%	122	18.2%
	1,252		660		1,292		672	
Education								
8th grade or less	152	12.1%	68	10.3%	158	12.2%	68	10.1%
Some high school	342	27.3%	186	28.2%	352	27.2%	190	28.3%
High school graduate	435	34.7%	257	38.9%	450	34.8%	265	39.4%
Some college	286	22.8%	120	18.2%	292	22.6%	120	17.9%
Four-yr. degree	31	2.5%	26	3.9%	34	2.6%	26	3.9%
>Four-yr. degree	*	<1%	*	<1%	*	<1%	*	<1%
	1,252		660		1,292		672	

Note: Asterisks in the table replace actual numbers as a mechanism to attempt to protect the confidentiality and anonymity of research subjects who are categorized in cells of exceptionally small cell size.

The primary independent variable, race concordance, is treated as a predisposing characteristic in this study. This variable provides the basis for assignment to the "treatment" and "comparison" groups in the propensity score matching procedure and was derived from the enrollee race and provider race variables. Respondents were deemed to be concordant if a white enrollee reported that his/her primary care provider was also white and if a black enrollee reported that his/her primary care provider was also black. By contrast, discordance occurred if a white enrollee reported that his/her provider was black or if a black enrollee reported his/her provider as white. Thus, race concordance is a binary variable with the discordant group serving as the comparison group.

The gender concordance variable was created in a similar manner. A value of 1 was assigned to female enrollees who reported a female primary care provider and to male enrollees who reported male primary care providers. All discordant pairs (female respondents with male primary care providers and male respondents with female primary care providers) were assigned a value of 0. The gender concordance variable is a dichotomous binary variable with the discordant group serving as the comparison category.

Data Analysis

The distributions of the dependent variables – primary care visits and emergency care visits – are count variables for reasonably rare events and ideally analyzed in terms of the Poisson distribution (Szklo & Nieto, 2000). Specialized Poisson regression models were required for this analysis because of the unique character of the distribution of these variables. On one hand, the upper-censored nature of these variables would require a method that accounts for the missing values at the upper-end of the scales of each of these variables. Conversely, the distributions of each variable are characterized by a relatively large number of zero values. In consideration of the large number of zero values for each variable, a zero-inflated poisson (ZIP) regression analysis with Vuong test was initially performed. The Vuong test compares the zero-inflated Poisson model with an ordinary Poisson regression model, with the ZIP model used when the z-score was significant (UCLA: Statistical Consulting Group, 2013). In the event that the z-score associated with the Vuong test was not significant, a right-censored Poisson regression was performed with the upper limit set at 5 (visits).

The independent variables were introduced as a single block of variables. A threshold of $p < 0.05$ was established to achieve statistical significance and the complete case approach was used to handle missing values. The propensity score matching procedures, the right-censored Poisson regression techniques, and the zero-inflated Poisson regression techniques were conducted using Stata/IC 12.1 for Mac.

FINDINGS/RESULTS

Causal Analysis of Primary Care Visits

Several predictor variables had a significant impact on primary care visits (Table 5). Among the independent variables constituting the predisposing

Table 5. Primary Care Visits, Zero-Inflated Poisson Regression.

	Rate Ratio	*p*-Value
Female**	1.1123	0.003
Age	1.0015	0.242
Black**	0.9031	0.006
Some high school	1.0048	0.922
High school graduate	0.9981	0.969
Some college	1.0337	0.525
Four-year degree	1.0209	0.827
>Four-year degree	0.8521	0.463
Gender concordance	0.9715	0.321
Race concordance	0.9904	0.793
Mountains	0.9563	0.297
Coastal Plain	1.0569	0.145
Tidewater	1.1054	0.113
Mixed urbanicity	1.0449	0.199
Rural	1.0521	0.243
Spanish	1.0446	0.900
Other language	1.6398	0.067
Health Status Index***	0.8145	0.000
Disease Management Program Enrollment Status	1.0332	0.376
Satisfaction Index**	0.9670	0.002
Trust Index*	1.0115	0.010
Vuong test of zip vs. standard Poisson: $z = 5.27$; $p = 0.0000$		

Note: $n = 1,912$; $^*p < 0.05$; $^{**}p < 0.01$; $^{***}p < 0.001$. (The regression output for primary care visits is expressed in terms of the incidence rate ratio, or the IRR, which is obtained by exponentiating the Poisson regression coefficient. Values of the IRR are appropriately interpreted by assuming that all other variables in the model are held constant.)

characteristics, two variables – the enrollee's gender and race – were statistically significant for predicting primary care use. Controlled for all other covariates, females had 11.2% more primary care visits than males. On the other hand, compared to whites, primary care visits among blacks were reduced by 9.7%. The remaining predictors among the pre-disposing characteristics – age, education, race concordance, and gender concordance – failed to achieve statistical significance.

Among the enabling resources, most of the predictors were expected to increase the rate for using primary care. The lone exceptions to this trend was the rate ratio for primary care visits among residents of the Mountain region who, compared to their Piedmont counterparts, experienced a 4.4% reduction in primary care visits. However, this and none of the other enabling resource variables achieved statistical significance.

One of the independent variables representing medical need was also a significant predictor of the use of primary care. Specifically, primary care visits were reduced by 18.6% for every one-unit increase in the health status index. In other words, higher levels of self-reported health status were expected to decrease the use of primary care. On the other hand, enrollment in one of the three disease management programs was not a significant predictor of primary care use.

Both of the variables that comprised the consumer satisfaction com-ponent of the Andersen framework were significant predictors of primary care use. In terms of the satisfaction index, a one-unit increase in this measure (i.e., higher levels of patients' satisfaction with their primary care providers) reduced primary care visits by 3.3%. The second component of consumer satisfaction – the trust index – was characterized by a one-unit increase in trust resulting in a rate 1.012 times greater for using primary care.

Causal Analysis of Emergency Care Visits

In a manner comparable to the primary care visits described in the previous section, the regression output for emergency care visits is expressed in terms of the incidence rate ratio (IRR) and interpreted by assuming that all other variables in the model are held constant. The entire list of predictor variables, rate ratios, and *p*-values appears in Table 6.

A number of predictor variables had an impact on emergency room use. Among the independent variables constituting the predisposing character-istics, four variables – the enrollee's gender, age, race, and education – were statistically significant for predicting emergency room use. Females had

Table 6. Emergency Room Use, Zero-Inflated Poisson Regression Analysis.

	Rate Ratio	*p*-Value
Female*	1.16468	0.038
Age***	0.98979	0.000
Black***	1.30955	0.000
Some high school	1.06809	0.516
High school graduate	0.93491	0.514
Some college*	0.76009	0.018
Four-year degree*	0.68499	0.049
>Four-year degree	0.13841	0.059
Gender concordance	1.00273	0.964
Race concordance	0.94460	0.428
Mountains	0.90527	0.275
Coastal Plain	0.89126	0.169
Tidewater	0.97090	0.823
Mixed urbanicity	1.05256	0.482
Rural*	1.19358	0.040
Spanish	0.73621	0.625
Other language**	3.68498	0.008
Health Status Index**	0.88395	0.008
Disease Management Program Enrollment Status***	1.32028	0.000
Satisfaction Index***	0.91924	0.000
Trust Index	0.99364	0.394
Vuong test of ZIP vs. standard Poisson: $z = 9.30$; $p = 0.0000$		

Note: $n = 1,964$; $^{*}p < 0.05$; $^{**}p < 0.01$; $^{***}p < 0.001$. (The regression output for emergency care visits is expressed in terms of the incidence rate ratio, or the IRR, which is obtained by exponentiating the Poisson regression coefficient. Values of the IRR are appropriately interpreted by assuming that all other variables in the model are held constant.)

16.5% more emergency care visits than males while blacks used 31% more emergency care services than whites. On the other hand, for every one-year increase in age, emergency care visits were reduced by approximately 1%. Additionally, compared to enrollees with an 8th-grade education or less, emergency room visits for those enrollees who had attended college but did not have a four-year degree and for those with a four-year degree were reduced and these reductions were statistically significant. Gender concordance and race concordance failed to achieve statistical significance for predicting emergency room use.

Among the enabling resources, two variables – urbanicity and language – were statistically significant for predicting emergency room utilization.

Compared to residents living in urban areas, enrollees who lived in rural areas used 19.4% more emergency care services. Moreover, compared to respondents who claimed that English was the primary language spoken in their homes, the small number of respondents who spoke a language other than English or Spanish used 3.685 times more emergency care services.

The independent variables representing medical need were also significant predictors of emergency care use. In terms of the health status index, a one-unit increase in the index decreased emergency room use by 11.6%. In other words, higher levels of self-reported health status were expected to decrease emergency room visits. On the other hand, enrollment in one of the three disease management programs increased emergency room use by 32%.

In terms of the consumer satisfaction component of the Andersen framework, the satisfaction index was a statistically significant predictor of emergency care utilization. Specifically, a one-unit increase in the satisfaction index (i.e., higher levels of patients' satisfaction with their primary care providers) reduced the use of emergency care by 8.1%. The second component of consumer satisfaction – the trust index – failed to achieve statistical significance.

Table 7 provides a summary of each of the significant predictors of primary care and emergency care use, including the direction of the effect (increased rate of use vs. decreased rate of use) and the magnitude of the statistical significance as measured by the p-value.

SUMMARY AND DISCUSSION

The stated aims of this research were twofold. The primary objective was to determine if race concordance had an effect on the utilization of primary care and emergency care visits. The second objective was to determine the impact that other variables in the Andersen model had on the utilization of primary and emergency care. The Poisson regression models presented here indicate that race concordance between patients and their primary care providers decreased the rate of primary care and emergency care visits, but that this direct effect was not statistically significant.

In terms of the second major goal of the study, a number of different variables within the study's theoretical framework were determined to be significant predictors of primary care and emergency care utilization. Compared to emergency care, fewer variables were significant predictors of primary care use. However, a number of the variables were significant predictors across both types of health service utilization. With respect to

Table 7. Summary of Impact and Statistical Significance Associated with Predictors of Primary Care and Emergency Care Visits.

	Primary Care	Emergency Care
Predisposing characteristics		
Female	↑↑	↑
Age		↓↓↓
Black	↓↓	↑↑↑
Some high school		
High school graduate		
Some college		↓
Four-year degree		↓
>four-year degree		
Gender concordance		
Race concordance		
Enabling resources		
Mountains		
Coastal Plain		
Tidewater		
Mixed urbanicity		
Rural		↑
Spanish		
Other language		↑↑
Need		
Health Status Index	↓↓↓	↓↓
Disease Management Program Enrollment Status		↑↑↑
Consumer satisfaction		
Satisfaction Index	↓↓	↓↓↓
Trust Index	↑	

↑ = increased rate of utilization and $p < 0.05$.
↑↑ = increased rate of utilization and $p < 0.01$.
↑↑↑ = increased rate of utilization and $p < 0.001$.
↓ = decreased rate of utilization and $p < 0.05$.
↓↓ = decreased rate of utilization and $p < 0.01$.
↓↓↓ = decreased rate of utilization and $p < 0.001$.

primary care utilization, females used this service at rates greater than their male counterparts. This finding is consistent with literature suggesting that women have higher medical care utilization than men (Bertakis, Azari, Helms, Callahan, & Robbins, 2000; McCormick, Fleming, & Charlton,

1995) and that men may be more inclined to dismiss their health care needs (Robertson, 2003; Tudiver & Talbot, 1999; White & Witty, 2009). Additionally, higher trust scores were associated with higher rates of primary care visits. This finding is consistent with the literature related to the race concordance hypothesis discussed in previous sections of this chapter. Conversely, individuals with better self-reported health status and individuals who were more satisfied with their primary care provider had lower rates of primary care use. These findings underscore the role that medical necessity plays in seeking medical care and the suggestion that satisfying encounters with one's health provider may translate to more productive, but fewer, visits to the doctor. Moreover, the study found that blacks used primary care at lower rates compared to whites, suggesting that blacks may have reported better health status in greater numbers than whites or that trust with one's provider may be lower among black respondents compared to white respondents.

The list of significant predictors for emergency care use was slightly longer and included variables inherent to each component of the Andersen framework. Interpretation of the predictive effects of these variables should be tempered by the possibility that without medical claims data to substantiate medical necessity, enrollees may have substituted emergency care visits for routine medical conditions amenable to primary care settings.

As was the case for primary care visits, females had higher rates of emergency room use compared to males while individuals with higher self-reported health status scores and those with higher satisfaction scores with their primary care providers had lower rates for emergency room visits. The explanations for these observations that appeared in the previous discussion of primary care use are likely to also apply to emergency care use.

A number of other variables also impacted the rate of emergency care use. Among the predisposing characteristics, age, education, and race were statistically significant. An increase in the enrollee's age was associated with lower rates of emergency room use. This effect may be partly attributable to the age distribution of the sampling frame, which excluded the elderly and included individuals in age groupings that may be more susceptible to the types of traumatic events that are typically cared for in the emergency setting. Compared to individuals with an 8th-grade education or less, enrollees who had attended some college and those who had attained a four-year college degree had lower rates of emergency room use. A possible explanation for this observation is the capabilities provided by higher education to discern what constitutes a true emergency and to take the necessary preventive and remedial measures to avoid emergency care visits.

Compared to whites, blacks had higher rates of emergency care, an outcome that might be explained by delaying seeking treatment until health conditions are exacerbated and there is no other recourse than the emergency room. This speaks to a central ambiguity in considering the sources of health utilization; do satisfaction and trust (both variables that are influenced by race concordance) *precede*, or *follow*, health care utilization? Obviously, both pathways are operative – satisfying doctor–patient interactions will lead to more appropriate utilization, but one must first have a primary care encounter to lead to such utilization. Only longitudinal data can answer this question.

Among the enabling resources, individuals who lived in rural areas had higher rates of emergency care use compared to their urban counterparts. This outcome may be due to difficulties in accessing primary care given longer distances to a medical provider, or difficulties with transportation. Additionally, the primary language spoken in the home was a statistically significant predictor of emergency care utilization with individuals speaking a language other than English or Spanish associated with higher rates of emergency care compared to those individuals who claimed that English was the primary language spoken in their households. While logical and expected, this observation should be tempered by the fact that so few cases in the data set fell into the category of "Other language."

Finally, with respect to variables that conceptualize the need for medical care, the individual's disease management program enrollment status was a significant predictor of emergency care use. Specifically, individuals who were formally enrolled in one of the three disease management programs that existed at the time that the survey was conducted had higher rates of emergency room use than individuals who were not enrolled in one of these programs. This can be explained by the fact that these individuals have chronic conditions – such as asthma and diabetes – that are subject to acute flare-ups, which, if inadequately managed, can escalate to full-scale emergencies.

Limitations and Strengths

There were several limitations associated with the study that limit its usefulness. One concern is related to the external validity of the study. Specifically, the sampling frame consisted of a non-elderly, adult Medicaid population living in the South Atlantic region of the United States that was enrolled in a specific type of managed care arrangement that excluded institutionalized long-term care enrollees. These factors limit the ability to generalize the study findings to other populations. Another liability is the possible introduction of sample bias as a result of the study's disproportionate stratified sampling strategy. This technique resulted in a disproportionate percentage of enrollees in each network who constituted the sample relative to the percentage of the total population of enrollees in each network. As a result, some networks were over-represented while others were under-represented. This situation might be especially problematic when conducting analysis on an aggregated statewide basis. However, the problem was neutralized to some degree by the propensity score matching techniques that were used to thwart the selection bias associated with self-selection into race-concordant and race-discordant groups.

The relatively low response rate of 27.1% may pose problems with respect to generalizing the study findings. Possible explanations for this observation were previously summarized in the Data and Methods section of this chapter. The developers of the CAHPS survey have recognized and acknowledged these difficulties and have suggested a desired range of 40–60% for response rates of surveys associated with Medicaid populations (U.S. Department of Health and Human Services, Centers for Medicare and Medicaid Services, 2002). Additionally, the American Association for Public Opinion Research (AAPOR) formula used to calculate the response rate is relatively conservative, with a number of dispositions included as terms in the denominator, which will drive response rates downward.

Data related to the primary language used by patients to communicate with their providers were not collected by the survey. As a result, the study was unable to control for language concordance, which plays a vital role in establishing effective communication between provider and patient. The language concordance variable would be especially useful to separate the effect of language from the effect of race or ethnicity. This point is emphasized by the work of Perez-Stable, Napoles-Springer, and Miramontes (1997), who reported that patient–provider language concordance might be more important than ethnic concordance with respect to patient reports of better well being and functioning. Subsequent studies of the impact of race concordance on the various forms of health services utilization might be improved by including additional survey items that operationalize language concordance.

The low interitem reliability scores for the satisfaction and trust indices may limit their value as predictors of health services utilization (Cronbach's alpha scores of 0.556 and 0.563 for satisfaction and 0.634 and 0.684 for trust). The low scores for these indices, particularly in the case of the

Satisfaction index, were attributable to the reluctance to use potential indicators from the survey that include a large number of missing values associated with the skip pattern(s) inherent to the survey instrument.

Despite these limitations, the study makes a valuable contribution in a number of ways. Perhaps most significantly is the knowledge added to the relatively small amount of literature dedicated to the study of the impact of race concordance on the utilization of health care services. The study attempted to comply with high standards of scientific rigor by employing credible quantitative methods – zero inflated Poisson regression and propensity score matching – to analyze the basic research questions. Moreover, the study provides a foundation upon which additional research can be conducted to expand our understanding of this phenomenon.

Additionally, by virtue of surveying a population of Medicaid enrollees, the study has the relatively unique ability to control for a very important variable that impacts health service utilization – an individual's health insurance status. This feature alone will not guarantee access to health care. Nonetheless, the benefit is extended to all enrollees thereby conveying some degree of analytical control for health insurance status.

CONCLUSION

Although race concordance failed to achieve statistical significance as a predictor of primary care or emergency care use, it is interesting to note the impact of the satisfaction and trust indices on these forms of health services utilization, given that there is considerable literature support for the role that each may play in the race concordance hypothesis. In theoretical terms, the findings of this study may point to satisfaction and trust as endogenous variables affected by race concordance in the context of a larger, more complex path model. Therefore, race concordance may have an indirect effect on the use of these health services by virtue of the direct effects of satisfaction and trust on the use of primary care and emergency care utilization, respectively. Clearly, both longitudinal data and in-depth qualitative data that enhance our understanding of the concepts of trust, satisfaction, and empowered decision-making can help clarify the role that race concordance plays in the utilization of health care services. In terms of the overall assessment of the Andersen model, the majority of the components identified by the model (predisposing characteristics, enabling resources, and need) as well as components of consumer satisfaction were shown to play an important role in predicting both primary care and emergency room visits. While the Andersen model is certainly a valid framework, it is important to recognize that satisfaction and trust both precede and follow patterns of health care utilization. Thus, the study's analytical framework and resultant findings are especially relevant in the larger sphere of reducing or eliminating race-based health disparities.

ACKNOWLEDGMENTS

This research received no specific grant from any funding agency in the public, commercial, or not-for-profit sectors. The authors wish to acknowledge the contributions of the following colleagues at the University of North Carolina at Charlotte for their contributions toward improving the quality of this manuscript: William P. Brandon, Metrolina Medical Foundation Distinguished Professor of Public Policy on Health, Department of Political Science and Public Administration; Jennifer L. Troyer, Department Chair and Professor of Economics in the Belk College of Business; and Joseph M. Whitmeyer, Professor of Sociology.

REFERENCES

American Association for Public Opinion Research. (2006). *Standard definitions: Final disposition of case codes and outcome rates for surveys* (4th ed.). Lenexa, KS: American Association for Public Opinion Research.

Andersen, R. (1995). Revisiting the behavioral model and access to medical care: Does it matter? *Journal of Health and Social Behavior, 36*(1), 1–10.

Atkinson, D. (1983). Ethnic similarity in counseling psychology: A review of research. *The Counseling Psychologist, 11*(3), 79–92.

Bertakis, K., Azari, R., Helms, L., Callahan, E., & Robbins, J. (2000). Gender differences in the utilization of health care services. *Journal of Family Practice, 49*(2), 147–152.

Boulware, L., Cooper, L., Ratner, L., LaVeist, T., & Powe, N. (2003). Race and trust in the health care system. *Public Health Reports, 118*(4), 358–365.

Brotherton, S., Stoddard, J., & Tang, S. (2000). Minority and nonminority pediatricians' care of minority and poor children. *Archives of Pediatrics and Adolescent Medicine, 154*(9), 912–917.

Brown, J., Nederend, R., Hays, R., Short, P., & Farley, D. (1999). Special issues in assessing care of medicaid recipients. *Medical Care, 37*(3, Supplement), MS79–MS88.

Cohen, A., Cantor, J., Barker, D., & Hughes, R. (1990). Young physicians and the future of the medical profession. *Health Affairs, 9*(4), 138–148.

Cooper, L., & Powe, N. (2004). *Disparities in patient experiences, health care processes, and outcomes: The role of patient-provider racial, ethnic, and language concordance.* New York, NY: The Commonwealth Fund. Retrieved from http://www.commonwealthfund. org/programs/minority/cooper_raceconcordance_753.pdf. Accessed on March 6, 2013.

Cooper, L., Roter, D., Johnson, R., Ford, D., Stienwachs, D., & Powe, N. (2003). Patient-centered communication, ratings of care, and concordance of patient and physician race. *Annals of Internal Medicine, 139*(11), 907–916.

Cooper-Patrick, L., Gallo, J., Gonzales, J., Vu, H., Powe, N., Nelson, C., & Ford, D. (1999). Race, gender, and partnership in the patient–physician relationship. *Journal of the American Medical Association, 282*(6), 583–589.

Diemer, J., & Bobyarchick, A. (2000). In D. M. Orr & A. W. Stuart (Eds.), *The North Carolina atlas: Portrait for a new century.* Chapel Hill, NC: The University of North Carolina Press.

Doescher, M., Saver, B., Franks, P., & Fiscella, K. (2000). Racial and ethnic disparities in perceptions of physician style and trust. *Archives of Family Medicine, 9*(10), 1156–1163.

Gray, B., & Stoddard, J. (1997). Physician–patient pairing: Does racial and ethnic congruity influence selection of a regular physician? *Journal of Community Health, 22*(4), 247–259.

Institute of Medicine. (2003). *Unequal treatment: Confronting racial and ethnic disparities in health care.* Washington, D.C.: National Academy Press.

Jöreskog, K. (2002). *Censored variables and censored regression.* Retrieved from http://www.ssicentral.com/lisrel/techdocs/censor.pdf Accessed on April 14, 2010.

Kaplan, S., Gandek, B., Greenfield, S., Rogers, W., & Ware, J. (1995). Patient and visit characteristics related to physicians' participatory decision-making style: Results from the medical outcomes study. *Medical Care, 33*(12), 1176–1187.

Keith, S., Bell, R., Swanson, A., & Williams, A. (1985). Effects of affirmative action in medical schools: A study of the class of 1975. *New England Journal of Medicine, 313*(24), 1519–1525.

King, W., Wong, M., Shapiro, M., Landon, B., & Cunningham, W. (2004). Does racial concordance between HIV-positive patients and their physicians affect the time to receipt of protease inhibitors? *Journal of General Internal Medicine, 19*(11), 1146–1153.

LaVeist, T., & Carroll, T. (2002). Race of physician and satisfaction with care among African-American patients. *Journal of the National Medical Association, 94*(11), 937–943.

LaVeist, T., & Nuru-Jeter, A. (2002). Is doctor–patient race concordance associated with greater satisfaction with care? *Journal of Health and Social Behavior, 43*(3), 296–306.

LaVeist, T., Nuru-Jeter, A., & Jones, K. (2003). The association of doctor–patient race concordance with health services utilization. *Journal of Public Health Policy, 24*(3–4), 312–323.

McCormick, A., Fleming, D., & Charlton, J. (1995). *Morbidity statistics from general practice. Fourth national study 1991-1992. OPCS series MB5 No. 3.* London: HMSO.

Meyer, P. (2006). *Online glossary of research economics.* Retrieved from http://www.econterms.com/econtent.html Accessed on April 14, 2010.

Moy, E., & Bartman, B. (1995). Physician race and care of minority and medically indigent patients. *Journal of the American Medical Association, 273*(19), 1515–1520.

Murray-Garcia, J., Garcia, J., Schembri, M., & Guerra, L. (2001). The service patterns of a racially, ethnically, and linguistically diverse house staff. *Academic Medicine., 76*(12), 1232–1240.

Perez-Stable, E., Napoles-Springer, A., & Miramontes, J. (1997). The effects of ethnicity and language on medical outcomes of patients with hypertension or diabetes. *Medical Care, 35*(12), 1212–1219.

Rabinowitz, H., Diamond, J., Veloski, J., & Gayle, J. (2000). The impact of multiple predictors on generalist physicians' care of underserved populations. *American Journal of Public Health, 90*(8), 1225–1228.

Robertson, S. (2003). Men managing health. *Journal of Men's Health*, *2*(4), 111–113.

Saha, S., Komaromy, M., Koepsell, T., & Bindman, A. (1999). Patient–physician racial concordance and the perceived quality and use of health care. *Archives of Internal Medicine*, *159*(9), 997–1004.

Saha, S., Taggart, S., Komaromy, M., & Bindman, A. (2000). Do patients choose physicians of their own race? *Health Affairs*, *19*(4), 76–83.

Smith, G. (2013). *The role of race concordance on prescription drug utilization among primary care case-managed Medicaid enrollees*. *Research in Social and Administrative Pharmacy*. Retrieved from http://dx.doi.org/10.1016/j.sapharm.2012.12.004. Accessed on March 15, 2013.

Sue, S. (1988). Psychotherapeutic services for ethnic minorities: Two decades of research findings. *American Psychologist*, *43*(4), 301–308.

Szklo, M., & Nieto, F. (2000). *Epidemiology: Beyond the basics*. Gaithersburg, MD: Aspen Publishers, Inc.

Traylor, A., Schmittdiel, J., Uratsu, C., Mangione, C., & Subramanian, U. (2010). Adherence to cardiovascular disease medications: Does patient–provider race/ethnicity and language concordance matter? *Journal of General Internal Medicine*, *25*(11), 1172–1177.

Tudiver, F., & Talbot, Y. (1999). Why don't men seek help? Family physicians' perspectives on help-seeking behaviour in men. *Journal of Family Practice*, *48*(1), 47–52.

UCLA: Statistical Consulting Group. (2013). *Stata data analysis examples: Zero-inflated poisson regression*. University of California at Los Angeles. Retrieved from http://www.ats.ucla.edu/stat/stata/dae/zip.htm Accessed on January 4, 2013.

U.S. Department of Agriculture. (2004). *Measuring rurality: Rural–Urban continuum codes*. U.S. Department of Agriculture, Economic Research Services. Retrieved from http://webarchives.cdlib.org/wayback.public/UERS_ag_1/20110913215735/, http://www.ers.usda.gov/Briefing/Rurality/RuralUrbCon/. Accessed on March 6, 2013.

U.S. Department of Health and Human Services, Agency for Health Research and Quality. (2008). *Instructions for analyzing data from CAHPS surveys: Using the CAHPS analysis program version 3.6*, CAHPS Survey and Reporting Kit 2008. Doc. No. 2015. Rockville, MD: Agency for Health Research and Quality.

U.S. Department of Health and Human Services, Centers for Medicare and Medicaid Services. (2002). *Administering or validating surveys: Two protocols for use in conducting Medicaid external quality review activities*. Washington, DC: U.S. Government Printing Office, 2002. Retrieved from http://www.dss.mo.gov/mhd/mc/pdf/p-surveyadmin.pdf. Accessed on September 27, 2012.

U.S. Department of Health and Human Services, Health Resources and Services Administration. (2006). *The rationale for diversity in the health professions: A review of the evidence*. U.S. Department of Health and Human Services, Health Resources and Services Administration, Bureau of Health Professions. Washington, DC: U.S. Government Printing Office. Retrieved from http://bhpr.hrsa.gov/healthworkforce/reports/diversityreviewevidence.pdf. Accessed on September 27, 2012.

Weitzen, S., Lapane, K., Toledano, A., Hume, A., & Mor, V. (2004). Principles for modeling propensity scores in medical research: A systematic literature review. *Pharmacoepidemiology and Drug Safety*, *13*(12), 841–853.

White, A., & Witty, K. (2009). Men's under use of health services – Finding alternative approaches. *Journal of Men's Health*, *6*(2), 95–97.

Xu, G., Fields, S., Laine, C., Veloski, J., Barzansky, B., & Martini, C. (1997). The relationship between the race/ethnicity of generalist physicians and their care for underserved populations. *American Journal of Public Health*, *87*(5), 817–822.

PART 4
CHRONIC CARE AND SERIOUS HEALTH PROBLEMS

A GENERATION SKIPPED: AN EXPLORATORY STUDY OF HIV/AIDS EDUCATION AND PREVENTION SERVICES FOR OLDER ADULTS

Ann Marie Wood

ABSTRACT

Purpose – *Older adults' sexual health is becoming an increasingly important component of healthy aging in the wake of the HIV/AIDS epidemic and rising infection rates among this age cohort. The increase in HIV/AIDS diagnoses in the older adult population ignites the need to understand the reasons why older adults are omitted from HIV/AIDS prevention education policy.*

Methodology/approach –*This chapter examines the social forces that influence HIV/AIDS policy at the state and community levels. Through qualitative methodology and analysis, including interviews with state policymakers and managers of AIDS service organizations in four Midwestern states (*n = 31*), I look for trends and patterns as to whether or not older adults are considered as an "at-risk" group for HIV infection.*

Social Determinants, Health Disparities and Linkages to Health and Health Care
Research in the Sociology of Health Care, Volume 31, 217–246
Copyright © 2013 by Emerald Group Publishing Limited
All rights of reproduction in any form reserved
ISSN: 0275-4959/doi:10.1108/S0275-4959(2013)0000031012

Findings – *Findings reveal that HIV/AIDS policy may be impacted by enduring sexual scripts about older adults. To some extent both state policymakers and AIDS service organization personnel adhere to stereotypes about older adults' sexuality and sexual activity, which is then implemented in their health promotion activities. The result is that gaps exist in HIV/AIDS prevention education for older adults, despite the fact that current trends show an increase in new HIV infections and AIDS diagnoses among people over the age of 50.*

Research limitations/implications – *While this is an exploratory study of the available HIV/AIDS prevention education and health promotion activities for older adults, as well as the viewpoints of state policymakers and AIDS service organization personnel, the findings do indicate the need for additional research on the potentially dangerous sexual behaviors – lack of HIV testing, low condom usage, multiple partners – exhibited by older adults. Future research involving interviews with older adults, physicians, and medical personnel may add new perspectives to the current research.*

Originality/value of chapter – *As the baby boomers continue to age and challenge cultural stereotypes of sexual behaviors among older adults, research in the area of sexual health and HIV/AIDS prevention education will remain an important component of healthy aging. This research begins what will ultimately be a necessary conversation.*

Keywords: Older adults; HIV; AIDS; prevention education; health promotion

The ferocity with which the HIV/AIDS epidemic spread in the 1980s among the disenfranchised created a socially constructed moral landscape for those with HIV/AIDS. Children, hemophiliacs, and blood-donor recipients were considered innocent victims, while those who contracted the virus through behavioral choices – sex, drugs, and other so-called illicit behaviors – were seen as deserving of their disease. The epidemic divided society between those who wanted to protect their own from the evil scourge of the diseased versus those who viewed it as a virus that did not discriminate. What is perhaps most fascinating about the HIV/AIDS epidemic is that there is nothing extraordinary about how it is spread. While some viruses, such as cholera or the flu, can move from host to host at a rapid rate, the HIV/AIDS virus is passed on from person to person through "established routines" (Johnson, 2006, p. 32). Having sex, injecting drugs, breastfeeding a child, receiving blood products – these are potential fatal mistakes with permanent repercussions. Commonplace life practices of ordinary people had an extraordinary impact that often caused divisions among the U.S. government, health officials, and the general public.

While epidemics in the United States traditionally are swift-moving and show physical manifestations early on in the infection period (cholera, for example, can kill within a matter of hours or a day), the HIV/AIDS epidemic differed. The virus's potential for a long incubation period and constant mutation meant that seemingly healthy people were unknowingly infecting others for years before showing any signs of the illness.This difference alone suggested that prevention education and testing were of the utmost importance in the fight against the HIV/AIDS epidemic. However, inadequate funding resulted in limited prevention education. Most prevention education is geared toward specific groups deemed "high risk," while other groups, despite having increasing numbers of new HIV infections and AIDS diagnoses, are not receiving focused prevention education.

One group in particular that does not perceive itself as being at risk is the older adult population, defined by researchers and public health organizations as those over the age of 50 (Cloud, Brown, Salooja, & McClean, 2003; Emlet, Tozay, & Raveis, 2010; Gott & Hinchliff, 2003; Orel, Wright, & Wagner, 2004). Once a seemingly taboo subject, the topic of older adults' sexual health is becoming an increasingly important component of healthy aging. The advent of the HIV/AIDS epidemic and the rising infection rates among this age cohort bring attention to what otherwise is an unmentionable subject for many. Individuals over the age of 50 will represent 50% of HIV/AIDS cases by 2015 (Brennan, Emlet, & Eady, 2011; Doyle et al., 2012; Frontini et al., 2012; Hughes, 2011; Jang, Anderson, & Mentes, 2011; Vance, Brennan, Enah, Smith, & Kaur, 2011); this large percentage of HIV/AIDS cases includes older adults who have aged with the disease, as well as those who contract the disease after the age of 50 (Emlet, 2008). However, little is known about the sexual behaviors of the over-50 population, despite the increasing incidence and prevalence of HIV and AIDS in older adults (Illa et al., 2008).

This chapter examines the social forces that potentially influence HIV/AIDS prevention education policies at the community and state levels in the Midwest. Of particular interest is how these forces impact the level of inclusion of older adults within HIV/AIDS prevention policies. In order to gather this data, I interviewed state policymakers and AIDS Service

Organization (ASO) personnel to determine whether or not HIV/AIDS prevention education extends to older adults, and the specific reasons for inclusion or exclusion of older adults in these policies.

Results fromthis paper are important, as this is an understudied – yet increasing – group within the HIV/AIDS community in the United States. Determining whether or not disparities in prevention education exist could influence future prevention education policy geared toward older adults.

The next section summarizes the literature on older adults and HIV/AIDS. Included in this section is literature on physician/medical personnels' influence over testing amongst older adults, as well as theoretical underpinnings of this research. The following two sections focus on the methods used to collect data as well as the results from the study. The final two sections provide conclusions from the study as well as the social and economic implications that are highlighted in this study.

RESEARCH AND THEORETICAL UNDERPINNINGS: OLDER ADULTS AND HIV/AIDS

White and Catania (1982) argued 30 years ago for the need for sex education interventions for older adults, yet older adults are almost universally excluded from sex-education campaigns (Stombeck and Levy, 1998) and risk reduction and prevention programs (Poindexter & Keigher, 2004). On the surface, these suggestions appear to have fallen on deaf ears, as the number of infected older adults is increasing. In fact, the fastest growing segment of the HIV population in the United States is people over the age of 50 (Sankar, Nevedal, Neufeld, Berry, & Luborsky, 2011). As these trends continue to show that older adults are at risk for infection, the need for research into the theories and assumptions held by service providers that might impede HIV prevention efforts among older adults is increasing (Coon, Lipman, & Ory, 2003).

While popular culture may see sexuality and old age as incompatible (Davidson & Fennell, 2002; Farrell & Belza, 2012; Gott, Hinchliff, & Galena, 2004), the rates of HIV infection and AIDS among older adults reveal disturbing trends. Historically, older adults were widely reported to have made up between an estimated 10% and 15% of the overall U.S. AIDS population during the early years of the epidemic. Recent studies show that this percentage increased to 18.9% in 2000 (Keigher, Stevens, & Plach, 2004) to 27% in 2006 (Karpiak, Shippy, & Cantor, 2006), to a full 50% by 2015

(Jang et al., 2011). Between the years of 1998 and 2002, new HIV infections among older adults increased a staggering 107% (Orel et al., 2004), while the cumulative amount of AIDS cases actually quintupled between 1990 and 2001 (Jang et al., 2011).

While these increases may be a surprise to some, medical experts tend to agree that older adults are among the most overlooked and vulnerable populations facing the HIV/AIDS epidemic, despite exhibiting the same risk behaviors as younger adults (Huffstutter, 2007). Overall, older adults by far are the age group that lacks the most knowledge about HIV/AIDS or their perceived risk for infection (Coon et al., 2003; Gallagher & Petersen,1992). In addition, older adults tend to not protect themselves against HIV infection through the use of condoms; the older adult cohort is the least likely by far of all age cohorts to use condoms in their previous sexual encounter, even when the encounter was casual and not part of a relationship (Substance Abuse & Mental Health Services Administration, 1997). One study on older adults and condom use revealed that 92% of older adults over the age of 50 never used condoms (Genke, 2000; Inelmen, Gasparini, & Enzi, 2005).

Risk

When analyzing an epidemic such as HIV/AIDS, dialogue about risk must always be at the forefront of any discussion. Risk is seen as the "potential for realization of unwanted, negative consequences of an event" (Tierney, 1999, p. 106). Risk and risk estimates are viewed as social constructions derived from social and cultural factors; risk is seen as the "likelihood or probability of some adverse effect of a hazard" and is scientifically measured and managed by both public and private domains (Short, Jr., 1984).The current trend (or, as Schiltz & Sandfort, 2000 call it, the prevailing sexual script) of promoting health and diminishing risk that public health officials use for the HIV/AIDS epidemic is recognizing that each individual has full responsibility over their own health via behavior modifications and risk management (Nettleton & Bunton, 1995). For example, individuals are given the tools at the community level – often through education and targeted outreach – to assess their own risk level for contracting HIV/AIDS. ASOs and state policymakers provide prevention education and it is up to individuals to decide whether or not to change their behaviors based on their risk perception.

The perception of not being at risk for HIV/AIDS is common among older adults. According to research (Cloud et al., 2003; Coon et al., 2003;

Ory & Mack, 1998), older adults have made fewer behavioral accommodations to avoid risk for HIV/AIDS infection because their risk perception is low. Additionally, it is taken for granted that older adults somehow cannot transmit the virus because they are not believed to be interested in sex (Riley & Riley, Jr., 1989). However, the number of new HIV infections and AIDS diagnoses among older adults tell us that they are at risk, either through sex or drug use (Heckman, Kochman, Sikkema, & Kalichman, 1999; Inelmen et al., 2005). Among the newly infected older adult population, heterosexual sex was the primary mode of transmission (ACRIA, 2006; Emlet, Tangenberg, & Siverson, 2002; Stombeck & Levy, 1998; THJKFF, 2007g). In fact, the largest percent of AIDS cases among any heterosexual group is in the older adult age group (Williams & Donnelly, 2002).

There are a few possible reasons why older adults do not correctly perceive their risk level. First, from the beginning of the HIV/AIDS epidemic, the media has powerfully influenced whom the public thought was at risk for infection and how citizens understood the AIDS epidemic (Holland, Ramazanoglu, & Scott, 1990). During the first two years of the epidemic, the mass media virtually ignored the outbreak of the new disease. When the first news report was published in the mainstream media (two years after the disease first appeared in five gay men), its title – "The Gay Plague" – not only set into motion the stigmatization of a subgroup of the population, but also set a precedent that AIDS was a strictly gay disease (Brennan et al., 2011). This left most of the United States feeling as though they were far removed from being at risk. Because older adults rarely are the focus of media depictions of people with HIV/AIDS, they may not identify themselves as being at risk.

Second, those who are part of older adult age cohorts (both pre-retirement and post-retirement ages) may have come of age during a time of strict moral sanctions, resulting in the reluctance to discuss any sexual issues in public or with their physician (Catania et al., 1989b; Genke, 2000). Discussion about sex and condoms may be an embarrassing subject for older adults, especially if they are talking to a younger physician. Further, older adults who use intravenous drugs or visit prostitutes might not be willing to admit this, and are therefore probably not going to get tested for HIV. Older adults, especially those in their later years, may be unwilling to discuss any behaviors seen as risky because of the stigma attached to these behaviors (ACRIA, 2004; Illa et al., 2008; Vance et al., 2011). This unwillingness to discuss risk behaviors also contributes to the difficulties that exist in finding representative samples and individuals willing to participate in HIV/AIDS research among older adults (Falvo & Norman, 2004).

Third, ageist attitudes and assumptions continue to dominate our culture. Not only does our society ignore the fact that older adults are sexual, but there is an assumption that older adults know how to avoid HIV infection simply by virtue of being older. Based on the increase in new infections among older adults, prevention education might not be reaching everyone in this particular age group. With the advent of sex-enhancing drugs for erectile dysfunction and hormone replacement therapy, the need for HIV/AIDS prevention education is even greater.

Sexual Scripts

Lingering stereotypes about older adults and sexuality that continue to dominate our culture are a result of the dominance of sexual scripts regarding this particular age group. To put it simply, sexual scripts guide sexual behavior (Lewis & Kertzner, 2003; Weinberg, Swensson, & Hammersmith, 1983). Each culture gives shape to unique sexual scripts through symbolic and learned aspects rather than biological drives (Bardella, 2002; Netting & Burnett, 2004). Cultural scenarios are instructional guides that influence an individual to become an active participant in shaping their own behaviors based on appropriate cultural scripts (Simon & Gagnon, 1984). Additionally, the social determinant of age in sexual domains exists, accompanied by expectations as well as limitations (Simon, 1986).

In the case of older adults, societal norms stipulate that they should be androgynous; sexuality is rarely anticipated in cultural scripts dealing with older adults. However, as researchers found, many older adults do not adhere to prevailing cultural sexual scripts that say they should be asexual as they grow older. There is some indication that our culture has not advanced very far in our acceptance of older adults as sexual, even as older adults ignore the cultural sexual scripts and continue to have sex. Altschuler, Katz, and Tynan (2004) argue that it is society's views and misconceptions about older adults that may be putting them at risk. They state (p. 122):

> Old people are no longer interested in sex; if they are interested, no one's interested in them; if they do have sex, it's within a monogamous, heterosexual relationship; they don't do drugs; and if they ever did, it's so long ago it doesn't matter.

The cultural and sexual scripts of older adults can be difficult to understand. On the one hand, society is telling older adults that they are not sexual beings, and therefore are not at risk for contracting HIV/AIDS. But on the other hand, physicians are prescribing Viagra, Cialis, and Levitra (erectile dysfunction drugs), and hormone replacement therapy in increasing numbers to older adults, and the television commercials for this classification of drugs are touting the positive side of regaining a once-lost sexual vitality. Researchers (Berkeley & Ross, 2003) point out that receiving this type of mixed message from the surrounding social world is considered one of the main reasons for adhering to risk-taking sexual behavior. If physicians, public health officials, and the media are not relaying the message that older adults are at risk for contracting HIV/AIDS, why would they stop exhibiting behaviors that put them at risk?

Physician Denial about Older Adults' Risk

Contracting HIV or AIDS is not what people necessarily think of as an older adult issue, and the denial about their potential to become infected is prevalent among many care providers (Coon et al., 2003; Hayes Taylor, 2004; Langley, 2006; Orsulic-Jeras, Shepher, & Britton, 2003). Physicians and health practitioners are also ignoring the sexual needs and, more importantly, the sexual education of older adults. In their research on whether or not physicians discuss issues related to sexuality with their older adult patients, Gott et al. (2004) found that physicians were more likely than not to hold stereotypes about older adults and sex. For example, the physicians they interviewed equated sexual health with younger people, resulting in their reluctance give any type of prevention advice to older adults (Gott et al., 2004). According to a study by the National Institutes of Health, only 38% of men and 22% of women over the age of 50 discussed sex with their physician (Huffstutter, 2007). Overall, sexual histories are not routinely included in patient assessments of older adults (Inelmen et al., 2005).

Other studies confirm these findings. Researchers found that, despite having more interactions with health care professionals than younger adults (Musa, Schulz, Harris, Silverman, & Thomas, 2009), primary care physicians are less likely to discuss HIV-risk reduction with their patients over the age of 50 than with patients under the age of 50 (Williams & Donnelly, 2002). Further, Falvo and Norman (2004) found that only 10.8% of persons over the age of 50 discussed HIV/AIDS with their physicians. Similarly, a study done by the Centers for Disease Control (CDC) revealed that, even though physicians are in an excellent position to provide HIV/AIDS prevention education to older adults, only 31% of doctors discuss condom use, 27% discuss sexual orientation, and 22% discuss the number of sexual partners an older adult has (Fitzpatrick, 2011; Stombeck & Levy, 1998). As Gott et al. (2004) explained:

Safe sex was not seen as a relevant topic to discuss with middle aged andolder patients, reflecting very clearly both policy priorities and wider societalbeliefs that it is *only* young people who engage in risky sexual practices (p. 2101).

Instead of viewing sexuality in the aged as a positive aspect of aging, some research suggests that medical professionals view it as something to be eliminated (Farrell & Belza, 2012; Schlesinger, 1996). This might not necessarily be the fault of physicians alone. Lindau et al. (2007) point out that no comprehensive or nationally representative population-based data are available to inform physicians about the sexual norms and problems of older adults. Medical personnel may also be lacking adequate training on the subject of older adults' sexual health (Farrell & Belza, 2012). Further, older adult patients are reluctant to initiate discussions about sex, perhaps due to the age differences between the patient and the physician (Brooks, Jr., 2003; Huffstutter, 2007; Kilgannon, 2007; Nusbaum, Singh, & Pyles, 2004; Siegel, Raveis, & Karus, 1998).

Among those who do become infected, there are challenges that older adults face that younger adults might not necessarily encounter. These include misdiagnosis, comorbidities – as high as 92% of HIV-positive older adults experience this – and mental health issues, specifically depression (Frontini et al., 2012). HIV-related illnesses can be very difficult to distinguish from other so-called "typical" age-related health issues. For example, research shows that age-related diseases such as Alzheimer's, arthritis, breast or prostate cancer, diabetes, vision/hearing loss, and high blood pressure all share common symptoms with HIV/AIDS (ACRIA, 2004; Avis & Smith, 1998; Fitzpatrick, 2011; Genke, 2000). This has become so common that Mack and Bland (1999, p. 687) labeled the disease in older adults as the "new great imitator" due to its resemblance to other conditions related to aging.

HIV/AIDS also has gender implications, as older adult women are over-whelmingly excluded from any type of HIV/AIDS research and intervention. This is especially dangerous for older women, who were among the fastest growing populations infected with HIV recent years. In fact, when looking at the numbers of new infections and diagnoses among women, the incidence of new cases actually increased with age (Brooks, Jr., 2003; Genke, 2000).

Additionally, racial and ethnic minorities in the older adult category are seeing higher rates of infection than white older adults (Harawa, Leng, Kim, & Cunningham, 2011). Brennan et al. (2011) report the rates of HIV diagnoses in older adult African-Americans is four times the overall rate for all older persons; this rate increases to sixfold when looking at older adults aged 65 and older. Among Hispanic older adults, the researchers found the rates of new HIV infections were 1.5 times greater than the rates for all older adults; this rate increased to twofold when looking at older adults aged 60 and older (Brennan et al., 2011). Among older adults who self-identify as mixed-race older adults the rates were lower than that of Hispanic older adults but higher than rates of HIV infection among American Indian, White, and Asian older adults (Brennan et al., 2011).These findings, along with Simone and Appelbaum's (2008) revelation that the death rate from AIDS-related illnesses among older adults was five times higher among older adult Hispanics and twelve times higher in older African Americans than in older white adults, indicates the need for increased prevention education among minorities.

Knowing the HIV/AIDS trends among older adults, I sought to uncover the level of inclusion of specific targeted prevention education by state policymakers and ASO personnel toward the older adult population. I collected information on prevention education policies, opinions on older adults' risk for HIV/AIDS, and other pertinent information related to my target age group. I analyzed the information gathered through interviews in order to determine if health disparities based on age exist within the HIV/AIDS prevention education policies of states and ASOs.

METHODS AND RESULTS

The crux of this research is based on the interviews conducted with Executive Directors, Prevention Directors, and/or Case Managers of ASOs, and state HIV/AIDS policymakers (State AIDS Directors, Prevention Directors, Surveillance Coordinators, Ryan White Titles Directors, etc.) in four states in the Midwest. Data was gathered in the Midwest for two reasons. First, the Midwest is certainly not a focus in much HIV/AIDS research, and there is very little mention of HIV/AIDS research being conducted in the Midwest, an area that remains significantly understudied. Second, the Midwest is a unique region to study for a few reasons. Surprisingly, the Midwest was the region with the largest percent of new AIDS diagnoses between 2001 and 2005. It is critical to focus on rural areas such as those located in the Midwest, because there is an increase in the number of individuals with HIV/AIDS and restricted care available for those who are infected (Preston et al., 2002).

In addition, rural service providers rely heavily on ASOs for prevention, education, and case management assistance more than they do in urban areas (Roeder, 2002).

ASOs provide counseling and testing services, case management services for HIV positive people or persons with AIDS (PWAs), and prevention education in the community in which they are located. They provide these direct services, as well as palliative care, and prevention education to a wide range of different populations (Barton-Villagrana, Bedney, & Miller, 2002). ASO personnel were interviewed because ASOs are the only organizations that devote 100% of their efforts to AIDS care and prevention education as compared to public health departments in which AIDS is just one of the many health concerns in which they focus. I was able to perform eighteen interviews at fourteen ASOs, or 78% of all the ASOs in the four-state region. I conducted thirteen interviews with state HIV/AIDS policymakers, which at the time of the interview process represented 92% of all of the state HIV/AIDS officials in the four states.

I employed a stratified purposeful sampling technique because of the relatively small number of potential participants. In order to find both the names and contact information for both sets of potential interviewees, I consulted the National Alliance of State and Territorial AIDS Directors (NASTAD, 2005) website and the "Local HIV/AIDS service organizations in the USA" page at AVERT.org (2005). A search of each state's Department of Health website and a search for "AIDS organizations" confirmed or corrected the contact information. Communication with the interviewees then took place either by e-mail or phone, and arrangements were made for the in-person interview.

The interviews were semi-structured in nature. I had a number of questions that were demographic, as well as questions that I asked of every one of the interviewees in order to compare answers. Each interview lasted between 45 minutes and 2 ½ hours. I interviewed participants at the ASOs in private offices or rooms for confidentiality, while the interviews with the state policymakers took place at their offices in the capital city of each state. After completion of the interviews, I transcribed the audiotapes of each interview, and reviewed the transcripts for accuracy.

I undertook the process of open coding in order to analyze the interviews. I used several rounds of coding, employing a constant comparative analysis and grounded theory to identify variations between the interviews both individually and categorically. For example, I looked for patterns across all of the interviews, between the two groups (ASO personnel and state HIV/ AIDS policymakers), between the four states, and then between the two groups within each state. Fortunately, strong patterns emerged on all levels, which I interpreted as reaching theoretical saturation.

Questions pertaining specifically to older adults' inclusion in HIV/AIDS prevention education were asked and are the focus of this chapter. I asked six questions that were exclusively about older adults; further, the answers to two other questions not specifically related to older adults were answered by some in such a way that they also focused on age-related issues. I grouped the answers to these particular questions I posed to the interviewees into three categories: *High-Risk Behaviors*, *Sexual Scripts*, and *Prevention Education*. The following are a synopsis of the answers, as well as the themes and trends that emerged from the respondents' answers. For purposes of confidentiality, I refer to the four states as "State A," "State B," "State C," and "State D." For the following answers, I also state whether the answer came from a state policymaker or from ASO personnel in order to ascertain if there are differences in responses from the two groups. Because ASO personnel are at the "ground level," so to speak, and have direct contact with members of their respective communities, I anticipated that there may have been differences in their responses versus those of state policymakers who have less community involvement.

RESULTS/FINDINGS

High-Risk Behaviors

I asked three questions that were specifically about the high-risk behaviors that older adults may or may not be exhibiting that put them at risk for HIV/AIDS. The first question was asked in the following manner: *Do you agree or disagree with this statement: "I believe that older adults in my community exhibit high-risk behaviors that make them susceptible to contracting HIV."* The overall consensus among most ($n = 9$) state policymakers and ASO personnel was that older adults do exhibit high-risk behaviors that make them susceptible to contracting the virus. When asked the same question, 18 ASO personnel said that older adults do exhibit high-risk behaviors that make them susceptible to contracting HIV; only one employee at an ASO said they were not sure if older adults exhibit high-risk behaviors or not. As one ASO Executive Director from State C explained, "Yes, I agree, and I don't think it is just [in] my community."

The second question I asked about the high-risk behaviors that older adults may or may not be exhibiting that put them at risk for HIV/AIDS was: *What are the activities or behaviors that older adults in your community exhibit that could put them at risk for HIV infection?* The answers I received were not mutually exclusive, and I was given anywhere between one and several answers from each respondent. The following themes emerged from the answers I received.

(1) *Older adults exhibit the same risk behaviors as other groups*: One policymaker and two ASO personnel stated that the behaviors exhibited by older adults that put them at risk are the same as other groups, especially engaging in sexual activity. As one ASO Executive Director from State B explained, "They are having sex. People think that you have to do some weird, unique thing to be at risk. No, you just have to have sex!"A state policymaker from State C provided further explanation:

> I guess the thought is why would we think that older adults would be different than other groups of people? They date, they have substance abuse problems, they have housing problems, they have mental illness … all of these factors that contribute to people acquiring HIV are the same factors in older adults.

(2) *Older adults are dating*: Similarly, two policymakers and nine ASO personnel said that dating, especially after divorce, was a risk behavior that older adults exhibit that may put them at risk for HIV infection. Once I probed the question a bit further, it became apparent that it was not necessarily dating, per se, which put them at risk, but was the fact that older adults were never socialized to think about safe sex (i.e., sexual scripts). The result was that older adults were entering the dating scene again without practicing safe sex. The following quote from an ASO Executive Director from State D describes this scenario.

> I think people who are maybe going through separations or going through life changes, they are not used to thinking in the safer sex category because when we were in our 20s, this didn't exist. Or we didn't know about it, and so if you've been married for 15 or 20 years or been in a relationship for 15 or 20 years and are just getting back out there, it's not something that is going to be at the forefront of your mind. (State D ASO Executive Director)

A few ASO policymakers also mentioned that "dating" also incorporated husbands who are cheating on their wives either with other women, but more likely with other men – a phenomenon often referred to as being on the "down low." An ASO Executive Director from State B explained that this occurs regularly in their community, and is the main transmission route for their female HIV population over the age of 45.

> Let me tell you, I regularly frighten married women. I don't mean to but … when you tell them, look … 30% of our [HIV-infected] population is women, and 80% of those

women were infected by men who [were] monogamous partner[s]. Guess what? That was
a man! That was a husband or a boyfriend. So it's an issue. People have a false idea that
marriage protects them from all sorts of things. (State B ASO Executive Director)

(3) *Older adults are using IV drugs*: Drug use/abuse or IV drug use was
listed by two state policymakers and five ASO personnel as being a risk
behavior that they view some older adults exhibiting. As one ASO Executive
Director from State D said, "Being 59 don't mean you don't use meth!" An
example of just how many older adults use drugs came from one of the
ASOs in the four-state Midwestern region which runs an underground
needle-exchange program out of their location. In one year's time, the
ASO's underground needle-exchange program exchanged 37,000 needles.
According to the Executive Director, "The people that we see on the
program are not young people ... we are talking about people in their 40s
and 50s. These are people who have been using for years."

Drug use as a risk behavior that older adults exhibit, thereby placing them
at risk for HIV infection, is not necessarily the use of illegal drugs. As a state
policymaker from State B stated, it could be a matter of sharing needles that
puts older adults at risk for contracting HIV.

Unprotected sex and drug use, needle sharing. It doesn't have to be drugs; it doesn't have
to be illegal drugs. It can be anything in which you are going to share paraphernalia with
someone who might be infected. We had a number of cases where an individual would
get needles from an older family member who is diabetic and giving themselves insulin
because those are good needles. The philosophy among some of these folks was "Aren't I
safer using Grandma's discarded needle than I am sharing with a bunch of friends?"
Yeah, you are right, but as times got tighter and tighter, Grandma might be using hers
two or three times. There was a lot of potential there. (State Policymaker State B)

(4) *Older adults exhibit dangerous sex behaviors*: Six state policymakers
and three ASO personnel stated that dangerous sex behaviors that some
older adults exhibit may be putting them at risk for HIV infection. The
behaviors mentioned include being swingers or attending sex parties, having
promiscuous sex or having multiple partners at one time, finding sex on the
Internet, and being a bug chaser, which is the term used to describe an
individual who seeks to be intentionally infected by someone who is HIV-
positive. Several respondents claimed that they knew many members of their
respective communities who were exhibiting these behaviors, and that it was
just a matter of time before these groups would experience an outbreak of
HIV or another sexually transmitted disease.

A few state policymakers commented that exhibiting dangerous sexual
behaviors could be a product of being risk takers as adolescents and not

modifying behaviors as they aged. As a state policymaker from State B stated:

> Some folks survive their youth and modify their behavior, but we are talking about human beings. Some people still may exhibit behaviors and risk taking. Sometimes the longer you live and you haven't had things happen to you...if you live a long time and think well nothing has really negatively impacted me, so you do the same risks. (State Policymaker State B)

Another state policymaker from State D believed that it was specifically the Baby Boomer generation who were at risk because they grew up exhibiting potentially dangerous sexual behaviors and did not learn to modify them or protect themselves against the risk to HIV infection.

> Sex, drugs, and rock and roll are all part of the life, particularly with Baby Boomers. They've grown up in a time, from the time of their adolescence, that was the 50s and 60s, and we all remember what was going on with the freedom of flow and things then. That's a part of their life that has just continued on. I know what it's been like and that's not going to change. They are not hearing the message at all. They, particularly heterosexual baby boomers, are just not going to hear the message and aren't seeing it as them. (StatePolicymakerState D)

(5) *Older adults adhere to sexual scripts*: Sexual scripts, which serve as a type of social regulation of sexual behavior via set standards and constructed norms, were seen as a possible risk that may increase older adults' chances for contracting HIV infection. While this was mentioned by only three state policymakers, seventeen ASO personnel's statements were coded as referring to the sexual scripts of older adults as being potential risk behaviors. Adhering to sexual scripts was, by far, seen as the biggest risk behavior that older adults exhibit. These sexual scripts which older adults adhere to included: not worrying about pregnancy due to menopause, and therefore not using protection; not asking about sexual history; and not discussing safe sex with partners. One ASO Executive Director from State C explained how older adults did not grow up in an era where talking about safe sex was a priority.

> You are no longer at risk for pregnancy, you didn't grow up in era when condom use was common, you're certainly not going to use it now that you aren't going to get pregnant. You are too polite to ask someone their sexual history, because we weren't raised that way. We didn't want to offend by suggesting a condom. (State C ASO Executive Director)

(6) *Older adults are not using protection*: Three state policymakers and five ASO personnel mentioned that not using protection during a sexual encounter was a risk behavior that older adults exhibit that may be putting

them at risk for HIV infection. The fact that a large percent of older adults do not use condoms is certainly supported by literature. However, a few of the respondents also spoke specifically about the lack of condom use within assisted living facilities and nursing homes, which has not been fully explored in research and literature on older adults and sexuality. One ASO Executive Director from State C relayed a story about an incident concerning condoms in a nursing home.

> We've actually been to [nursing home] and talked to people there several times. One of the meetings we went to there was this 90-year-old lady and she was very outspoken and was grabbing a lot of condom packets, and she said, "These are for my grandkids" and we said, "That's okay, take as many as you want." And she said, "But I'm here to tell you that we have sex." And I said, "Yes, that's why we are here to talk to you guys." And she said, "No, I'm telling you that people my age have sex." And I said, "Okay, well, take those condom packs and distribute them to whoever." She keeps telling me that "I don't think you understand, these people in this room do have sex." And I said, "I understand, that's why we are going to talk to you." So she sees this guy out in the hallway and she went up to him and said, "You should have been here! This talk was about HIV!" So a lot of people saw it was very important. That was pretty powerful for those people, too, but I don't think you can get people in that age group to understand that starting over again or finding other partners, that you really have to talk about these things, you can't just assume that they aren't going to get it. (State C ASO Executive Director)

The fact that older adults have a very low level of testing, and therefore do not know their HIV status was only mentioned by one state policymaker as being a behavior that puts older adults at risk for HIV infection. This was not listed by any ASO personnel as being a high-risk behavior, despite the vast amount of literature and research that shows it is a dangerous trend among older adults. Additionally, one state policymaker and two ASO personnel mentioned that being a man who has sex with a man (MSM) was a high-risk behavior that puts older adults at risk for HIV infection. This is both surprising and a step in the right direction. It is surprising that being an MSM was only mentioned as being a high-risk behavior that puts older adults at risk for infection by three respondents, considering how HIV/AIDS risk was defined during the formative years of the epidemic. But it is also reassuring that it was mentioned as an individual behavior rather than as a matter of group membership, dispelling the long-standing myth that a person is at risk for infection if they are gay.

In addition to the questions I asked that were specific to older adults, I also asked general questions about HIV/AIDS. One of these questions was: *Who do you see as being at-risk for HIV infection?* It should be noted that I asked this question before I asked specific questions pertaining to older adults. Three of the interviewees, one state policymaker and two ASO personnel, mentioned that older adults are specifically at-risk for HIV infection. An ASO Executive Director from State D mentioned that there are probably older adults who are infected and do not know it because they are not being tested for HIV, which is supported in the literature.

> I think that we are probably going to see a couple of different trends in *****. One is definitely the elder population because I think that what we know about HIV is that it can live inside your body for up to ten years without showing any signs or symptoms, and I think that there are folks who are probably infected who will find that out later on. (State D ASO Executive Director)

Sexual Scripts

I asked the interviewees a question related to sexual scripts, specifically the sexual scripts about older adults to which our society adheres. The question was listed as follows: *How do you think our culture views older adults and sexuality?* Additionally, I used the following prompts to elicit additional responses: *In a positive or negative light, as something to embrace or fear, as something to talk about or ignore? Do you think there are certain rules or expectations that exist concerning older adults being sexual?* The answers provided by the respondents ranged from denial that older adults are even sexual to the thought of older adults being sexual seen as being humorous, disgusting, or shocking. Only a few referred to how sexual scripts about older adults are changing as sexuality is being discussed more openly.

The most common answer given by five state policymakers and four ASO personnel was that our culture views older adults as not being sexual beings at all. As one state policymaker from State C explained:

> That [older adults having sex] doesn't exist. I was at a training once, and somebody stood up and said people past 25 don't have sex. People will always think of younger people when they talk about sex and injection drug use, they really don't think about the older population. (State Policymaker State C)

Several respondents echoed a statement made by a state policymaker from State D stated. According to this state policymaker, "We just pretend it [older adults and sex] doesn't happen. Our mothers and fathers never had sex." This is a common belief that seems to permeate our culture, regardless of the age of our parents.

If any thought is given to older adults and sexuality, cultural views, according to the respondents, are generally that of humor or disgust. The

humor tends to surround older men, as an ASO Executive Director from
State C explained:

> They think it is humorous. Object of humor. "Why that old fart, what's he thinking
> about?" You don't talk about it. They don't talk about sex, and if they do, it's
> funny...hahahaha. "Grandpa had a woody." (ASO Executive Director State C)

Additionally, an ASO Director from State A pointed out that some of the
jokes commonly used in our culture pertaining to older adults and sexuality
focus on shame and disgust at the thought of older people engaging in
sexual activities.

> There's too many jokes about being disgusted by people who are old and having sex,
> whatever "old" is. There's a disbelief that older people do have sex. It's like, it doesn't
> happen, so we probably don't have to worry about it. Or they are being "naughty" if
> they are having sex. Shame involved. People who are older should be ashamed if they are
> having sex. And so there is no need for education, there is no need to have chats about it.
> Seems to be in our culture. (ASO Director State A)

Prevention Education

In order to ascertain whether or not older adults were viewed as being at risk
for HIV/AIDS infection, I asked all of the interviewees about the types of
prevention education that was made available to older adults. Specifically,
I asked: *What types of health promotion, prevention services, or education
for HIV/AIDS do you provide to the older adult population?* As a prompt,
I followed this question with: *Do you offer any education or information
specifically geared toward older adults?* All of the state policymakers
responded that they provide the same prevention education to older adults
as they do to all other populations. Twelve of the ASO personnel also stated
that they provide the same types of health promotion and prevention
education to older adults as they do to anyone else.

However, three of the ASO personnel did offer age-specific HIV/AIDS
information and prevention education for older adults. An ASO Executive
Director and Education Specialist from State D both mentioned the fact
that they were just beginning to offer age-specific HIV/AIDS information to
older adults, and they were targeting the 55+ age group. This was due to a
specific request they received from the community to provide prevention
education to seniors who lived in senior housing. Another ASO Executive
Director and a Volunteer Coordinator from State A mentioned that they

display information at health fairs that are specifically for seniors in order to reach that particular population.

Out of the thirty-one interviews I conducted, only one – an ASO Director from State A – had actual HIV/AIDS educational materials that were specifically for older adults. This ASO Director noticed that some of the population they were seeing coming in for HIV tests and HIV information were in the older adult age cohort. Because the ASO Director was not able to find any educational materials that were specifically geared toward older adults, they made their own flyers and brochures. When I asked about these materials, the ASO Director replied:

> I think it's in my health fair box. I have something called "Older Americans and HIV." I have it in a box I take to [health] fairs. I noticed that, if I'm sitting at the table, they [older adults] do not pick them up. If I'm not sitting there, if I'm talking to the person next to me, they definitely take the pamphlets up if nobody is watching. They rarely stop and talk. (ASO Director State A)

Even though this particular population is one of the fastest rising populations of new HIV infections, they are not considered a target group by most of the ASOs. When I asked why older adults are not being targeted, an ASO Volunteer Coordinator from State A answered bluntly in a sarcastic tone that "Older adults, older gay people don't matter. They have no value. They are invisible. Because of that, what it says is so what if you die when you are 40?" Further, a state AIDS Director from State D stated that, even if the ASOs and the state provided prevention education to older adults, the message would not necessarily be received unless it was a member of the older adult community who was spreading that message.

> There needs to be people in older populations that are helping to carry that message. You need a little old lady to go in and talk to the Red Hat club…that's the only people that are going to get in there to talk to them. It's not going to be a young woman, a young man, it's got to be a little old lady that looks like them. (StateAIDS DirectorState D)

A few answers to the question on availability of HIV/AIDS prevention/ education for older adults resulted in some discussion of physicians and medical personnel. For example, an ASO Executive Director from State C stated that doctors in their area were not trained to talk to older adults about safe sex. They said that "They [doctors] aren't comfortable doing that because they haven't been trained and they don't know what to say." This sentiment was also communicated by another ASO Executive Director in State C, who pointed out that "Grandpa and Grandma aren't having sex. I can't imagine doctors are asking older adults about their sexual habits."As mentioned, research reveals that doctors do not talk to older adults about their sexual habits, and therefore are not in a position to provide HIV/AIDS prevention education to older adults. A state HIV/AIDS Surveillance Director from State B relayed their own personal experience with this subject by stating "I'm 54, and I don't think any physician I've ever visited has asked me about my sexual history or status or those kinds of things."

ASO personnel from two states provided examples of how physicians act as barriers against HIV/AIDS prevention education and health promotion. An ASO Executive Director from State B told a story of having an older female client who requested an HIV test due to physical symptoms she was exhibiting, but her doctor told her she did not need a test.

> Sure and that's still out there [physician ignorance], and we still have rural providers...we had an older client who kept going because she had real funky stuff, and she asked the doctor if she needed an AIDS test, and he said "No, good girls don't get AIDS". A month later she is in the hospital half dead because he didn't think she needed an AIDS test. (ASO Executive Director State B)

This was not the only example provided by the respondents of a physician acting as a gatekeeper (in their opinions) to HIV/AIDS prevention education. An ASO Volunteer Coordinator from State A gave the example of their mother being denied an HIV test by her doctor, even though she admitted to him that she was exhibiting behaviors that put her at risk for HIV infection.

> I think it's generational... they don't talk about it for one thing. But living in small towns, everybody knows everybody else's business so they talk about it, but it's not openly talking about it. My mother went to the doctor and she was in her 60s at the time and having unprotected sex, and so I told her to say to her doctor that she would like an HIV test, because my son has talked to me about this and I've been participating in high-risk behaviors. He wouldn't do it. He said, "You are *SO* not a risk for me to do it." In rural areas, doctors are such authority figures, especially with the older generations who do not ignore the doctor. If he tells you something, you do it. (ASO Volunteer Coordinator State A)

DISCUSSION

In the case of HIV/AIDS, deciphering risk level is based on an assessment of specific behaviors exhibited and whether or not they have the potential to result in infection. Because risk estimates are socially constructed, we must keep in mind that other social factors – particularly stereotypes and sexual scripts – might be influencing who is seen as being at risk for HIV/AIDS infection. Responses from state policymakers and ASO personnel indicate that the respondents did, in fact, believe that older adults exhibited behaviors that put them at risk for HIV infection. The respondents exhibited a high level of knowledge concerning possible transmission routes for HIV infection and behaviors that are considered high risk for infection.

While the respondents were well aware that older adults within their communities exhibit certain behaviors that potentially could result in contracting HIV, overall this did not translate to recognizing this population as a whole as being at risk. This disconnect was puzzling given the fact that the respondents readily agreed that older adults in their communities were exhibiting behaviors that were considered high-risk for infection. But somehow being cognizant of the high-risk behaviors exhibited by older adults did not mean that they viewed the whole older adult population as being at risk. I can only conjecture that the older adults the respondents thought were exhibiting high-risk behaviors were considered outliers in the older adult population of the respondents' particular state, and that the rest of this population was not at risk. However, even if this is a true statement, the typical protocol of public health is to target a population who exhibit dangerous or risky behaviors and then provide interventions or behavioral modifications (Gazmararian, Curran, Parker, Bernhardt, & DeBuono, 2005; Morgan &Tyler, 1971). The fact that these older adults who are at risk for infection are not receiving any interventions or prevention education is still perplexing.

The behaviors that put older adults at risk for HIV/AIDS infection – having sex, not getting tested, adhering to sexual scripts that do not include frank and open discussion about safe sex, and protection, etc. – are essentially the same behaviors that younger adults exhibit. Several state policymakers and ASO personnel pointed out these behaviors but later associated HIV risk with specific populations, such as gay men, minorities, and younger adults, but rarely with older adults. If the behaviors that older adults are exhibiting are the same as those exhibited by younger adults, gay men, and minorities, why is it that state policymakers and ASO personnel do not associate HIV risk with older adults?

I expected to answer this question by explaining that state policymakers and ASO personnel were adhering to existing sexual scripts about older adults. However, the fact that the interviewees listed specific behaviors that older adults exhibited that could put them at risk for HIV infection caused me to consider other possible explanations. The state policymakers and ASO personnel were not necessarily supporting sexual scripts about older adults which indicate that older adults were asexual or not at risk for HIV.

In fact, both groups were open to the possibility that older adults did exhibit risk behaviors that could result in new infections. In an effort to explain why older adults were excluded from HIV/AIDS prevention education, I did find that sexual scripts were, in fact, a guiding force, though not in the way I had anticipated.

Sexual Scripts

Our culture's stereotyping and sexual scripts about older adults as asexual and therefore not exhibiting risk behaviors is anything but rare, as is evident from the literature I analyzed. In this study, I found that state policymakers and ASO personnel are aware that society holds stereotypes and sexual scripts about older adults. A number recognized that our culture views older adults as not being sexual beings, or are subjects of humor or disgust. As a whole, most interviewees answered questions in such a way that indicated they were critical of society's views of older adults and sexuality.

The respondents were also aware that older adults themselves adhere to society's sexual scripts which tell them that they are not at risk for infection for various reasons (past childbearing stage, do not use condoms because they grew up in an era when condom use was not common, do not discuss sexual history, etc.). As a group, state HIV/AIDS policymakers and ASO personnel were also cognizant of the fact that the disease itself is laden with stereotypes and misconceptions. For example, only three respondents mentioned that being an MSM was a high-risk behavior that puts older adults at risk for infection. This is most certainly a departure from society's view of HIV/AIDS as being a risk to only gay men.

This is not to say that cultural sexual scripts about older adults did not have any influence over the respondents' views. Some of the state policymakers and ASO personnel who were critical of society's views of older and sexuality also exhibited signs of adhering to society's sexual scripts of older adults. For example, an ASO volunteer who helped to hand out condoms while sitting at an HIV/AIDS educational table did not consider that older single men need condoms to practice safe sex while back on the dating scene. The assumption may have been that these older men were not sexual, or knew how to practice safe sex and therefore did not need any condoms (which the literature (Altschuler et al., 2004, for example) says is highly unlikely). Either way, they were overlooked as candidates for HIV/AIDS prevention education.

Physician Influence

I had anticipated that I would hear references to physicians being reluctant to discuss issues of sexuality with older adults, but I had not expected to learn that physicians and other medical personnel were acting as gatekeepers for patients' receiving HIV prevention education. Some respondents believed that physicians (especially in smaller towns and rural areas) could also serve as barriers against testing, even if the older adult requests an HIV test or prevention education. Something I heard repeatedly during the interviews was that physicians held a large amount of influence over older adults, who often took the physicians' word as authority. If older adults were told by their physicians that they were not at risk and therefore did not need to be tested or receive HIV/AIDS prevention education, there was nothing the ASO personnel could do to provide prevention education to this population. Further, several interviewees voiced frustration with having to educate physicians and medical personnel about HIV/AIDS at the same time as trying to work in partnership with them to help provide prevention education to the communities.

Based on this information, there could be a pattern in which physicians in these four Midwestern states hold stereotypes and adhere to sexual scripts about older adults. Because of this, older adults are less likely to receive HIV/AIDS prevention education from medical personnel. This could be a dangerous trend, as older adults are probably more likely to speak to their doctor about such intimate information than a stranger at an ASO. However, I can only hypothesize that this is a trend and explore it further in future research.

CONCLUSIONS AND IMPLICATIONS

The findings from this research suggest that state HIV/AIDS policymakers and ASO personnel fail in their efforts to provide much needed information that would reduce the HIV/AIDS infection rate among older adults. However, it is not simply that they are adhering to sexual scripts about older adults, which influence them to believe that older adults are not at risk for infection for various reasons. While at times this is certainly the case, there are also other social factors at play that result in older adults being left out of HIV/AIDS prevention education and health promotion in the Midwest.

This research also uncovered hints of physician influence over older adults, especially when it comes to HIV testing and prevention education.

This is an important finding, given that older adults in the conservative Midwest would most likely be reluctant to seek out HIV/AIDS prevention education on their own unless it came from a medical authority figure with which they had a past history. Further, the fact that state policymakers and ASO personnel have to educate physicians and medical personnel about HIV/AIDS is a surprising revelation. If older adults are not being educated about their risk of HIV/AIDS infection when being prescribed Viagra or when discussing their sexual or drug histories with their physicians, they are probably not going to make an effort to seek out this information from an ASO or state agency. Physicians and other medical personnel certainly need to be educated about HIV/AIDS – especially how it manifests itself as normal signs of aging in older adults – in order to avoid misdiagnosing those who may already be infected, as well as to provide some form of prevention education to their patients if this epidemic has any chance of being slowed.

What became obvious as this research progressed was the interconnectedness of political, social, and economic factors with the HIV/AIDS epidemic. Perhaps due to the enduring stigma of the disease, federal and state governments and governmental agencies appear reluctant to expand funding to subgroups that are not the typical marginalized groups that are often associated with the epidemic (i.e., gay men, IDUs, and minorities). It is easier to provide funds to already-stigmatized groups than to admit that an older adult may need HIV/AIDS prevention education because he or she is having unprotected sex or injecting drugs. Because of this situation and the trickle-down effect of HIV/AIDS funding, ASOs have to restrict to whom they are able to provide prevention education. So if ASOs are not able to provide HIV/AIDS prevention education to older adults due to funding restrictions, and a large number of physicians are either refusing or are not educated enough about HIV/AIDS to provide education, from what source will older adults receive prevention education? This question remains unanswered.

Addressing these needs is important because of the social and financial implications of the increasing rates and numbers of HIV/AIDS cases among older adults. While many HIV-positive individuals are experiencing great success with their HIV drug cocktails, they are facing the extreme financial burden of their disease. This epidemic is different than previous epidemics in U.S. history because illness has the potential to linger on for years before death, resulting in extreme financial costs. Given the fact that the AIDS epidemic is still a relatively young epidemic, the number of infections and deaths, as well as the cost to society, are staggering. As the lifetime costs of treating HIV/AIDS continues to rise – from $119,300 in 1993 to $618,900 in 2006 (the most recent available data on cost of treating

HIV/AIDS) – the importance of funding is not diminishing (Farnham, 2010; Schackman et al., 2006).

The social cost and degree of suffering is also high with HIV/AIDS, and the disability-adjusted life-years of this particular disease – the age of the infected, the degree of disability, and the number of deaths – all have had the highest health-care costs and loss of productivity to society of any disease in modern history. HIV/AIDS remains the only disease in which states and institutions are receiving grants and reimbursements to help coordinate both inpatient services and services in the community (Fox, 1988). These grants and reimbursements are necessary as HIV/AIDS is a disease that has the potential to linger for several years, thereby costing more than other diseases. Due to the expense associated with HIV/AIDS drugs and treatments, federal funds are unable to cover all related expenses.

Older adults utilize more health care dollars than any other age group, and there are predictions that increasing numbers of older adults with HIV/AIDS will cause an even bigger strain on the nation's health care industry (Orel, Spence, & Steele, 2005). According to research (ACRIA, 2006), the aging HIV/AIDS population faces a system of health care and social supports that is not prepared to meet its needs. Further, older adults may find fewer HIV/AIDS community support systems available to them than those available to younger adults, which may explain why older adults as a whole are not accessing ASOs or getting tested for HIV/AIDS (Avis & Smith, 1998; Neundorfer et al., 2004).

The impact of HIV/AIDS on public and private finances is but one concern that researchers and medical personnel will continue to face as the U.S. HIV/AIDS population continues to age and increase.The HIV/AIDS epidemic has been complicated by social constructs – prevailing sexual scripts, the enduring stigma of HIV/AIDS, and the construction of risk groups. The lack of federal and state funding, enduring sexual scripts, risky sexual behavior, and the continuing stigma associated with HIV/AIDS combine as a force that continues to challenge ASO personnel, state policymakers, and medical personnel.The "problem" of older adults and HIV/AIDS is a bureaucratic and social predicament with a looming challenge to the U.S. public health system.

ACKNOWLEDGMENT

IRB Approval (University of Kansas) #15942. Research funded by The Horowitz Foundation for Social Policy.

REFERENCES

ACRIA (AIDS Community Research Initiative of America). (2004). (AIDS Community Research Initiative of America). Over 50 with HIV. *Newsletter*, *13*(3). New York, NY: AIDS Community Research Initiative of America.

ACRIA (AIDS Community Research Initiative of America). (2006). *Research on older adults with AIDS: Final report*. New York, NY: AIDS Community Research Initiative of America.

Altschuler, J., Katz, A., & Tynan, M. (2004). Developing and implementing an HIV/AIDS educational curriculum for older adults. *The Gerontologist*, *44*, 121–126.

Avert.org. (2005). Local HIV/AIDS service organizations in the USA. *Internet*. Retrieved from http://www.avert.org/hiv_usa.htm. Accessed on October 26, 2005.

Avis, N., & Smith, K. (1998). Quality of life in older adults with HIV disease. *Research on Aging*, *20*, 822–846.

Bardella, C. (2002). Pilgrimages of the plagued: AIDS, body and society. *Body and Society*, *8*, 79–105.

Barton-Villagrana, H., Bedney, B., & Miller, R. (2002). Peer relationships among community-based organizations (CBO) providing HIV prevention services. *The Journal of Primary Prevention*, *23*(2), 215–234.

Berkeley, D., & Ross, D. (2003). Strategies for improving the sexual health of young people. *Culture, Health & Sexuality*, *5*, 71–86.

Brennan, D. J., Emlet, C. A., & Eady, A. (2011). HIV, sexual health, and psychosocial issues among older adults living with HIV in North America. *Ageing International*. doi:10.1007/s12126-011-9111-6

Brooks, C., Jr. (2003). Older adults and HIV. *The New Social Worker*, *10*, 23.

Catania, J., Turner, H., Kegeles, S., Stall, R., Pollack, L., & Coates, T. (1989b). Older Americans and AIDS: Transmission risks and primary prevention research needs. *The Gerontologist*, *29*, 373–381.

Cloud, G., Brown, R., Salooja, N., & McClean, K. (2003). Newly diagnosed HIV infection in an octogenarian: The elderly are not 'immune'. *Age and Ageing*, *32*(3), 353–354.

Coon, D. W., Lipman, P. D., & Ory, M. G. (2003). Designing effective HIV/AIDS social and behavioral interventions for the 50 plus population. *Journal of AIDS Research*, *33*(S2), S194–S205.

Davidson, K., & Fennell, G. (2002). New intimate relationships in later life. *Ageing International*, *27*, 3–10.

Doyle, K., Weber, E., Atkinson, J. H., Grant, I., Woods, S. P., & The HIV Neurobehavioral Research Program (HNRP) Group. (2012, January 14). *Aging, prospective memory, and health-related quality of life in HIV infection*. AIDS Behavior. [Epub ahead of print]. Retrieved from http://www.springerlink.com/content/b34832414k27006k/. Accessed on June 1, 2012.

Emlet, C. (2008). Truth and consequences: A qualitative exploration of HIV disclosure in older adults. *AIDS Care*, *20*, 710–717.

Emlet, C., Tangenberg, K., & Siverson, C. (2002). A feminist approach to practice in working with midlife and older women with HIV/AIDS. *Affilia*, *17*, 229–251.

Emlet, C., Tozay, S., & Raveis, V. (2010). I'm not going to die from the AIDS": Resilience in aging with HIV disease. *The Gerontologist*, *51*(1), 101–111.

Falvo, N., & Norman, S. (2004). Never too old to learn: The impact of an HIV/AIDS education program on older adults' knowledge. *Clinical Gerontologist, 27*, 103–117.

Farnham, P. G. (2010). Do reduced inpatient costs associated with highly active antiretroviral therapy (HAART) Balance the overall cost for HIV treatment? *Applied Health Economics and Health Policy, 8*(2), 75–88.

Farrell, J., & Belza, B. (2012). Are older patients comfortable discussing sexual health with nurses? *Nursing Research, 61*(1), 51–57.

Fitzpatrick, L. K. (2011). Routine HIV testing in older adults. *Virtual Mentor, 13*(2), 109–112.

Fox, D. M. (1988). AIDS and the American health polity: the history and prospects of a crisis of authority. In E. Fee & D. M. Fox (Eds.), *AIDS: The burden of history* (pp. 316–344).

Frontini, M., Chotalia, J., Spizale, L., Onya, W., Ruiz, M., & Clark, R. A. (2012). Sex and race effects on risk for selected outcomes among elderly HIV-infected patients. *Journal of the International Association of Physicians in AIDS Care (JIAPAC), 11*, 12–15.

Gallagher, T., & Petersen, J. (1992). Patterns of HIV-AIDS knowledge and attitudes among Michigan adults: Implications for public health education. *Sociological Practice Review, 3*, 251–257.

Gazmararian, J., Curran, J., Parker, R., Bernhardt, J., & DeBuono, B. (2005). Public health literacy in America: An ethical imperative. *American Journal of Preventive Medicine, 28*, 317–322.

Genke, J. (2000). HIV/AIDS and older adults: The invisible ten percent. *Care Management Journals, 2*, 196–205.

Gott, M., & Hinchliff, S. (2003). How important is sex in later life? The views of older people. *Social Science and Medicine, 56*, 1617–1628.

Gott, M., Hinchliff, S., & Galena, E. (2004). General practitioner attitudes to discussing sexual health issues with older people. *Social Science and Medicine, 58*, 2093–2103.

Harawa, N. T., Leng, M., Kim, J., & Cunningham, W. E. (2011). Racial/ethnic and gender differences among older adults in nonmonogamous partnerships, time spent single, and human immunodeficiency virus testing. *Sexually Transmitted Diseases, 38*(12), 1110–1117.

Hayes Taylor, K. (2004). *More seniors crushed by HIV, AIDS. Global Action on Aging.* Retrieved from http://www.globalaging.org/health/us/2004/hiv.htm. Accessed on June 26, 2007.

Heckman, T., Kochman, A., Sikkema, K., & Kalichman, S. (1999). Depressive symptomatology, daily stressors, and ways of coping among middle-age and older adults living with HIV disease. *Journal of Mental Health and Aging, 5*, 311–322.

Holland, J., Ramazanoglu, C., & Scott, S. (1990). AIDS: from panic stations to power relations sociological perspectives and problems. *Sociology, 25*, 499–518.

Huffstutter, P.J.(2007). A warning on safe sex at any age. *Los Angeles Times*, November 26. Retrieved from http://www.latimes.com/news/nationworld/nation/la-na-safesex26nov 26,0,4906332.story?page=1&coll=la-home-center

Hughes, A. K. (2011). HIV knowledge and attitudes among providers in aging: Results from a national survey. *AIDS Patient Care and STDs, 25*(9), 539–545.

Illa, L., Brickman, A., Saint-Jean, G., Echenique, M., Metsch, L., Eisdorfer, C., … Sanchez-Martinez, M. (2008). Sexual risk behaviors in late middle age and older HIV seropositive adults. *AIDS and Behavior, 12*, 935–942.

Inelmen, E. M., Gasparini, G., & Enzi, G. (2005). HIV/AIDS in older adults: A case report and literature review. *Geriatrics, 60*(9), 26–30.

Jang, H., Anderson, P. G., & Mentes, J. C. (2011). Aging and living with HIV/AIDS. *Journal of Gerontological Nursing, 37*(12), 4–7.

Johnson, S. (2006). *The ghost map: The story of London's most terrifying epidemic – And how it changed science, cities, and the modern world.* New York, NY: Riverhead Books.

Karpiak, S., Shippy, R. A., & Cantor, M. H. (2006). *Research on older adults with HIV.* New York, NY: AIDS Community Research Initiative of America.

Keigher, S., Stevens, P., & Plach, S. (2004). Midlife women with HIV: Health, social, and economic factors shaping their futures. *Journal of HIV/AIDS and Social Services, 3,* 43–58.

Kilgannon, C. (2007). Greatest generation learns about great safe sex. *New York Times,* February 14. Retrieved from http://www.nytimes.com/2007/02/14/nyregion/14sex.html?ex = 1185422400&en = a3b6559a17af61e0&ei = 5070. Accessed on February 14, 2007.

Langley, L.(2006).Sex and the single septuagenarian. *Salon.com,* December 4. Retrieved from http://www.salon.com/mwt/feature/2006/12/04/senior_std/index1.html. Accessed on June 26, 2007.

Lewis, L., & Kertzner, R. M. (2003). Toward improved interpretation and theory building of African American male sexualities. *The Journal of Sex Research, 40.*

Lindau, S. T., Schumm, L. P., Laumann, E., Levinson, W., O'Muircheartaigh, C., & Waite, L. (2007). A national study of sexuality and health among older adults in the U.S. *New England Journal of Medicine, 357*(8), 762–774.

Mack, K., & Bland, S. (1999). HIV testing behaviors and attitudes regarding HIV/AIDS of adults aged 50–64. *The Gerontologist, 39,* 687–694.

Morgan, L., & Tyler, E. (1971). Is public health education community development? *Community Development Journal, 6,* 28–37.

Musa, D., Schulz, R., Harris, R., Silverman, M., & Thomas, S. B. (2009). Trust in the health care system and the use of preventive health services by older black and white adults. *American Journal of Public Health, 99*(7), 1293–1299.

National Alliance of State and Territorial AIDS Directors. (2005). *NASTAD list of directors.* Washington, DC. Retrieved from http://nastad.org/News/NASTADDirectory.htm. Accessed on October 26, 2005.

Nettleton, S., & Bunton, R. (1995). Sociological critiques of health promotion. In R. Bunton, S. Nettleton & R. Burrows (Eds.), *The sociology of health promotion: critical analyses of consumption, lifestyle and risk* (pp. 41–59). London: Routledge.

Netting, N., & Burnett, M. (2004). Twenty years of student sexual behavior: Subcultural adaptations to a changing health environment. *Adolescence, 39,* 19–39.

Neundorfer, M. M., Camp, C. J., Lee, M. M., Skrajner, M. J., Malone, M. L., & Carr, J. R. (2004). Compensating for cognitive deficits in persons aged 50 and over with HIV/AIDS: A pilot study of a cognitive intervention. *Journal of HIV/AIDS and Social Services, 3,* 79–97.

Nusbaum, M. R. H., Singh, A. R., & Pyles, A. A. (2004). Sexual healthcare needs of women aged 65 and older. *Journal of the American Geriatric Society, 52,* 117–122.

Orel, N., Spence, M., & Steele, J. (2005). Getting the message out to older adults: Effective HIV health education risk reduction publications. *Journal of Applied Gerontology, 24*(5), 490–508.

Orel, N., Wright, J., & Wagner, J. (2004). Scarcity of HIV/AIDS risk-reduction materials targeting the needs of older adults among state departments of public health. *The Gerontologist, 44*, 693–696.

Orsulic-Jeras, S., Shepher, J. B., & Britton, P. (2003). Counseling older adults with HIV/AIDS: A strength-based model of treatment. *Journal of Mental Health Counseling, 25*, 233–244.

Ory, M., & Mack, K. (1998a). Middle-aged and older people with AIDS: trends in national surveillance rates, transmission routes, and risk factors. *Research on Aging, 20*, 653–665.

Preston, D. B., D'Augelli, A. R., Cain, R. E., & Schulze, F. (2002). Issues in the development of HIV-preventive interventions for men who have sex with men (MSM) in rural areas. *The Journal of Primary Prevention, 23*(2), 199–214.

Poindexter, C., & Keigher, S. (2004). Inclusion of 'older' adults with HIV. *Journal of HIV/ AIDS & Social Services, 3*, 3–8.

Roeder, K. (2002). Rural HIV/AIDS services: Participant and provider perceptions. *Journal of HIV/AIDS & Social Services, 1*(2), 21–42.

Riley, M. W., & Riley, J., Jr. (1989). The lives of older people and changing social roles. *Annals of the American Academy of Political and Social Science, 503*, 14–28.

Sankar, A., Nevedal, A., Neufeld, S., Berry, R., & Luborsky, M. (2011). What do we know about older adults and HIV? A review of social and behavioral literature. *AIDS Care, 23*(10), 1187–1207.

Schackman, B., Gebo, K., Walensky, R., Losina, E., Muccio, T., Sax, P., ... Freedberg, K. (2006). The lifetime cost of current human immunodeficiency virus care in the United States. *Medical Care, 44*(11), 990–997.

Schiltz, M. A., & Sandfort, Th. G. M. (2000). HIV-positive people, risk and sexual behavior. *Social Science and Medicine, 50*, 1571–1588.

Short, J., Jr. (1984). The social fabric at risk: Toward the social transformation of risk analysis. *American Sociological Review, 49*(6), 711–725.

Siegel, K., Raveis, V., & Karus, D. (1998). Perceived advantages and disadvantages of age among older HIV-infected adults. *Research on Aging, 20*, 686–712.

Simon, W. (1986). Sexual scripts: Permanence and change. *Archives of Sexual Behavior, 15*, 97–120.

Simon, W., & Gagnon, J. (1984). Sexual scripts. *Society, 22*, 53–60.

Simone, M., & Appelbaum, J. (2008). HIV in older adults. *Geriatrics, 63*(12), 6–12.

Stombeck, R., & Levy, J. (1998). Educational strategies and interventions targeting adults age 50 and older for HIV/AIDS prevention. *Research on Aging, 20*, 912–937.

Substance Abuse and Mental Health Services Administration. (1997).*National household survey on drug abuse: Population estimates, 1996*. Series H-4. Washington DC.: Substance Abuse and Mental Health Services Administration. Retrieved from http://www.oas.-samhsa.gov/trends.htm. Accessed on January 31, 2006.

Tierney, K. (1999). Toward a critical sociology of risk. *Sociological Forum, 14*, 215–242.

The Henry J. Kaiser Family Foundation. (2007, August 31). *Health officials, policymakers should implement HIV prevention measures aimed at older adults, letter to editor says.* Report.. Washington, DC.: The Henry J. Kaiser Family Foundation. Retrieved from http://www.kff.org. Accessed on October 31, 2007.

Vance, D., Brennan, M., Enah, C., Smith, G., & Kaur, J. (2011). Religion, spirituality, and older adults with HIV: Critical personal and social resources for an aging epidemic. *Clinical Intervention Aging, 6*, 101–109.

Weinberg, M., Swensson, R. G., & Hammersmith, S. K. (1983). Sexual autonomy and the status of women: Models of female sexuality in U.S. sex manuals from 1950 to 1980. *Social Problems, 30,* 312–324.

White, C., & Catania, J. (1982). Psychoeducational intervention for sexuality with the aged, family members of the aged, and people who work with the aged. *International Journal of Aging and Human Development, 15,* 121–138.

Williams, E., & Donnelly, J. (2002). Older Americans and AIDS: Some guidelines for prevention. *Social Work, 47,* 105–112.

THE SOCIOLOGY OF CHRONIC ILLNESS AND SELF-CARE MANAGEMENT

Mark Tausig

ABSTRACT

Purpose – *The purpose of this chapter is to use sociological theory and research to develop an explanation for how chronic illnesses are managed at home and to thereby suggest some ways in which a sociological perspective can be applied to improve health care for persons with chronic illnesses. Self-care illness management is crucial to the prevention of and reduction of morbidity and mortality from chronic illness.*

Methodology/approach – *Review and synthesis of research literature.*

Findings – *Sociological research and theory suggest two important insights that should inform health care services aimed at improving self-care; chronic illness care occurs in the context of the household, neighborhood, and community and, therefore, the "patient" (i.e., the object of health services) is really the caregiving social network around the patient, and because the risk of chronic illness and the resources available to deal with it are socially (and unequally) distributed, "health care" interventions need to take account of disparities in risks and resources that will affect the patient's ability to successfully comply with self-care regimens.*

Social Determinants, Health Disparities and Linkages to Health and Health Care
Research in the Sociology of Health Care, Volume 31, 247–272
Copyright © 2013 by Emerald Group Publishing Limited
All rights of reproduction in any form reserved
ISSN: 0275-4959/doi:10.1108/S0275-4959(2013)0000031013

Research limitations/implications – *The review does not include an examination of the clinical research literature. It does, however, suggest that sociologists need to explicitly study chronic illness and health care related to it.*

Originality/value of chapter – *The chapter links the long history of research on family caregiving to the concern with the success of self-management of chronic illness. It also links concerns about that success to social disparities in the distribution of social resources and hence to morbidity and mortality disparities.*

Keywords: Chronic illness; self-care management; caregiving; support networks

Improvements in the treatment and control of infectious disease and the general increase in life span have made chronic illness more prevalent worldwide. The health care system, however, still struggles to promote and sustain self-care illness management that is crucial to prevention and the reduction of morbidity and mortality from chronic illness. Self-care occurs largely out of the view of the health care system in the household and general community. As a result, studies of medical (non-)compliance or (non-)adherence with self-care protocols designed to minimize the daily and long-term impact of chronic illness indicate that we do not possess a full understanding of how routine compliance with medical advice can be obtained (Van Dulmen et al., 2007).

The purpose of this chapter is to employ sociological theory and research to explain how such illnesses might be managed at home and to thereby suggest some ways in which a sociological perspective can be applied to improve health care for persons with chronic illnesses. While the health care system has not developed an adequate, effective method to assure self-care management of chronic illness, neither have medical sociologists provided an explanation for variations in the quantity and quality of self-care management resources that might inform the efforts of health care providers to develop effective methods to promote self-care management of chronic illness. The health care system and medical sociology have both adapted prior models of care and theoretical accounts of the health practitioner–patient relationship to deal with chronic illness but these adaptations can be shown to be insufficient both medically and sociologically.

I will argue that sociological research and theory suggest two important insights that should inform health care services aimed at improving self-care; chronic illness care occurs in the context of the household, neighborhood, and community, and, therefore, the "patient" (i.e., the object of health services) is really the caregiving social network around the patient, and, because the risk of chronic illness and the resources available to deal with it are socially distributed, "health care" interventions need to take account of disparities in risks and resources that will affect the patient's ability to successfully comply with self-care regimens.

The ideal relationship between doctors (and other health care providers) and patients (and those involved in caregiving roles) when a chronic illness is the basis for the relationship requires finding a method to impart the practical knowledge held by medical providers to patients, their families, and the community in such a way that formal health services and informal self-care minimize the health risk associated with the illness. It does not appear, however, that such a relationship has been institutionalized into health care practice as evidenced by the vast literature on patient "compliance" or "adherence." For its part, medical sociology has not fully moved away from the physician–patient model that was originally articulated to describe this relationship in instances of acute illness or injury (Parsons, 1951). While this theoretical specification has been critiqued (Gallagher, 1976), sociologists have not developed a separate sociological model of the health practitioner–patient relationship in chronic illness that is based on the sociology *of* medicine (vs. the sociology *in medicine*). As a result, theoretical and practical insights regarding chronic illness have been piecemeal.

I will review health delivery models for the treatment of chronic illnesses and sociological approaches to explain chronic illness management in order to extract a critique that addresses the weaknesses of existing models of the health care system–patient relationship and sociological accounts of that relationship. The end result of this exercise also addresses health disparities and health services disparities.

MEDICAL MODELS OF CHRONIC ILLNESS AND CARE

We start by noting the historical shift in the societal disease burden in advanced industrial societies from acute illness to chronic illness. In Table 1 we see that deaths from infection (pneumonia, influenza, tuberculosis, diarrhea, etc.) held the top spot among the causes of death in 1900 in the United States but that these have been replaced by more chronic conditions

Table 1. Leading Causes of Death in the United States in 1900 and 2010.

1900	2010
Pneumonia and influenza	Diseases of the heart
Tuberculosis	Malignant neoplasms
Diarrhea, enteritis and ulceration of the intestines	Chronic lower respiratory diseases
Diseases of the heart	Cerebrovascular diseases
Intracranial lesions of vascular origin	Accidents
Nephritis	Alzheimer's disease
All accidents	Diabetes mellitus
Cancer and other malignant tumors	Nephritis
Senility	Influenza and pneumonia
Diphtheria	Intentional self-harm (suicide)

CDC (2012); Murphy, Jiaquan, and Kochanek (2012).

(diseases of the heart, malignancies, and chronic respiratory diseases) in 2010. These changes are generally attributed to improvements in sanitation and surveillance of epidemic disease, antibiotics, and the aging of the population that results from control of infectious disease.

The health care enterprise has adapted to this shift in the disease burden. But, it has done so in the context of a hospital-based medical model that still centers care systems on a "top-down" approach in which expert knowledge is imparted to patients. Moreover, the system is an individualized one in which the practitioner–patient relationship is the core of service provision. The attempt by the health care system to adapt to the need to treat chronic illnesses is embodied in the development of "extended care" models and variants. Although not the first to propose such a model, the essay by Wagner, Austin, and Von Korff (1996) that systematically described the elements of "high-quality chronic illness care" made an important contribution to policy and practice in health care systems. Wagner, Austin, and Von Korff (1996, p. 513) pointed out that, "Medical practices, especially in primary care, are generally organized to respond to the acute and urgent needs of their patients." However, they argue that the effective management of chronic health conditions "requires that they receive appropriate clinical care while they and their families appropriately cope with the illness and its therapies" (p. 512). The self-management tasks for patients are those outlined by Clark et al. (1991); engage in activities that promote health and build physiological reserve, such as exercise, proper nutrition, social activation, and sleep; interact with health care providers and systems and adhere to recommended treatment protocols;

monitor one's own physical and emotional status and make appropriate management decisions on the basis of symptoms and signs; and manage the impact of the illness on the ability to function in important roles, on emotions and self-esteem, and on relations with others. Wagner, Austin, and Von Korff (1996, p. 514) then assess the health care system as generally failing to include services that address and facilitate these self-management tasks. Moreover, they hypothesize that deficiencies in the health care system result in "failures in self-management of the illness or risk factors as a result of patient passivity or ignorance stemming from inadequate or inconsistent patient assessment, education, motivation, and feedback." All of this led to the description of a model for effective chronic illness care (Wagner, Davis, Schaefer, Von Korff, & Austin, 1999) that came to be known as the chronic care model (CCM) (Wagner et al., 2001) and to several modifications, extensions, and improvements (Barr et al., 2003; Glasgow et al., 2002; Ministry of Health and Long-term Care, 2007).

These extended chronic care models are complex and appreciate many of the factors that affect chronic care management. The expanded CCM (Barr et al., 2003), for example, makes the case that chronic care services need to account for the social, economic, and community-level factors that affect the success of functional and clinical-related outcomes. The expanded chronic care model thus adds a population health perspective to the clinical model proposed by Wagner et al. (1999). Indeed it is suggested that adding a population health model reflects the recognition that "the most significant determinants of health are social and economic factors" and that the "gradient nature of health status suggests that it is embedded in collective factors of society" (Barr et al., 2003, p. 75). And, while these suggestions are consistent with a sociological perspective on health and health care, actual health care delivery remains focused on clinical and educational interventions. *It is precisely this disjuncture between the recognition that social conditions affect self-care and illness conditions and the absence of any systematic incorporation of health care interventions that address social conditions which arguably makes many current clinical interventions relatively ineffective.*

Instead, the health care literature, in the effort to understand the relative ineffectiveness of health care services and organization intended to address chronic illness, has produced a vast literature on patient compliance/adherence. The focus of this literature and the service system recommendations that follow from it is to improve the ability of patients to comply with (or adhere to) the recommendations of medical professionals without reference to larger social and economic contexts. Lorig (1996) and Lorig et al. (1999), for example, argue that the health care system response to chronic illness management has not paid sufficient attention to the need for patient self-management and she proposes a model that "assists patients in gaining skills and, more important, in gaining the confidence to apply these skills on a day-to-day basis" (Lorig, 1996, pp. 677–678). The Chronic Disease Self-Management Program (CDSMP) is designed to educate patients regarding the management of their disease(s) and to give them the confidence (self-efficacy) to act on their own behalf (Lorig et al., 1999).

Patient self-management models, however, have been criticized on a variety of levels. Thorne and Paterson (2001) note that such programs assume that there is a linear relationship between health-related education, trust between the patient and practitioner, and effective self-management. Gately, Rogers, and Sanders (2007) noted that the relationship between self-management education and the use of health services is not well-understood. Paterson, Russell, and Thorne (2001), Newman, Steed, and Mulligan (2004), and Delamater (2006) note the complexity of the objectives of self-care interventions. There are social, physical, logistical, and economic barriers to self-care (Bayliss, Steiner, Fernald, Crane, & Main, 2003). Kendall and Rogers (2007) argued that the CDSMP program ignores the social context in which it is embedded. Thorne, Paterson, and Russell (2003) argue that not much is known about everyday decision-making by patients regarding their illnesses.

While "extended care" models of treatment recognize both the limitations of the role that health care professionals can play and the public health components of prevention and maintenance, they are still largely centered on the old-fashioned physician (as expert)–patient(as nonexpert) relationship. Ironically the "expert-patient" movement that seeks to reorient the physician–patient relationship by trying to equalize knowledge across actors actually represents recognition that the physician–patient relationship is generally one of medical dominance. The expert patient perspective recognizes two elements of the physician–patient relationship that are different in dealing with chronic illness. First, it is intended to acknowledge that both health care providers and patients contribute relevant information about the disease state and factors affecting the disease state (Greenhalgh, 2009; Ministry of Health and Long-term Care, 2007). Second, it recognizes that much of the management of the disease occurs in day-to-day activities and decisions that are beyond the health care system to monitor and interpret (Bodenheimer, Lorig, Holman, & Grumbach, 2002).

The intention of the expert patient movement is to reduce paternalistic practices on the part of physicians and to develop self-esteem and self-efficacy among patients. The expert patient notion is clearly an attempt to equalize the status of medical practitioners and the patient. But, harkening back to the critique leveled by Wagner, Austin, and Von Korff (1996), all of these efforts to expand the modes of health care delivery and to recognize the need to consider details of patient behavior continue to reside within the hospital-based biomedical model of treatment. That model is still, at base, an acute care model that places the physician in the dominant position in the provider–patient relationship. The empowerment of patients through access to knowledge is intended to equalize the participation of physicians and their patients but even when this training of patients is conducted by "lay" trainers, research does not show that attempts to alter the relationship improves health outcomes, improves self-management, or reduces health care costs (Greenhalgh, 2009). Sociologists have also studied self-help groups, many of which are organized around specific chronic illness conditions. Such groups are often formed to bolster patient knowledge and self-efficacy relative to the formal medical system (Borkman, 1990). The internet has also become a possible mechanism that conditions the relationship between the health care system and the individual (Lemire, Sicotte, & Paré, 2008).

Reviews of patient compliance/adherence research suggest that all of the above efforts have produced limited results (Wagner et al., 1999; Vermeire, Hearnshaw, Van Royen, & Denekens, 2001; van Dulmen et al. (2007). These reviews uniformly note the low rates of compliance/adherence by community-residing patients *despite* efforts by health care practitioners to educate and support patients, to decrease the status differences between doctors and patients, or to decentralize health services. Although there are certainly examples of programs that are effective (van Dulmen et al., 2007; Wagner et al., 1999), the overall assessment of medical programs designed to increase patient compliance/adherence is that they are largely ineffective and that there is little theoretical understanding of the fundamental issues related to effective patient self-management. "The problem of non-adherence to medical treatment remains a challenge for the medical profession and social scientists. Efforts to explain and improve patient adherence often appear to be ineffective. Although successful adherence interventions do exist, half of interventions seem to fail and adherence theories lack sufficient explaining power. As a result of the widespread problem of poor adherence, substantial numbers of patients do not get the maximum benefit of medical treatment, resulting in poor health outcomes, lower quality of life, and increased health care costs. In spite of many advances made in adherence research, nonadherence rates have remained nearly unchanged in the last decades" (Van Dulmen et al., 2007, p. 2).

Summary: Despite considerable effort to develop effective models of self-care by health care providers, such services are disappointingly ineffective. The focus on proximal care issues may limit the system's ability to understand what needs to be done and how. Reviews and critiques (Bury, 2004; Bury, Newbould, & Taylor, 2005) are consistent in identifying the practitioner–patient interaction as the key relationship that is not understood well-enough, and is thus, relatively ineffective. Because the doctor–patient relationship has been a core concern of medical sociologists for so long, we now turn to the sociological literature to see how sociologists have conceptualized the problem and to look for insights that might apply to the relationship in the context of chronic illness.

SOCIOLOGICAL MODELS OF CHRONIC ILLNESS AND CARE

Talcott Parsons (1951) provided the theoretical account of the physician–patient relationship that still influences sociological conceptualizations of the relationships between health care providers and patients. Part of that description is based on the patient sick role and, in terms of its immediate relevance, the obligation of the patient to comply with medical treatment and advice as a condition for retaining access to the sick role and its exemptions from normal social role obligations. In health care, this notion is clearly analogous to the notion of compliance/adherence. Compliance/ adherence is a marker that patients are acting within the sick role, and failure to comply with care recommendations of health care practitioners is seen as a sign of patient deviance that reinforces the Parsonian description of the doctor–patient relationship as it was outlined with an acute care model of health care in mind.

It is helpful here to consider the discussion contributed by Gallagher (1976) regarding "The Parsonian Sociology of Illness." Gallagher notes that Parsons was not attempting to explain health practices so much as he was trying to develop general social theory using health care as an exemplar. This orientation partly accounts for the limitations of the Parsonian view, including the following points made by Gallagher (1976, p. 209): "the deviance conception fails to account for the situation of the patient with a chronic somatic illness or disability. It fails to account for preventative health care or health maintenance, and it presents a relatively undifferentiated picture of the *social structure of health care* (italics in the original). It pays little attention to the possibility that the varied types of physician role, coupled with variations in the setting of medical practice, may induce systematic differences in patient performance and expectations."

In short, Gallagher (1976) identified all of the theoretical limitations of the Parsonian view relative to the sociology *of* medicine that I also argue have not yet been adequately addressed concerning a sociology of chronic illness. Gallagher notes that the conception of illness as deviance *ala* Parsons is not easy to apply to chronic illnesses because of the indefinite/lifelong duration of such illnesses. Moreover, he notes that the objective in treating chronic illness is not recovery but adaptation. Gallagher notes that, "the treatment of chronic illness draws upon elements of family and lay social support which require more theoretical recognition (Gallagher, 1976, p. 210). He explains that, "the patient must come to accept his condition and to manage his own treatment and rehabilitation within the limits of what the physician can delegate to lay implementation" (Gallagher, 1976, p. 210). With these observations, Gallagher is able to specify the missing elements of a sociological theory of chronic illness. Such a theory must accord a substantial autonomous component to the role of the patient; there must be a greater scope for the patient's values and resources, differences in adaptation based on physical and social setting need to be considered, including households as physical and temporal environments that supply resources, and the theory must more accurately account for the therapeutic impact of the family and other lay supportive systems. Finally, he notes that the "blind spot in professional practice stems directly from the nature of medical practice and the social structure of medical care, both of which place heavy emphasis upon the cognitive understanding of disease process" (Gallagher, 1976, p. 213).

Medical sociologists reading the argument above should immediately recognize that each of these observations has led to separate and productive lines of research (e.g., family caregiving, social support and health, support groups and health). What has not developed is a theoretical account that incorporates Gallagher's observations and thus directly addresses the inadequacy of the Paronsian theoretical description of the doctor–patient relationship in acute illness and care as it would apply to chronic illness. Indeed, these areas of research (caregiving, social support and health, support groups and health) have largely progressed without reference to the general context of chronic illness!

To the extent that caregiving within a family represents the lay response to the presence of chronic health conditions and the need to manage these in the household, everyday context, then caregiving and its effects on care-recipient health represents one of the ways that sociologists study chronic illness and its health consequences. If the object of caregiving is to sustain the care-recipient so that chronic health conditions do not deteriorate as quickly as they might and the care-recipient avoids health complications that result in increased need for formal health care services and or hospitalization or institutionalization, then caregiving studies can be seen as addressing the management of patient health needs within the family. The vast majority of caregiving research focuses on care to older family members. I do not mean to imply that aging is equivalent to a chronic illness, of course. I am making the argument that caregiving and the resultant health outcomes for care-recipients can, however, be viewed as one way that sociologists have studied the (self)-management of chronic illness. That most studies of caregiving are focused on health or psychological outcomes for caregivers rather than care-recipients also does not negate the argument I make about those studies that focus on care-recipient outcomes. Horowitz (1985a, b) describes the functions of caregiving in terms of care-recipient benefits which include emotional support, direct service provision, linkages with the formal service sector, and financial assistance.

Caregiver–care-recipient studies are, in fact, largely concerned with the dyadic or individual consequences of this relationship. Mostly the physician– "patient" or health care system–"patient" relationship is not considered simultaneously with the dyadic relationship (but, see Rosow (1981) or Haug (1994) for discussions of the health care triad or Noelker and Bass (1989) or Litwak (1985) for a discussion of service specialization or supplementation of informal care by formal care providers). Caregiver–care-recipient studies can be helpful to medical practitioners nevertheless because they generate insights into the largely invisible (for health care providers) arena of family assistance to persons with chronic health conditions. So, while much of the caregiving literature is conceptualized in ways that have nothing to do with self or family assisted management of chronic illness as an adjunct to formal medical care, this is one way sociologists have ended up studying chronic illness management. Family caregivers and caregiving networks are clearly understood to exist for the purpose of managing the care-recipient's daily physical and emotional needs by mobilizing resources (mostly those of the caregiver and/or the family of the care-recipient) to assist with daily living and long-term health problems. And, notwithstanding the fact that the vast majority of caregiving studies are concerned with caregiver stress outcomes, high levels of caregiver stress are also related to care-recipient institutiona- lization, and thus are relevant to the study of lay management of chronic illness (Aneshensel, Pearlin, & Schuler, 1993; Gaugler, Kane, Kane, &

Newcomer, 2005; McKinlay, Crawford, & Tennstedt, 1995; Miller & McFall, 1991; Newman, Struyk, Wright, & Rice, 1990).

There are sociological perspectives that address the problem from the point of view of the sociology *of* medicine and that have a broader potential to affect how chronic illness is understood and how it might be managed. Strauss and Corbin (1988) approach this problem from a phenomenological perspective. They argue that in order for the health care system to develop an appropriate treatment system for chronic illnesses, it is necessary to understand the challenges of chronic illness from the perspective of those with chronic illnesses. They suggest that the health care system can use this understanding to construct a system that functions in a way that is compatible with the lived experience of chronic illness and maximizes quality of life. Certain principles of their trajectory model are important to note, although I will suggest that they be applied in a different manner than suggested by Strauss and Corbin (1988, pp. 47–48). The trajectory model asserts that: home is the central site where lifelong illness is managed, the major concern of the ill is not managing illness but maintaining quality of life, and lifelong illness requires lifelong work to manage. While there are other elements of the trajectory framework, I will note that these particular components of the model are completely compatible with the caregiver–care-recipient approach and the social-support approach that otherwise represents the sociological study of chronic illness. These aspects of the model also focus our attention on the patient support network as a crucial element in the understanding of and development of services designed to promote the self-management of chronic illness.

If caregiving is seen as a form of social support, there is also a line of research that directly relates social support to adherence to self-care regimens and medical treatment. While the caregiving literature is largely focused on caregiving to impaired elders, the research on social support and adherence with health protocols is most often based on self-care management among persons with diabetes or heart disease (Toljamo & Hentinen, 2001). This research recognizes the immediate social context as relevant to patient behavior (adherence), and therefore broadens the physician–patient relationship to include the family (mostly) as a social context in which patients function (Gallant, 2003). Both Gallant (2003) and DiMatteo (2004) reviewed studies of the relationship between social support and patient adherence. DiMatteo (2004, p. 212) concluded that: " Social support may buffer stress and allow an individual to engage in more adaptive sick-role behaviors ... The presence of close others may result in the direct or indirect control of behavior, facilitating adherence through internalization of norms and the provision of sanctions for deviating from behavior that is conducive to health."

The role of support groups and now, the internet, as sources of social support and information have been studied extensively by sociologists (particularly the role of support/self-help groups for "patient" health). These studies highlight the role of network resources beyond those composed of family and friends who most often comprise the proximal caregiving and support resources for the "patient." In general, social networks provide access to material and emotional resources that augment personal resources. The widespread availability of self-help and support groups (often formed around specific disease entities) provides access to information and personal supportive resources that increase the personal expertise of "patients" and affects the power dynamic between the physician and patient (Adamsen & Rasmiussen, 2001; Borkman, 1990; Gottlieb, 1983; Levy, 1978; Stewart, 1990; Trojan, 1989). These studies also recognize that health professionals can and do interact with self-help groups to directly and indirectly help patients (Adamsen & Rasmiussen, 2001; Borkman, 1990; Stewart, 1990).

The use of the internet to obtain health information also represents the use of network resources (albeit not interpersonal network resources) by patients as part of their personal health care. Such use is also seen as a challenge to the existing health provider expert knowledge monopoly and as a boon to patient empowerment (Hardey, 1999; Lemire et al., 2008; McMullan, 2006). There is now evidence that those who obtain health information online may differ from those who obtain information offline. Online users have been found to be better educated and to have higher incomes (Cotten & Gupta, 2004). Such findings suggest that we will observe differences in the use of social and information networks by patients and families based on social status differences that will be discussed later.

To the extent that caregiving studies, social support, support group, and internet use studies represent sociological approaches to the study of the management of chronic illness; they represent approaches within the sociology *in* medicine tradition. The conclusions drawn at the end of these studies are insights into the practical day-to-day management of chronic illness that can be very helpful to health care professionals as they design services to promote patient adherence.

Summary: The major conclusion that can be drawn from sociological studies of caregiving, social support, and health, etc. is that the patient–physician relationship is not descriptive of the actual way that patients come to manage illness. The more accurate relationship would be specified as the physician–"patient nexus" relationship. The medical system focus on patients – perhaps useful for acute illness – may not be the best way to conceptualize the patient-in-the-community. Hence, health services addressed solely to patients may founder on the failure to recognize the caregiving/social support structures that seem to affect patients' ability to manage (as a result of family, friend and social network interaction) their illness. In other words, the sociological literature on caregiving and social support suggests that chronic illness management is probably not *self*-care. It is household/social network/community care management. As such, health providers need to be directed toward the caregiving/support networks of persons with chronic illnesses.

A sociological approach to understanding the social context of the patient response to chronic illness will center on personal (family and friends) and social network resources (the patient nexus) that represent the household and community context of social relationships. These resources are reflected in the notions of caregiving and also of social support. These resources will be mobilized to manage a lifelong, chronic strain/condition. Hence, a sociological understanding of chronic illness care will focus on the social resources (including access to caregivers, family, and network support) that are available to a person with a chronic illness and the social structural conditions that affect the quantity and quality of those social resources.

The previous critique of the medical model approach as represented by extended care models for treating chronic illness noted that such models recognize the importance of social and economic context but do not incorporate these analytic levels into the actual services proposed for delivery. Also, the extended care model is still a model based on the health provider–*patient* relationship. The sociological study of caregiving and social support related to health has thus far made it clear that focusing on the "patient" as the recipient of health services is likely to be inadequate because it fails to also recognize that multiple individuals and groups (the patient nexus) contribute to care and care decisions.

I have chosen to use the term "patient nexus" to represent the object of physician (or health care provider) relationships and suggest that this term should replace "patient" when addressing matters of chronic illness management. The term "nexus" is meant to encompass the relevant set of family, friends, and other ties that might affect the consequences of health care interventions. It is also meant to include generalized access to social capital and resources. The medical definition of nexus includes the notions of connection, links, and groups, and is thus perfectly compatible with a sociological notion of nexus.

SOCIAL STRUCTURE, CHRONIC ILLNESS, AND
SELF-CARE MANAGEMENT RESOURCES

To the extent that the patient nexus is recognized by health care providers in any form (e.g., the extended care model), it refers to the proximal level of association where medical practitioners deal directly with service provision and the patient nexus. From this proximal perspective we cannot truly generate a sociological understanding of the levels of caregiving and/or social support, social resources, or social capital that are available to a given individual with a chronic illness. In this case we need to move to a more distal level to understand how the health burden arises and what resources are available to manage that burden at the proximal level. Indeed, I will suggest that the poor outcomes of medical education/training programs that aspire to assist patients with the self-management of their illnesses can only be understood by taking a more distal perspective on the problem. The argument would be that the patient nexus will contain more or fewer resources depending on social status characteristics of the patient and that understanding the success or failure of patient chronic illness management needs to account for these distal effects on resource distribution.

Chronic health conditions are not uniformly distributed within U.S. society. Indeed, one might argue that the meaning of health disparities is partly specified by morbidity patterns such as those displayed in Table 2. Except for the racial/ethnic distribution of respondent–reported heart disease, for all three chronic illnesses listed there are racial/ethnicity, education, and income gradients such that lower status groups have higher prevalence rates of chronic illness. This is an observation that is yet unaccounted for by sociological studies of caregiving and social support generally. This is why the sociology *of* medicine needs to stand apart from and be carried out by investigators who are not part of the medical system (Straus, 1999). To understand the gradient in chronic illness we need to stand back from observations of particular caregiver or social support study populations and develop a theoretical account that factors in the effects of the social gradient that cuts through any particular study sample.

Chronic illness management clearly requires the mobilization of the patient nexus and the resources that the nexus can provide. As sociologists have studied them, social support, caregiving, and support groups are examples of resources. But taking a broader social epidemiological perspective such as implied in Table 2 suggests that the outcome of caregiving or social support resource mobilization might be a function of the quantity and

Table 2. Prevalence of Selected Chronic Health Conditions in the United States by Gender, Race/Ethnicity, Education, and Income.

	Diabetes[a] (%)	Hypertension[b] (%)	Heart Disease[c] (%)
Male	8.1	30.6	12.8
Female	7.7	28.7	10.3
White	7.0	28.8	11.6
Black	11.0	42.6	11.0
Asian	8.2	–	6.7
Hispanic	10.7	25.5[d]	8.3
Less than HS	11.8	37.3	14.5
HS	9.0	35.6	12.7
More than HS	6.2	31.6	12.2
Poor	11.7	32.6	14.5
Near Poor	10.4	32.7	12.8
Middle Income	8.3	29.7	11.8
High Income	5.5	27.4	10.0

[a]Age-adjusted prevalence of medically diagnosed diabetes among adults aged ≥ 18 years, National Interview Survey, United States, 2008. Beckles, Zhu and Moonesinghe (2011).
[b]Age-adjusted percentage of hypertension among adults aged ≥ 18 years, National Health Examination Survey, United States, 2005–2006. Keenan and Rosendorf (2011).
[c]Respondent-reported prevalence of heart disease among adults 18 years of age and over, United States, average annual 2009–2010. U.S. Department of Health and Human Services (2012).
[d]Category is Mexican Americans, only.
Note: HS = high school.

quality of social resources available by dint of social structure. At the social epidemiological level, we observe a gradient in the prevalence of chronic illnesses but we also know that there is a gradient in the distribution of social resources, and the two gradients are likely related (see Berkman, Glass, Brissette, & Seeman, 2000; Bury et al., 2005; Sorensen et al., 2003).

Having suggested a link between the social gradient in the prevalence of chronic illness and the gradient in the distribution of social resources that might be used to manage illness, we can now ask how we can relate the distribution of social resources to the distribution of health disorders and management of those disorders.

Dealing with chronic illness requires a broader recognition of the causes and mediators of chronic illness in order to manage it. Recognition that the immediate context in which patients live affects their ability to comply/adhere with medical protocols and to adapt to health conditions and that the broader context of public health influences individual ability to manage health leads now to the consideration of the sociological contributions to the understanding of this problem. The recognition that the family/household/social network (the patient nexus) is involved in the management of chronic illness makes it clear that we need an explanation of how the social resources associated with a given caregiving network are established and maintained. The structure and function of caregiver/support/ resource networks is partially determined by social statuses, especially socioeconomic status (SES), gender, and race/ethnicity. Therefore, services need to be understood in this context as well and may consist of efforts to introduce social resources into caregiver/support/resource networks.

Sociologists have been successful in linking social status to disease morbidity and mortality (Berkman et al., 2000; House, Landis, & Umberson, 1988; Link & Phelan, 1995; Phelan, Link, Diez-Roux, Kawachi, & Levin, 2004). The "fundamental causes" argument (Link & Phelan, 1995) is that differences in social statuses such as SES, race/ethnicity, and gender systematically expose individuals to different levels of health risk and provide access to different levels of resources to either minimize exposure to risk or to the consequences of exposure. This explanation accounts for the widely observed social gradient in health by asserting that risk factors and resources related to health are unequally distributed as a function of social status differences and that this distribution is logically distal from the immediate "causes" of illness such as smoking, drinking, obesity, and lack of exercise. Phelan et al. (2004, p. 267) note, "These resources directly shape individual health behaviors by influencing whether people know about, have access to, can afford, and are motivated to engage in health-enhancing behaviors."

Such an explanation can be used to account for the differences in chronic illness prevalence observed in Table 2. And, although the general discussions of the fundamental cause argument do not distinguish between acute and chronic illnesses, the fundamental cause argument is seen to apply most appropriately to illness conditions that are preventable and/or treatable (Phelan et al., 2004). Mortality associated with chronic conditions such as cerebrovascular diseases, diabetes mellitus, and congestive heart failure are rated as relatively "preventable" (Phelan et al., 2004), and as such represent health conditions that can be affected by treatment and/or care management presumably including family or network caregiving and social support. The argument is made explicit by Berkman et al 2000. These authors develop a model that links social structural conditions (including socioeconomic factors) to the structure and characteristics of social networks, the quantity and quality of social support (and other resources), and health behaviors and health outcomes. They also note that the social networks that are conditioned by socioeconomic and other social status characteristics provide four types of resources: social support, social influence, social engagement and attachment, and access to resources and material goods. *It is precisely these resources that determine the quality of "self"-management of chronic illness.*

All of these socially structured network resources are relevant to the explanation for the gradient observed for chronic illnesses *and* for the health outcomes related to the patient nexus (i.e., successful management of chronic illnesses). I argue that the assertion above by Phelan et al. (2004) that "…resources directly shape individual health behaviors by influencing whether people know about, have access to, can afford, and are motivated to engage in health-enhancing behaviors…" applies equally to the patient nexus. That is, for chronic illness management, it is appropriate to conceptualize the relationship between health care services and the patient in terms of health care services and the patient nexus, and to reason that the resources in the nexus are socially distributed as well. The structure and function of the patient nexus is partly determined by the social status characteristics of the patient as these affect access to and quality of social resources (social support, social influence, social engagement and attachment, and access to material goods) that can be engaged to deal with a chronic health condition. Hence, effective health services for chronic illness involve assessing and working with the social resources available in the patient nexus. This may include modifying those resources to address the consequences of differences in the social distribution of those resources.

To support this assertion we use a perspective on social capital developed by Lin (2001). Lin's notion of social capital is that it is best understood as embedded resources in social networks. In this respect it differs from the notion of social capital as the stock of trust, civic engagement, and norms of reciprocity in a community (Ahern & Hendryx, 2005; Kawachi, Subramanian, & Kim, 2008). However, it is the more appropriate conceptualization here because of its emphasis on social networks (patient nexus) and the social gradient in network resources that is central to this conceptualization of social capital. Social capital as a community or neighborhood-level indicator of trust and/or cohesion has been shown to be related to community health, mostly in a preventive context (Cohen, Finch, Bower, & Sastry, 2006; Kawachi et al., 2008). Social capital in this sense can affect rates of "bad" health behaviors such as alcohol and drug consumption, cigarette smoking, and physical activity at the community or neighborhood level (Lindstrom, 2008). Certainly the social environment beyond the patient nexus can be understood to affect individual health behavior and norms related to health. While a sociological theory of chronic illness must account for these community or neighborhood effects and variations based on SES and/or race, I will not develop this part of the argument here because part of my objective is to outline ways in which health care providers can adapt their services to the immediate needs of person with chronic illnesses.

Lin's notion of social capital and its distribution is key to understanding the potential strengths and weaknesses of the patient nexus and provides guidance on how to align health care services that contribute to the ability of the patient nexus to support the self-management of chronic illness. The best way to envision Lin's conception is to imagine an individual who has been diagnosed with a chronic illness and told to practice self-care activities. The individual's ability to cope with the demands for self-care will be a function of the ability of that individual to draw instrumental and expressive resources from family and friends and more distant relationships (weak ties, for example) as well as information and normative values from the patient nexus. Individuals (patients) are embedded in social networks (in this case, specifically, the patient nexus) from which they draw resources with which to cope with the demands of self-care. Not all patient nexus structures are equal in their ability to provide the patient with access to the resources needed to deal with chronic illness. Part of the reason for the variability in patient nexus resources is due to the effects of social gradients that affect the resources that are available.

Lin argues that both ascriptive and achieved statuses locate individuals in resource hierarchies and that positions in these hierarchies determine the structure and content of social networks. To the extent that individuals interact with persons like themselves (e.g., family and friends), they interact with others who are in similar locations in resource hierarchies and thus have access to resources that are similar. That is, people are likely to interact with others who have similar education, information, values, and financial assets. Hence, persons in lower status positions interact with others with similar lower amounts of social resources while persons in higher status positions interact with others who also have higher amounts of useful social resources. Note that this proposition, by definition, puts individuals with chronic illnesses into different patient nexus structures based on the patient's location in social status systems. This observation applies mainly to instrumental resources. Kith and kin are always the best source of expressive support.

The drawback to lower social status, however, extends to the ability to acquire resources from members of the network who have access to different (and better) resources than those who are socially similar to the patient. This proposition applies mostly to instrumental resources such as information, entrée to services and specialists. Persons in lower social statuses have less access to better instrumental network resources because their "weak" ties are themselves less likely to be of much higher status than the patient him/herself.

These propositions not only clarify the reasons why education-based self-care training is differentially successful, but also why there is a social gradient associated with this success. The prevalence of chronic health problems is associated with a social gradient, and so too is the ability to mobilize the resources of the patient nexus to deal with the demands of the chronic illness. Therefore, health services need to account for these variations and how they may be altered to improve the likely quality of self-care.

Berkman et al. (2000) argue that social networks operate through four pathways: provision of social support, social influence, social engagement and attachment, and access to resources and material goods. In turn these supportive resources impact health by affecting health behaviors, psychological coping, and well-being and physiologic conditions. Services to the chronically ill patient, then, would be directed toward enhancing social network structures and the social resources that can be derived from them. When network structures and resources are optimized so too are health and self-management conditions: exactly the goals of treating chronic illness. The recognition that not all social networks associated with patient care (the patient nexus) are adequately structured to provide sufficient social resources indicates that services could be addressed to enhancing either network structures and/or access to resources via the network. This notion is what the sociology of chronic illness contributes to the provision of services to persons with chronic illnesses.

In the context of the distal influence of social status on both the likelihood of experiencing a chronic illness and possessing the resources to manage one's care, the outlines of health services (and their objectives) become clarified. Health care services that enable self-management of chronic illness would be designed to develop, support, and maintain a patient nexus that provides adequate expressive and instrumental support to the patient for managing self-care activities. Moreover, this nexus will also transmit and support behavioral norms that make management of chronic illness a priority and that motivate the individual to take care of him/herself. In addition, the recognition that the extent and quality of social support, social influence, social engagement and attachment, and access to resources and material goods varies by (at least) social status characteristics means that "medical" services may require different types of "service" to differently positioned patients vis-à-vis social statuses.

This is clearly a different set of services than those nominally specified by extended care models intended to facilitate self-care. They are aimed at the part of the health care system–patient relationship that is currently largely invisible to health care providers but which is crucial to the self-management of chronic illness and the ability of patients to comply/adhere with/to recommended health protocols. These services have two objectives: the organization and activation of effective patient nexus care networks and the development of patient network resources in the context of socially determined variations in network assets. These are not necessarily (or even primarily) medical interventions in the traditional sense of biophysical intervention but they enable patients to more effectively incorporate traditional medical intervention and education into day-to-day life.

Summary: A sociological model of chronic illness management, derived from a sociology *of* medicine, highlights the social causes of health disparities and provides a context for sociological research on caregiving, social support and health, and support groups and health. It emphasizes the social epidemiology of chronic illness, the importance of the patient nexus (as opposed to the patient) as the context for management of chronic illness, and the simultaneous influence of social status on the prevalence of chronic illness and access to resources to manage chronic illness.

THE CONVERGENCE OF MEDICAL AND SOCIOLOGICAL MODELS AND CLUES TO A SOLUTION

The patient is embedded in personal and community networks that reinforce adherence norms and provide practical assistance. In part, these networks arise because of the same status differences (SES, race/ethnicity, gender) that explain morbidity and mortality patterns. Patient autonomy notwithstanding, the idea is to create and maintain networks that reinforce behavior norms and facilitate adherence. This is clearly not solely the job of the health care system but it also implies that the health care system itself needs to consider the implications of this broader conception of chronic illness self-care for the kinds of services offered and their method of delivery.

Health care services will need to take into account the structure and capacity of the patient nexus. The nexus can range from nonexistent for a physically and emotionally isolated patient to one that is rich in both emotional and material supportive resources. In fact this understanding is not necessarily foreign to health care providers. The concern (and poor treatment outcomes) arises because the condition of the patient nexus is either not subsequently addressed or because the origins of poor patient nexus resources is not sufficiently understood. Hence, some "medical" services need to be directed toward developing and maintaining the structure and content of the patient nexus that is related to good self-care practices.

Services that benefit the "patient" may need to be delivered to the patient nexus rather than directly to the patient. The nexus may need to add members and/or be restructured. The members of the nexus may need to be educated about the illness and the relationship between care and morbidity. The nexus may require access to a wider range of informational and material resources. The nexus is also a normative context for patient behavior. As such, the value of good health and attention to self-care protocols may need to be developed within the nexus value system in order to place normative pressure on the patient to "adhere" to protocols. In essence, these types of health care services are directed toward the redress of differences in social network structure and function that arise, in part, because of social status variations (Sorensen et al., 2003). Part of the reason that chronic illnesses are distributed on a social gradient and that morbidity and mortality that is associated with chronic illness is also associated with an identical social gradient is that the structure and content of social networks of individuals are also affected by this social gradient (Link & Phelan, 1995). In turn, because of social network characteristics, some individuals are at greater risk of developing chronic illness and will have a lesser ability to minimize the consequences of chronic illness because of the structure and function of their social networks (Cornwell & Waite, 2012). Health policy and services that influence social and economic inequalities are therefore health care policies and health services (Freese & Lutfey, 2011).

In this chapter I began by noting the increasing prevalence of chronic illness and the relatively low levels of successful chronic illness self-management. I argued that the health care system and medical sociologists have yet to develop a useful understanding of the origins and progression of chronic illness and that that limits the success of medical system services to persons with chronic illnesses. The health care system has developed care models for chronic illness and intervention that reflect the acute care medical model. While these models recognize the important differences in disease management required for chronic illness in contrast to acute care models, none of the models successfully reduce chronic illness morbidity and mortality.

Medical sociologists do not appear to have specifically recognized the increased relevance of chronic illness as an indicator of health condition(s) and its implications for understanding health status. Sociologists have, however, studied caregiving, social support, and support groups as these are related to health status and, indirectly, to the role of social networks for health. I have shown that medical sociologists have not yet developed an understanding of the origins and function of patient support (the patient nexus) that can improve or maintain successful adaptation to chronic illness. In other words, sociologists have not yet provided health service providers with insights about self-care.

My analysis leads to the assertion that health care services to persons with chronic illnesses must focus on the patient nexus as a source of support and caregiving rather than just the patient. If the family and household represent a blind spot to the formal health care system, then this argument is intended to improve that vision. Chronic illness and care resources are distributed based on social status such that persons with lower social status are at more risk of developing chronic health conditions and of having ineffective providers of informal health care and/or network support. Thus, more effective means to deal with chronic illness by improving self-care must account for the disparate distribution of social resources and social capital based on social status differences. From the perspective of the health care system if we think about the quality of self-care illness management in terms of compliance or adherence, then the analysis provided here indicates that improving compliance/adherence requires working with the patient nexus and includes redressing the consequences of status difference effects on the structure and function of social resources available to a given patient. Health care providers will correctly argue that some services either implicitly or explicitly recognize these issues, but generally they do not. What I hope comes from the discussion here is a helpful basis for the development of health care approaches that more systematically account for the structure and function of self-care support networks. That the issue of compliance/adherence is both substantial and arguably unimproved over the last several decades suggests that a theoretically based account of compliance/adherence resources and their distribution in society may offer a useful opening for addressing this broad concern.

REFERENCES

Adamsen, L., & Rasmiussen, J. M. (2001). Sociological perspectives on self-help groups: Reflections on conceptualization and social processes. *Journal of Advanced Nursing, 35*(6), 909–917.

Ahern, M. M., & Hendryx, M. S. (2005). Social capital and risk for chronic illness. *Chronic Illness, 1,* 183–190.

Aneshensel, C. S., Pearlin, L. I., & Schuler, R. H. (1993). Stress, role capacity, and the cessation of caregiving. *Journal of Health and Social Behavior, 34*(March), 54–70.

Barr, V. J., Robinson, S., Marin-Link, B., Underhill, L., Dotts, A., Ravensdale, D., & Salivaras, S. (2003). The expanded chronic care model: An integration of concepts and strategies from population health promotion and the chronic care model. *Hospital Quarterly, 7*(1), 73–82.

Bayliss, E. A., Steiner, J. F., Fernald, D. H., Crane, L. A., & Main, D. S. (2003). Descriptions of barriers to self-care by persons with comorbid chronic diseases. *Annals of Family Medicine, 1*(1), 15–21.

Beckles, G. L., Zhu, J., & Moonesinghe, R. (2011, January 14). Diabetes: United States, 2004–2008. *Morbidity and Mortality Weekly Report, 60,* 90–93.

Berkman, L. F., Glass, T., Brissette, I., & Seeman, T. E. (2000). From social integration to health: Durkheim in the new millennium. *Social Science and Medicine, 51,* 843–857.

Bodenheimer, T., Lorig, K., Holman, H., & Grumbach, K. (2002). Patient self-management of chronic disease in primary care. *JAMA, 288*(19), 2469–2475.

Borkman, T. (1990). Self-help groups at the turning point: Emerging egalitarian alliances with the formal health care system. *American Journal of Community Psychology, 18*(2), 321–332.

Bury, M. (2004). Researching patient-professional interactions. *Journal of Service Reesarch Policy, 9*(Suppl 1), 48–54.

Bury, M., Newbould, J., & Taylor, D. (2005). *A rapid review of the current state of knowledge regarding lay-led self-management of chronic illness.* U.K: National Institute for Health and Clinical Excelence.

CDC (Center for Disease Control). (2012). Retrieved from http://www.cdc.gov/nchs/data/dvs/lead1900_98.pdf

Clark, N. M., Becker, M. H., Janz, N. K., Lorig, K., Rakowski, W., & Anderson, L. (1991). Self-management of chronic disease by older adults: A review and questions for research. *Journal of Aging Health, 3,* 3–27.

Cohen, D. A., Finch, B. K., Bower, A., & Sastry, N. (2006). Collective efficacy and obesity: The potential influence of social factors on health. *Social Science and Medicine, 62,* 769–778.

Cornwell, E. Y., & Waite, L. J. (2012). Social network resources and management of hypertension. *Journal of Health and Social Behavior, 53*(2), 215–231.

Cotten, S. R., & Gupta, S. S. (2004). Characteristics of onlline and offline health information seekers and factors that discriminate between them. *Social Science and Medicine, 59,* 1795–1806.

Delamater, A. M. (2006). Improving patient adherence. *Clinical Diabetes, 24*(2), 71–77.

DiMatteo, M. R. (2004). Social support and patient adherence to medical treatment: A meta-analysis. *Health Psychology, 23*(2), 207–218.

Freese, J., & Lutfey, K. (2011). Fundamental causality: Challenges of an animating concept for medical sociology. In B. Pescosolido, J. K. Martin, J. D. McLeod & A. Rogers (Eds.), *Handbook of the spciology of health, illness, and healing* (pp. 67–81). New York, NY: Springer.

Gallagher, E. B. (1976). Lines of reconstruction and extension in the parsonian sociology of illness. *Social Science and Medicine, 10*, 207–218.

Gallant, M. P. (2003). The influence of social support on chronic illness self-management: A review and directions for research. *Health Education & Behavior, 30*(2), 170–193.

Gately, C., Rogers, A., & Sanders, C. (2007). Re-thinking the relationship between long-term condition self-management education and the utilisation of health services. *Social Science and Medicine, 65*, 934–945.

Gaugler, J. E., Kane, R. L., Kane, R. A., & Newcomer, R. (2005). Unmet care needs and key outcomes in dementia. *Journal of the American Geriatrics Society, 53*, 2098–2105.

Glasgow, R. E., Funnell, M. M., Bonomi, A. E., Davis, C., Beckham, V., & Wagner, E. H. (2002). Self-management aspects of the improving chronic illness care breakthrough series: Implementation with diabetes and heart failure teams. *Annals of Behavioral Medicine, 24*(2), 80–87.

Gottlieb, B. H. (1983). *Social support strategies: Guiidelines for mental health practice.* Beverly Hills, CA: Sage Publications.

Greenhalgh, T. (2009). Chronic illness: Beyond the expert patient. *British Medical Journal, 338*, 629–631.

Hardey, M. (1999). Doctor in the house: The internet as a source of lay health knowledge and the challenge to expertise. *Sociology of Health and Illness, 21*(6), 820–835.

Haug, M. R. (1994). Elderly patients, caregivers, and physicians: Theory and research on health care triads. *Journal of Health and Social Behavior, 35*(March), 1–12.

Horowitz, A. (1985a). Family caregiving to the frail elderly. *Annual Review of Gerontology and Geriatrics, 5*, 194–246.

Horowitz, A. (1985b). Family caregiving to the frail elderly. In C. Eisdorfer (Ed.), *Annual review of gerontology and geriatrics.* New York, NY: Springer.

House, J. S., Landis, K. R., & Umberson, D. (1988). Social relationships and health. *Science, 214*, 540–545.

Kawachi, I., Subramanian, S. V., & Kim, D. (2008). Social capital and health: A decade of progress and beyond. In I. Kawachi, S. V. Subramanian & D. Kim (Eds.), *Social capital and health* (pp. 1–28). New York, NY: Springer Science + Business Media.

Keenan, N. L., & Rosendorf, K. A. (2011, January 14). Prevalence of hypertension and controlled hypertension-United States, 2005–2008. *Morbidity and Mortality Weekly Report, 60*, 94–97.

Kendall, E., & Rogers, A. (2007). Extinguishing the social? State sponsored self-care polcy and the chronic disease self-mamangement programme. *Disability and Society, 22*(2), 129–143.

Lemire, M., Sicotte, C., & Paré, G. (2008). Internet use and the logics of personal empowerment in health. *Health Ploicy, 88*, 130–140.

Levy, L. H. (1978). Self-help groups viewed by mental health professionals: A survey and comments. *American Journal of Community Psychology, 6*(4), 305–312.

Lin, N. (2001). *Social capital: A theory of social structure and action*. Cambridge, UK: Cambridge University Press.

Lindstrom, M. (2008). Social capital and health-related behaviors. In I. Kawachi, S. V. Subramanian & D. Kim (Eds.), *Social capital and health* (pp. 215–238). New York, NY: Springer Science + Business Media.

Link, B. G., & Phelan, J. C. (1995). Social conditions as fundamental causes of disease. *Journal of Health and Social Behavior*, Extra Issue, 80–94.

Litwak, E. (1985). *Helping the elderly: The complementary roles of informal networks and formal systems*. New York, NY: Guilford Press.

Lorig, K. (1996). Chronic disease self-management: A model for tertiary prevention. *American Behavioral Scientist*, *39*(6), 676–683.

Lorig, K. R., Sobel, D. S., Stewart, A. L., Brown, B. W., Bandura, A., Ritter, P., & Holman, H. R. (1999). Evidence suggesting that a chronic disease self-management program can improve health status while reducing hospitalization: A randomized trial. *Medical Care*, *37*(1), 5–14.

McKinlay, J. B., Crawford, S. L., & Tennstedt, S. L. (1995). The everyday impactcs of providing informal care to dependent elders and their consequences for the care recipient. *Journal of Aging and Health*, *7*(4), 497–528.

McMullan, M. (2006). Patients using the internet to obtain health information: How this affects the patient-health professional relationship. *Patient Education and Counseling*, *63*, 24–28.

Miller, B., & McFall, S. (1991). The effect of caregiver's burden on change in frail older person's use of formal helpers. *Journal of Health and Social Behavior*, *32*, 165–179.

Ministry of Health and Long-Trem Care. (2007). *Preventing and managing chronic disease: Ontario's framework*. Ontario, Canada.

Murphy, S. L., Jiaquan, X., & Kochanek, K. D. (2012). Deaths: Preliminary data for 2010. *National Vital Statistics Reports*, *60*(4).

Newman, S., Steed, L., & Mulligan, K. (2004). Self-management interventions for chronic illness. *The Lancet*, *364*, 1523–1537.

Newman, S. J., Struyk, R., Wright, P., & Rice, M. (1990). Overwhelming odds: Caregiving and the risk of institutionalization. *Journal of Gerontology*, *45*, S173–S183.

Noelker, L. S., & Bass, D. M. (1989). Home care for elderly persons: Linkages between formal and informal caregivers. *Journal of Gerontology*, *44*(2), S63–S70.

Parsons, T. (1951). *The social system*. Glencoe,IL: Free Press.

Paterson, B. L., Russell, C., & Thorne, S. (2001). Critical analysis of everyday self-care decision making in chronic illness. *Journal of Advanced Nursing*, *35*(3), 335–341.

Phelan, J., Link, B. G., Diez-Roux, A., Kawachi, I., & Levin, B. (2004). Fundamental causes" of social inequalities in mortality: A test of the theory. *Journal of Health and Social Behavior*, *45*(3), 265–285.

Rosow, I. (1981). Coalitions in geriatric medicine. In M. R. Haug (Ed.), *Elderly patients and their doctors* (pp. 137–146). New York, NY: Springer Publishing.

Sorensen, G., Emmons, K., Hunt, M. K., Barbeau, K., Goldman, R., Peterson, K., & Berkman, L. (2003). Model for incoporating social context in health behvaior interventions: Applications for cancer prevention for working-class, multiethnic populations. *Preventive Medicine*, *37*, 188–197.

Stewart, M. J. (1990). Professional interface with mutual-aid self-help groups: A review. *Social Science and Medicine*, *31*(10), 1143–1158.

Straus, R. (1999). Medical sociology: A personal fifty year perspective. *Journal of Health and Social Behavior*, *40*(June), 103–110.

Straus, A., & Corbin, J. M. (1988). *Shaping new health care system: The explosion of chronic illness as a catalyst for change.* San Francisco, CA: Jossey-Bass Publishers.

Thorne, S. E., & Paterson, B. L. (2001). Health care professional support for self-care management in chronic illness: Insights from diabetes research. *Patient Education and Counseling, 42,* 81–90.

Thorne, S., Paterson, B., & Russell, C. (2003). The structure of everyday self-care decision making in chronic illness. *Qualitative Health Research, 13*(10), 1337–1352.

Toljamo, M., & Hentinen, M. (2001). Adherence to self-care and social support. *Journal of Clinical Nursing, 10,* 618–627.

Trojan, A. (1989). Benefits of self-help groups: A survey of 232 members from 65 disease-related groups. *Social Science and Medicine, 29*(2), 225–232.

U.S. Department of Health and Human Services. (2012). *Health, United States, 2011.* Washington, D.C: Centers for Disease Control and Prevention, National Center for Health Statistics.

Van Dulmen, S., Sluijs, E., Van Dijk, L., de Ridder, D., Heerdink, R., & Bensing, J. (2007). Patient adherence to medical treatment: A review of reviews. *Health Services Research, 7,* 55–67.

Vermeire, E., Hearnshaw, H., Van Royen, P., & Denekens, J. (2001). Patient adherence to treatment: Three decades of research. A comprehensive review. *Journal of Clinical Pharmacy and Therapeutics, 26,* 331–342.

Wagner, E. H., Austin, B. T., & Von Korff, M. (1996). Organizing care for patients with chronic illness. *The Milbank Quarterly, 74*(4), 511–544.

Wagner, E. H., Davis, C., Schaefer, J., Von Korff, M., & Austin, B. (1999). A survey of leading chronic disease management programs: Are they consistent with the literature? *Managed Care Quarterly, 7*(3), 56–66.

Wagner, E. H., Glasgow, R. E., Davis, C., Bonomi, A. E., Provost, L., McCulloch, D., & Sixta, C. (2001). Quality improvement in chronic ilnness care: A collaborative approach. *Journal on Quality Improvement, 27*(2), 63–80.

SOCIAL CAPITAL, GATEKEEPING, AND ACCESS TO KIDNEY TRANSPLANTATION

Nancy G. Kutner and Rebecca Zhang

ABSTRACT

Purpose – *Disparities in transplant rates across social categories provide limited information about gatekeeping processes in access to kidney transplantation. We hypothesized that early opportunities for discussion of kidney transplantation potentially generate social capital that serves as a resource for patients as they navigate the transplantation pathway.*

Methodology – *A national sample of first-year dialysis patients was surveyed and asked if kidney transplantation had been discussed with them before and after starting dialysis treatment. Associations between reported discussion and patient-specific clinical and nonclinical (socio-demographic) indicators of attributed utility for transplantation were investigated, and the association of reported transplant discussion with subsequent transplant waitlisting was analyzed.*

Findings – *Time to placement on the kidney transplant waiting list was significantly shorter for patients who reported that transplantation had been discussed with them before, as well as after, starting dialysis. Likelihood of reported discussion varied by patient age, employment and*

Social Determinants, Health Disparities and Linkages to Health and Health Care
Research in the Sociology of Health Care, Volume 31, 273–296
Copyright © 2013 by Emerald Group Publishing Limited
ISSN: 0275-4959/doi:10.1108/S0275-4959(2013)0000031014

insurance status, cardiovascular comorbidity burden, and perceived health status; in addition, women were less likely to report early discussion.

Research limitations – *It would be valuable to know more about the nature of the transplant discussions recalled by patients to better understand how social capital may be fostered through these discussions.*

Practical implications – *Indicators of attributed utility for successful transplantation were associated with transplant discussion both before and after starting dialysis, potentially contributing to observed disparities in access to kidney transplantation.*

Social implications – *Predialysis nephrology care and patient participation in discussion of kidney transplantation may foster social capital that facilitates navigating the transplantation pathway.*

Keywords: Gatekeeping; health disparities; kidney transplant; social capital

INTRODUCTION

Disparities in access to kidney transplantation provide a fertile area for examination of heath disparities in the United States (U.S.). Transplantation is the treatment of choice for patients with kidney failure, offering the promise of longer survival and better quality of life than the other available option, chronic dialysis. However, there is a large body of evidence that the equitable distribution of kidney transplants among adults and children is suboptimal across persons, space, and time (Powe & Boulware, 2002).

The majority of persons who develop kidney failure initiate treatment on dialysis. If transplantation is desired and a living donor is not available, patients who pursue the option of receiving a deceased donor transplant must be referred to a transplant center and undergo an evaluation to determine suitability and readiness for transplantation, after which the transplant center decides to place the individual on a waiting list and the individual's "active" status on the list is confirmed at regular intervals. These processes constitute steps on the pathway to receipt of a transplant (Petrou, 2011). Gatekeeping may influence candidate selection at any of these points, based on nonclinical as well as clinical factors. Receipt of health care at early stages of the individual's decline in kidney function, especially receipt of nephrology specialist care, also serves as an early gatekeeping exposure. Earlier and more frequent predialysis nephrology visits reported by patients in a large national survey were associated with greater access to the kidney transplant waiting list and a higher rate of transplantation (Winkelmayer, Mehta, Chandraker, Owen, & Avorn, 2007).

Early information can help an individual become interested in kidney transplantation as a therapy option and understand what actions to take to increase the opportunity to receive a transplant (Petrou, 2011). The value of early exposure to transplant information was formally recognized in a 2010 policy directive by the Centers for Medicare and Medicaid Services (CMS). Kidney disease education for patients nearing kidney failure (defined as stage-four chronic kidney disease, with stage five representing the need for renal replacement therapy) was added as a Medicare Part B covered benefit. The goal was to promote opportunity for patients to know about the advantages and disadvantages of all therapy options pre-kidney failure and to actively participate in the choice of their therapy, including kidney transplantation. However, implementation of the benefit was delayed and its impact on transplant access remains unknown (Zuber, Davis, & Rizk, 2012).

In a 2005–2007 survey of a national sample of first-year dialysis patients, participants were asked if kidney transplantation had been discussed with them (a) before dialysis start and (b) since their dialysis start. We analyzed the association of clinical and nonclinical patient characteristics with these reported discussions and investigated the association of reported discussions with subsequent transplant waitlisting as recorded in the national registry of patients with end-stage renal disease (ESRD) that is maintained by the National Institutes of Health (NIH). We refer to clinical and nonclinical patient characteristics, including age, gender, race, socioeconomic status (SES), and social support, as "indicators of attributed utility" for successful transplantation. Race and SES are especially prominent in discussions of barriers and disparities in access to kidney transplantation (e.g., Johansen, Zhang, Huang, Patzer, & Kutner, 2012; Kasiske, London, & Ellison, 1998; Keith, Ashby, Port, & Leichtman, 2008; Patzer et al., 2012).

Participation in discussion of kidney transplantation potentially generates social capital that serves as a resource for patients as they navigate the transplantation pathway. As summarized by a transplant nephrologist: "… our ability to deliver the promise of kidney transplantation to all those who would clearly benefit … begins with *routine identification of impending kidney failure early enough to allow early education* and, when feasible, the very best of alternatives: preemptive transplantation" (Gaston, 2009, p. 17, italics added). While this statement acknowledges the value of early education, it is important to note that the health care goal is phrased as providing access to transplantation "to all those who would clearly benefit." The challenge of balancing utility and equity is a pervasive tension (Courtney & Maxwell, 2009), as this statement by another transplant nephrologist indicates: "…it is important for the transplant community to focus on patients who are better prepared through education and adequate resource as suitable recipients and caretakers of a newly transplanted organ…many would argue that transplanting patients better prepared to be the steward of the gifted organ will ultimately serve all patients best. In rendering daily clinical care, we cannot be expected to address all socio-demographic inequities, but rather we must strive for the best patient-centered clinical outcomes" (Peters, 2012, p. 911).

According to the allocation algorithm for patients waitlisted to receive a standard criteria donor kidney, as specified by the United Network for Organ Sharing (UNOS), candidates receive one point for each year of waiting time and another point for matching at each of two human leukocyte antigen loci. However, the totality of transplantation decision-making takes place within a complex organizational system. Both of the physician statements quoted above emphasize making patient education widely available, while at the same time defending the need for optimal utilization of a scarce resource. Our objective was to explore the role of social capital that is presumably generated through exposure to transplant discussion, within the context of the tension between utility and equity (non-disparity) that surrounds access to kidney transplantation.

GATEKEEPING AND DISPARITIES IN KIDNEY TRANSPLANT ACCESS

Increasing sophistication of transplant technology over time has facilitated significant improvement in survival of both the graft (the transplanted kidney) and the organ recipient, making transplantation a potential therapeutic treatment option for all patients with kidney failure. Organ transplantation is severely limited by availability of transplantable organs, however. In the most recent calendar year for which data are available, fewer than 17,000 kidney transplants were performed but more than 400,000 persons with kidney failure received dialysis (USRDS, 2012). About four times more patients are waitlisted than receive a kidney each year.

Patients may receive an organ from a living donor or from a deceased donor, but the majority of transplanted kidneys come from deceased donors. For most patients, it is necessary to be placed on a waiting list to receive a deceased donor organ. UNOS, a not-for-profit organization, maintains a computerized national list of patients waiting for deceased donor organ transplants. The length of time a patient has been on the waitlist is a criterion used in regional and national allocation of donated organs to transplant candidates, with one point being awarded for each year of waiting time. Risks of graft failure and reduced survival increase with length of pretransplant dialysis time. Therefore, waitlisting and transplantation would ideally occur as early as possible (Vamos, Novak, & Mucsi, 2009).

"Preemptive" transplantation, that is, transplant as the first form of therapy without having to first spend a period of time undergoing dialysis, is viewed as a valuable therapy option (Abecassis et al., 2008). A preemptive transplant usually requires having an available living donor who is willing to provide a kidney. The proportion of patients who receive preemptive transplants is approximately 2.4% of all incident ESRD patients but is higher, 14%, among pediatric (age < 18 years) ESRD patients (Patzer et al., 2013; USRDS, 2012).

Placement on a waiting list to receive a donated organ reflects gatekeeping that sorts potential recipients with respect to their transplant "merit," consistent with a utility perspective. Deceased donor organs are a scarce societal resource, and the goal of waitlisting from a functionalist perspective is to identify candidates who can be expected to make the "best use" of this scarce resource. The candidate's clinical status influences decision-making about transplantation eligibility, but placement on a waiting list reflects judgments of merit based on nonclinical factors as well. Important economic and psychosocial resources include the individual's ability to afford costly medications that are prescribed post-transplant to prevent rejection and the individual's likelihood of medication compliance and returning for transplant follow-up evaluations.

Variables associated with observed disparities in kidney transplantation are multifactorial and multilevel. Disparities are recognized with regard to persons (age, gender, race and ethnicity, socioeconomic indicators, available social support), but also with regard to "space" (dialysis clinic affiliation, organ procurement region, geographic location as measured by state and rural/urban residence, and neighborhood poverty) and "time" (e.g., current trends in donation, and policy changes influencing organ allocation). These disparities often overlap and have cumulative influence on transplant access, as, for example, in the concentration of low rates of early specialist care in certain geographic regions (McClellan et al., 2009).

Major contributors to disparities in kidney transplantation are briefly summarized below:

- *Age.* The percentage of patients who receive a transplant or are placed on the waiting list within one year of starting treatment for kidney failure is approximately 60% for those aged 0–17, 40% for those aged 18–34, 25% for those aged 35–49, 15% for those aged 50–64, and 2% for those aged 65 and older. The average age of people starting dialysis is steadily increasing, and the majority of older people who could benefit from a transplant never receive one (Grams et al., 2012; O'Hare, 2012).
- *Gender.* Garg, Furth, Fivush, and Powe (2000) concluded that female patients of all ages face barriers to obtaining a kidney transplant, even though they constitute the majority of living kidney donors and tend to have better survival than men following transplantation (Jindal, Ryan, Sajjad, Madhukiran, & Baines, 2005). Gender disparity in kidney transplantation does not seem to be explained by gender differences in income/insurance coverage (Zeier, Dohler, Opelz, & Ritz, 2002), but gender differences in employment status and perceived earning potential (physician bias) and compliance (men tolerate dialysis less well and are less compliant) may contribute (Kutner & Brogan, 1990).
- *Race and ethnicity.* Minority race, that is, black, is associated with reported delay in patients' early assessment for transplantation (Johansen et al., 2012) and with reduced access to transplant referral, to the national deceased donor waiting list, and to transplantation following waitlisting (Hall, Choi, Xu, O'Hare, & Chertow, 2011; Patzer et al., 2009, 2012). Some physicians may perceive blacks and persons of lower SES more negatively (likely risk behaviors and noncompliance) compared to their majority or higher SES counterparts (Ayanian et al., 2004; Eggers, 2009; Powe & Melamed, 2005; van Ryn, 2002; van Ryn & Burke, 2000), and there is often an added burden of race, over and above SES, that is linked to disparities (Williams, 2012). Physicians' views of reasons for racial differences in access to kidney transplantation may affect how they present this treatment option to their patients (Ayanian et al., 2004). Minority patients (blacks and others) may lack trust in providers and the health care system, may fear being "cut on" for a transplant, or may feel that transplantation is not compatible with their religious views (Gordon, 2001; Powe & Boulware, 2002). Graft survival presents immunologic challenges in the black population (Young & Gaston, 2011), and patients may be discouraged from considering transplantation when they know other patients whose transplants failed (Gordon, 2001). Lower rates of

living organ donation among minorities may reflect many of these same factors.

- *Socioeconomic indicators: Income, private insurance, employment, education.* Higher annual income and educational level were found to be associated with a higher score on the Test of Functional Health Literacy in Adults (Grubbs, Gregorich, Eliseo, & Hsu, 2009), defined by the NIH as the "degree to which individuals have the capacity to obtain, process, and understand basic health information and services needed to make appropriate health decisions" (IOM, 2004). Transplant candidates' financial resources must be adequate to cover an ongoing regimen of required immunosuppressive medications following transplantation. In addition to financial advantages associated with higher educational level, well-educated persons report a greater sense of control over their lives and their health and are more likely to be aware of the benefits of a healthy lifestyle (Ross & Wu, 1995). In a nationally representative sample of more than 3,000 new dialysis patients, college graduates experienced three times greater rates of waitlisting and kidney transplantation compared with patients who lacked a high school degree (Schaeffner, Mehta, & Winkelmayer, 2008).
- *Social support.* Social support (living with others vs. living alone; being married) is expected to enhance patients' ability to comply with post-transplant regimens (Chisholm-Burns, Spirvey, & Wilks, 2010).
- *Dialysis clinic affiliation.* The proportion of patients considered eligible for transplantation varies widely across dialysis facilities (Alexander & Sehgal, 2002; Johnson, Firth, Bird, & Mander, 2001). Patients may be less likely to be informed about transplantation if their dialysis clinic is a for-profit facility that benefits by maintaining a high dialysis patient census (Balhara, Lucirka, Jarr, & Segev, 2012; Kucirka, Grams, Balhara, Jaar, & Segev, 2012).
- *Organ procurement region and available transplant center(s).* Effectiveness of local kidney recovery, algorithms used for organ distribution, and a relatively smaller number of transplant candidates per region or center influence candidates' opportunity to receive deceased donor organs (Healy, 2004; Mathur, Ashby, Sands, & Wolfe, 2010; Sanfilippo et al., 1992). Some transplant centers list patients sooner than others in an effort to transplant more patients (Kasiske et al., 1998).
- *Geographic location.* Tonelli, Klarenbach, Rose, Wiebe, and Gill (2009) concluded that remote or rural residence was not associated with increased time to kidney transplantation, although O'Hare, Johansen, and Rodriguez (2006) found that blacks living in rural areas were less

likely than their urban counterparts to undergo kidney transplantation. Impoverished neighborhoods may be associated with social fragmentation (Cattell, 2001), providing limited social network support to help patients through the transplant process, including less availability of living donors.

SOCIAL CAPITAL AND HEALTH

"Capital" refers to resources for investment. Social capital can be defined as those features of social structures that function as resources. Social capital reflects the quality of social relations among individuals and the impact of these social relations on the lives of participants (Coleman, 1990). The processes comprising these interactions take place through different stages (Bankston & Zhou, 2002). Thus, rather than being located at any one level of analysis, social capital emerges across different levels of analysis.

Demographic characteristics, such as race and SES, can be viewed as components of the social capital process (Bankston & Zhou, 2002). For example, privileged SES can be a source of norms and values consistent with productive goal-oriented behavior. Ethnic or racial group membership may be a basis for systems of social relations. Holders of social capital derive advantages and opportunities that accrue through membership in certain communities (McClenaghan, 2000).

In the context of public health, social capital is manifest in actors who view themselves as gaining maximum benefits from their investment in themselves, calculate their behavior according to individual risk assessment, and direct their action toward the generation of trust in order to become an accepted partner within relationships that are beneficial for those involved (Erben, Franzkowiak, & Wenzel, 2000). Mutual trust and information channels are hallmarks of social capital (Wan & Lin, 2003). Network connections foster social capital when they involve goal-oriented interactions "of sufficient frequency and depth to produce and maintain productive normative orientations" (Bankston & Zhou, 2002, p. 287). Browne (2011) observed evidence for this process in her study of 228 black dialysis patients in Chicago. In addition to patients with higher income, black patients who got information from their dialysis team, and patients who had people in their social network with information about kidney transplant, were more likely to be seen at a kidney transplant center. Wan and Lin (2003) maintain that health services utilization has received limited attention in studies focusing on social capital and that incorporating social capital in studies of health services utililzation can improve understanding of individual choice.

We hypothesized that social capital, as measured by reported participation in discussion of kidney transplantation predialysis and soon after dialysis start, is associated with access to kidney transplantation as measured by placement on a transplant waiting list. We viewed receipt of specialist care prior to the need to start renal replacement therapy as an additional opportunity to acquire social capital relevant to the goal of kidney transplant access.

METHODS

Data Source and Sample Selection

Data for this study are taken from registry files maintained by the United States Renal Data System (USRDS) and from participant responses obtained in the Comprehensive Dialysis Study (CDS), which was a survey conducted by the USRDS of ESRD patients who started chronic dialysis 2005–2007 in dialysis facilities located across the U.S. This study focuses on 1,634 CDS participants who provided answers to questions about whether kidney transplantation had been discussed with them (Fig. 1). All respondents provided informed consent.

Selection of the CDS sample began with identification of outpatient dialysis units from a sampling frame of 4,410 clinics listed by CMS, excluding pediatric facilities and facilities located outside the 50 states and the District of Columbia. The list was sorted by ESRD Network, adjacent states within Network, and number of annual incident patients per facility (SAS PROC SURVEYSELECT). A sample of 335 facilities was selected using equal probability systematic random sampling. Use of systematic random sampling in conjunction with the sorted facility list yielded implicit geographical stratification (Network and state within Network). The selected units matched the total population of clinics closely on number of patients and dialysis stations, facility type (free-standing, hospital-based), dialysis chain/non-chain affiliation, types of dialysis offered, and ESRD Network (geographically defined administrative units by which CMS oversees the ESRD Program of Medicare).

Patients aged > 18 who initiated dialysis between June 1, 2005 and June 1, 2007 at one of the selected dialysis clinics were reported to the USRDS

282   NANCY G. KUTNER AND REBECCA ZHANG

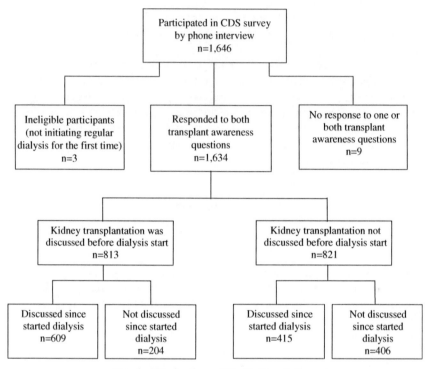

Fig. 1. Derivation of Study Population.

Coordinating Center by the CMS Standard Information Management System when they had been receiving chronic dialysis for at least two months but no more than three months. Study eligibility required that participants had no prior transplantation or other renal replacement therapy before their current start of dialysis as their regular treatment for ESRD. Patient lists were provided monthly to the USRDS Coordinating Center, which then contacted patients to request their participation in the study. Patients who consented were asked to participate in a structured interview administered by professional interviewers using a computer-assisted telephone interviewing system. CDS participants ($n = 1643$) were affiliated with 296 different dialysis clinics, located across all 18 ESRD Networks and in all states except Alaska and Vermont (Kutner et al., 2009).

Social Capital Indicators

Transplantation Discussion(s)

Two survey questions provided indicators of patients' opportunity for social capital: (a) "Was kidney transplantation discussed with you before you started your regular treatment for kidney failure?" and (b) "Has kidney transplantation been discussed with you since you started dialysis?" These questions were asked at different points in the interview in order to minimize a response set bias. Responses were categorized as 1 = yes; 0 = no/not sure.

Predialysis Nephrology Care

Providers are required to report at the initiation of renal replacement therapy: "prior to ESRD therapy, was patient under care of a nephrologist?" This information is included in the Medical Evidence file of the USRDS database. Responses were categorized as 1 = yes; 0 = no.

Indicators of Attributed Utility for Transplant Candidacy

Sociodemographic indicators of attributed utility for transplantation included younger age at treatment start (categorized as > 65/65 + years), male gender, nonblack race, working full or part time, and private health insurance as reported by patients and also recorded in the USRDS Medical Evidence file. Highest education level completed (categorized as high school graduate or higher vs. less than high school graduate/) and living alone (no/ yes) were reported by the patient in the phone interview.

A substantial literature addresses transplant candidacy considerations relative to clinical risk factors, especially diabetes, cardiovascular status, obesity, and smoking (Thomas et al., 2003). In this study, clinical/health status indicators of attributed utility for transplantation included body mass index (BMI); diabetes; burden of cardiovascular comorbidity as measured by congestive heart failure, atherosclerotic heart disease, other cardiac disease, cerebrovascular disease, and peripheral vascular disease; and started treatment on hemodialysis (HD) or on peritoneal dialysis (PD). Data for these variables were available from the USRDS Medical Evidence file. In addition, CDS participants were asked about their smoking history and to complete the Medical Outcomes Study Short Form-12 (MOS SF-12) health status survey. The SF-12 yields a Physical Component Summary (PCS) score (range 0–100) that provides a summary physical health status score.

The PCS is normalized to a general population mean of 50 and an SD of 10 (Ware, Kosinski, & Keller, 1994).

Time and Organizational Context

Calendar year of the participant's dialysis start (2005, 2006, 2007) was of interest because of potential changes in national or regional transplantation policy and candidate assessment priorities. Dialysis chain ownership of the patient's dialysis facility was identified in the CMS database that was used for sample selection. At the time of the survey this ownership was concentrated in three large dialysis organizations, or "LDOs," which are defined by the USRDS as including 100 or more free-standing dialysis clinics located in more than one state. Patients whose dialysis facility was not included in one of the LDOs were in facilities owned by independent providers, units affiliated with academic medical centers, and small dialysis organizations in which 20 or more units are owned and/or operated by a corporation that controls fewer than 100 total units. The three LDOs were assigned random codes LDO1–LDO3; patients whose dialysis facility was not affiliated with an LDO were considered to be in a non-LDO.

Data Analyses

To assess the representativeness of the study population compared with the overall patient population, patient characteristics available from the USRDS national ESRD patient registry were compared for the study population and all other incident patients who started dialysis in the U.S. in the same time period (Table 1).

Characteristics of CDS participants who reported that transplantation was discussed with them before they started dialysis ($n=813$) were compared with characteristics of patients who did not report that transplantation was discussed with them before they started dialysis ($n=821$), using t test (continuous variables) and χ^2 analysis (categorical variables). Variance estimation accounted for stratification by ESRD Network and patient clustering within dialysis facilities (Table 2).

Logistic regression analysis was used to estimate predictors of patient-reported discussion of transplantation *after* starting dialysis (yes vs. no, or not sure), including in the model patient-reported predialysis discussion (yes vs. no or not sure) and indicators of clinical and nonclinical attributed utility listed in Table 2. The model also included two clinical variables that

Table 1. Characteristics of The Study Cohort and of The Overall Population Who Started Treatment for Kidney Failure During The Same Time Period.

	Study Population ($n = 1,634$)	U.S. Patients Who Started Treatment 5/1/05–4/30/07 ($N = 211,637$)
Age < 65 years, %	61.8	50.4
Male, %	54.8	55.7
Black, %	28.3	28.8
Working full or part time, %	12.9	10.4
Private health insurance, %	27.2	26.2
BMI, mean (SD), kg/m^2	29.8 (8.0)	28.4 (7.6)
Diabetes, %	52.6	51.2
Cardiovascular comorbid condition categories, mean (SD)	0.9 (1.1)	1.0 (1.1)
Had predialysis nephrology care, %	72.3	65.2

Note: BMI = body mass index.

Table 2. Characteristics of Study Participants Who Reported, and Did Not Report, That Kidney Transplantation Was Discussed with Them *Before Dialysis Start.*

Characteristics	Reported That Kidney Transplantation Was Discussed Before Dialysis Start ($n = 813$)	Did Not Report That Kidney Transplantation Was Discussed Before Dialysis Start ($n = 821$)
**Had predialysis nephrology care, %	80.8	63.5
**Age < 65 years, %	67.8	55.8
*Male, %	57.4	52.1
Black, %	26.8	29.7
**Working, %	16.2	9.5
**Private health insurance, %	32.2	23.3
High school graduate, %	78.7	76.0
Living alone, %	20.5	24.5
BMI, mean (SD), kg/m^2	29.6 (7.8)	30.0 (8.3)
Diabetes, %	51.8	53.5
**Cardiovascular comorbid condition categories, mean (SD)	0.8 (1.1)	1.0 (1.)
Ever smoked, %	60.1	61.3

Note: BMI = body mass index. $^*p < 0.05$, $^{**}p < 0.001$.

became relevant once the patient started dialysis, that is, current dialysis treatment modality (HD vs. PD) and reported PCS score, as well as indicators of time and organizational context, that is, calendar year of dialysis start and provider chain affiliation of the patient's dialysis unit (Table 3).

We constructed a four-level categorical variable to summarize patient-reported participation in transplantation discussion, as follows: (1) before as

Table 3. Predictors of Transplant Discussion *After Dialysis Start,* From Logistic Regression.

	Odds Ratio	(95% CI)	p
Social capital indicators			
Transplant discussed with patient before starting dialysis	2.59	(2.03, 3.30)	<0.001
Had predialysis nephrology care	1.21	(0.90, 1.64)	0.21
Utility indicators: nonclinical			
Age <65 years	2.96	(2.24, 3.90)	<0.001
Male	1.04	(0.81, 1.34)	0.76
Black race	0.96	(0.66, 1.39)	0.82
Working	2.34	(1.43, 3.82)	<0.001
Private health insurance	0.93	(0.66, 1.30)	0.67
High school graduate	0.98	(0.76, 1.26)	0.85
Living alone	0.85	(0.65, 1.12)	0.25
Utility indicators: clinical/health status			
BMI	1.01	(0.99, 1.02)	0.48
Diabetes	1.19	(0.93, 1.53)	0.17
Cardiovascular comorbidity burden	0.94	(0.84, 1.07)	0.36
HD (vs. PD)	0.63	(0.36, 1.12)	0.12
Ever smoked	0.83	(0.66, 1.06)	0.13
SF-36 PCS score	1.02	(1.00, 1.03)	<0.01
Time and organizational context			
Calendar year of dialysis start			
2005	0.99	(0.64, 1.51)	0.79
2006	0.89	(0.66, 1.20)	0.33
2007 (referent)	1.00		
Dialysis facility ownership			
LDO1	0.94	(0.64, 1.37)	0.38
LDO2	0.78	(0.52, 1.17)	0.55
LDO3	0.69	(0.36, 1.33)	0.38
Non-LDO (referent)			

Note: CI, confidence interval; BMI, body mass index; SF-36 PCS, Short Form-36 Physical Component Summary; LDO, large dialysis organization.

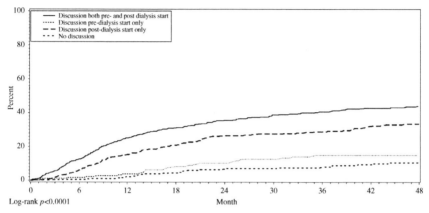

Fig. 2. Kaplan–Meier Analysis of Kidney Transplant Awareness and Time to Waitlisting in Months.

well as after dialysis start, (2) before dialysis start only, (3) after dialysis start only, and (4) neither before nor after dialysis start. The association of this variable with waitlisting from dialysis start to September 30, 2011 was described using a Kaplan–Meier plot (Fig. 2). The analysis start date was defined as date of first regular dialysis, and patients who were placed on the waiting list before they started dialysis were excluded, consistent with other researchers (Winkelmayer et al., 2007). The study end date was the latest date for which event dates were available in the USRDS database. Patients were censored at death and the end of follow-up. Statistical analyses were carried out using SAS 9.3 (SAS Institute, Cary, NC, USA).

RESULTS

Sample Characteristics

At the time they were interviewed, patients had been on dialysis for an average of approximately four months (median = 122 days; mean = 129 days). CDS participants did not differ statistically from other U.S. incident patients who began dialysis during the same time period with respect to sex, race, or diabetic status, but the sample included patients who were younger and "healthier" in several ways compared to all other new dialysis patients.

CDS participants were more likely to be younger than 65 years old, to be working, and to have private health insurance, and they had fewer cardiovascular comorbid conditions. They were also more likely to have been under the care of a nephrologist prior to initiating dialysis (Table 1).

Opportunity for Social Capital Acquisition: Participation in Transplantation Discussions

Approximately half of the study population reported that kidney transplantation had been discussed with them before they initiated dialysis. An additional 415 patients reported that transplantation had been discussed with them since they had started dialysis (Fig. 1). Thus, 1,228/1,634 (75%) of the study population said that kidney transplantation had been discussed with them at one or both time points.

Study participants who reported that kidney transplantation was discussed with them predialysis were more likely to be younger than age 65, male, currently employed, and to have private health insurance. They also had a lower burden of cardiovascular comorbidity and were more likely to have received predialysis nephrology care. No race or education differences were evident, however (Table 2).

Compared with those who did not report having predialysis discussion of kidney transplantation, patients who reported that kidney transplantation was discussed predialysis were more than twice as likely to report that this was discussed with them after dialysis start. As was true of predialysis transplant discussion, younger patients and those who were currently working were more likely to report kidney transplantation discussion after dialysis start. A higher PCS score, reflecting patient reported health status, was also associated with greater likelihood of reported transplantation discussion after dialysis start (Table 3).

Transplant Discussion Participation and Placement on a Kidney Transplant Waiting List

A total of 62 patients were placed on a transplant waiting list before they started dialysis, and 333 wait list events occurred after patients started dialysis with a median follow-up time of 21.7 months. A Kaplan–Meier analysis showed that waitlisting after dialysis start varied by transplant discussion category (log rank $p < 0.0001$), with patients who reported that kidney transplantation had been discussed with them both before and after starting dialysis being most likely to be wait listed (Fig. 2).

DISCUSSION

We conceptualized kidney transplantation discussions as social interactions that may promote social capital useful for navigating the pathway to kidney transplantation. Compared to patients who reported no participation in discussions of transplantation as a treatment option, time to placement on the transplant waiting list was significantly shorter for patients who reported that transplantation had been discussed with them before, as well as after, starting dialysis. We also found that patients who reported having predialysis discussion of kidney transplantation were more likely to report that transplantation was discussed with them after starting dialysis.

Predialysis nephrology specialist care is also an opportunity for social interactions that promote social capital (Stack & Martin, 2005). Significantly more patients who reported early discussion had received early nephrology care. There is an extensive literature on the importance of care by a kidney specialist for patients who are in the early stages of declining kidney function, providing a compelling argument for referral to kidney specialists by primary care providers. Early care from a specialist can help to preserve remaining kidney function and to maximize individuals' health status, for example, by addressing the electrolyte and metabolic imbalances that accompany declining kidney function. Individuals who receive this care are therefore not only more likely to be knowledgeable about potential treatment options when they reach kidney failure but are also more likely to develop coping skills and to present with optimal health status in subsequent health care treatment contexts (Powe, 2003).

Mutual trust and information channels are key elements of social capital (Wan & Lin, 2003). As early as possible, kidney patients need adequate information about risks and benefits of transplantation. For example, patients may believe that dialysis must precede transplantation or that transplantation is a "last resort." They may not know that there is a survival benefit associated with transplantation compared to dialysis. Finding out about transplantation early allows patients to seek a kidney donated by a relative or friend. If patients cannot find a living donor, they can at least "get in line" for a kidney from a deceased donor as soon as possible. There is evidence that when educated about transplantation as a therapeutic option, most patients want to be referred to a transplant center (Ayanian, Cleary, Weissman, & Epstein, 1999).

Improved access to transplantation requires, as part of the educational process, skilled attention to acknowledging and addressing patient fears and reservations about the transplant procedure and life with a transplant (Gaston, 2005; Gordon, 2001). In a survey conducted by the National Kidney Foundation, having a one-on-one discussion with a physician was the preferred option for receiving education, but other agents, such as patient navigators and nurse advocates, can work in conjunction with the referring physician to connect patients with the transplant center and with needed resources (Coorey, Paykin, Singleton-Driscoll, & Gaston, 2009). These interactions ideally increase not only patients' level of information and understanding but also their sense of personal agency and control.

Patients with whom transplantation is discussed early may have an opportunity not only for earlier waitlisting but also for preemptive transplantation. Receiving a transplant instead of starting dialysis is increasingly viewed as the ideal treatment option (Abecassis et al., 2008), and because preemptive transplantation usually involves a living donor this does not add another candidate to the lengthy deceased donor waiting list. No patients with transplants were surveyed in the CDS because the study design required that participants were receiving maintenance dialysis as their first renal replacement therapy. However, 62 incident patients who participated in the CDS had been waitlisted for a kidney transplant before they started dialysis. All pre-listed patients reported that transplantation had been discussed with them before dialysis start, as would be expected.

Our data showed that patients who reported having predialysis transplantation discussion but no follow-up discussion after starting dialysis had no waitlisting advantage compared to patients who reported no discussion at either time point. There are several possible explanations for this. First, these patients' health status may have declined between the time of the predialysis discussion and the start of dialysis, altering their clinical suitability for transplantation once on dialysis. Second, patients may have elected not to pursue transplantation after the early discussion (Gordon, 2001). If an individual receives a transplant but is not a "good" candidate for clinical or nonclinical reasons, that individual may be at elevated risk for graft failure (Epstein et al., 2000). This is not a desirable outcome for the patient or for society.

Previous surveys, using slightly different questions to estimate early transplantation awareness, have shown that patients for the most part have limited early exposure to information (Ayanian et al., 1999; Coorey et al., 2009; Mehrotra, Marsh, Vonesh, Peters, & Nissenson, 2005). Unlike earlier surveys, we used a population-based sampling design and were able to link responses from a national cohort with transplant waiting list registration in the USRDS database. Survey participants' educational level was similar across the four transplant awareness categories, suggesting that early discussion was not merely a surrogate indicator of formal education level.

It would be valuable to know more about the nature and source of the transplant discussion recalled by patients to better understand how social capital may be fostered through these discussions. A previous study showed that the amount of time spent in discussing treatment options, and patient satisfaction with the information presented, influenced patient decision-making about dialysis treatment options (Mehrotra et al., 2005). We also acknowledge that recall error is always possible in survey responses.

Indicators of attributed utility for successful transplantation were associated with transplant discussion both before and after starting dialysis, suggesting an important avenue by which disparities in access to kidney transplantation arise (Fig. 3). Younger age, employment, private health insurance, low cardiovascular comorbidity burden, and higher perceived health status may be viewed as justifiable metrics for judging transplant eligibility relative to the goal of maximizing successful post-transplant

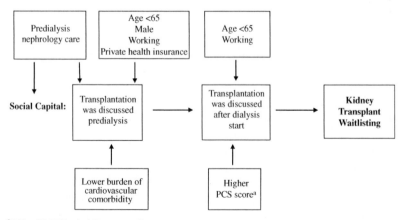

[a]PCS = SF-36 Physical Component Summary

Fig. 3. Social Capital and Gatekeeping Prior to Kidney Transplant Waitlisting.

outcomes. However, we also found that male gender was associated with having kidney transplantation discussed before dialysis start. There is no clear evidence of a gender difference in likelihood of successful post-transplant outcomes. In this study, patient-reported discussion of transplantation before dialysis start was an early point at which gender disparity was evident.

We observed no association between patient race and transplant discussion. Similar proportions of blacks and whites reported that transplantation had been discussed with them before dialysis start. The social capital implications of this finding for black patients are less clear, however, given that racial disparities in access to kidney transplantation at later steps are well documented, involving likelihood of referral to a transplant center, waiting list registration after dialysis start, waiting time, matching criteria, and organ offers and acceptance (Eggers, 2009). Patient/provider interactions that determine the content and context of transplantation discussion both before and after dialysis start may differentially shape social capital opportunity for patients of different races.

CONCLUSION

We view discussion of kidney transplantation with patients as goal-directed interaction that can promote social capital with respect to kidney transplant access. Social capital and attributed utility are conceptually important for the processes that characterize kidney transplant gatekeeping and resulting disparities. The goal of optimal benefit from each organ and the goal of providing a fair opportunity for everyone in need to receive a transplant compete with each other (Courtney & Maxwell, 2009). For example, arguments favoring increased transplantation among older persons, who now comprise a growing proportion of patients placed on the waiting list for a kidney transplant, increasingly pose ethical dilemmas (O'Hare, 2012). Disparities in transplant *rates* across groups and social categories provide limited information about gatekeeping at successive stages of access to kidney transplantation. Viewing access to transplantation as a *process* with multiple potential gatekeeping points influenced by considerations of attributed utility, and recognizing the potential role that social capital may play in promoting individuals' access to desired health outcomes, offers insight into the dynamics of kidney transplant allocation and observed disparities in health care.

ACKNOWLEDGMENTS

Contracts N01-DK-1-2471 and N01-DK-7-5004 from the National Institutes of Health provided research support. The participation of CDS respondents is gratefully acknowledged. An earlier version of this paper was presented at the 2010 annual meetings of the American Sociological Association.

REFERENCES

Abecassis, M., Bartlett, S. T., Collins, A. J., Davis, C. L., Delmonico, F. L., Friedewald, J. J., ... Gaston, R. S. (2008). Kidney transplantation as primary therapy for end-stage renal disease: A national kidney foundation/kidney disease outcomes quality initiative (NKF/KDOQI) Conference. *Clinical Journal of the American Society of Nephrology, 3*, 471–480.

Alexander, G. C., & Sehgal, A. R. (2002). Variation in access to kidney transplantation across dialysis facilities: Using process of care measures for quality improvement. *American Journal of Kidney Diseases, 40*(4), 824–831.

Ayanian, J. Z., Cleary, P. D., Keogh, J. H., Noonan, S. J., David-Kasdan, J. A., & Epstein, A. M. (2004). Physicians' beliefs about racial differences in referral for renal transplantation. *American Journal of Kidney Diseases, 43*(2), 350–357.

Ayanian, J. Z., Cleary, P. D., Weissman, J. S., & Epstein, A. M. (1999). The effect of patients' preferences on racial differences in access to renal transplantation. *New England Journal of Medicine, 341*, 1661–1669.

Balhara, K. S., Lucirka, L. M., Jarr, G. G., & Segev, D. L. (2012). Disparities in provision of transplant education by profit status of the dialysis center. *American Journal of Transplantation, 12*, 3104–3110.

Bankston, C. L., III., & Zhou, M. (2002). Social capital as process: The meanings and problems of a theoretical metaphor. *Sociological Inquiry, 72*(2), 285–317.

Browne, T. (2011). The relationship between social networks and pathways to kidney transplant parity: Evidence from black Americans in Chicago. *Social Science and Medicine, 73*, 663–667.

Cattell, V. (2001). Poor people, poor places, and poor health: The mediating role of social networks and social capital. *Social Science and Medicine, 52*(10), 1501–1516.

Chisholm-Burns, M. A., Spirvey, C. A., & Wilks, S. E. (2010). Social support and immunosuppressant therapy adherence among adult renal transplant recipients. *Clinical Transplantation, 24*, 312–320.

Coleman, J. S. (1990). *Foundations of social theory.* Cambridge: Harvard University.

Coorey, G. M., Paykin, C., Singleton-Driscoll, L. C., & Gaston, R. S. (2009). Barriers to preemptive kidney transplantation. *American Journal of Nephrology, 109*, 28–37.

Courtney, A. E., & Maxwell, A. P. (2009). The challenge of doing what is right in renal transplantation: Balancing equity and utility. *Nephron Clinical Practice, 111*, c62–c68.

Eggers, P. W. (2009). Racial disparities in access to transplantation: A tough nut to crack. *Kidney International, 76*, 589–590.

Epstein, A. M., Ayanian, J. Z., Keogh, J. H., Noonan, S. J., Armistead, N., Cleary, P. D., ...
    Conti, R. M. (2000). Racial disparities in access to renal transplantation—Clinically
    appropriate or due to underuse or overuse?. *New England Journal of Medicine, 343*,
    1537–1544.
Erben, R., Franzkowiak, P., & Wenzel, E. (2000). People empowerment vs. social capital.
    From health promotion to social marketing. *Health Promotion Journal of Australia, 9*(3),
    179–182.
Garg, P. P., Furth, S. L., Fivush, B. A., & Powe, N. R. (2000). Impact of gender on access to
    the renal transplant waiting list. *Journal of the American Society of Nephrology, 11*(5),
    958–964.
Gaston, R. S. (2005). Improving access to renal transplantation. *Seminars in Dialysis, 18*,
    482–486.
Gaston, R. S. (2009). Must health literacy be a prerequisite for kidney transplantation? *Clinical
    Journal of the American Society of Nephrology, 4*, 16–17.
Gordon, E. J. (2001). Patients' decisions for treatment of end-stage renal disease and their
    implications for access to transplantation. *Social Science and Medicine, 53*, 971–987.
Grams, M. E., Kucirka, L. M., Hanrahan, C. F., Montgomery, R. A., Massie, A. B., & Segev,
    D. L. (2012). Candidacy for kidney transplantation of older adults. *Journal of the
    American Geriatrics Society, 60*, 1–7.
Grubbs, V., Gregorich, S. E., Eliseo, J. P-S., & Hsu, C-y. (2009). Health literacy and access
    to kidney transplantation. *Clinical Journal of the American Society of Nephrology, 4*,
    195–200.
Hall, Y. N., Choi, A. I., Xu, P., O'Hare, A. M., & Chertow, G. M. (2011). Racial ethnic
    differences in rates and determinants of deceased donor kidney transplantation. *Journal
    of the American Society of Nephrology, 22*, 743–751.
Healy, K. (2004). Altruism as an organizational problem: The case of organ procurement.
    American Sociological Review, 69, 387–404.
Institute of Medicine (IOM). (2004). *Health literacy: A prescription to end confusion.*
    Washington, D.C.: The National Academies Press.
Jindal, R. M., Ryan, J. J., Sajjad, I., Madhukiran, H. M., & Baines, L. S. (2005). Kidney
    transplantation and gender disparity. *American Journal of Nephrology, 25*, 474–483.
Johansen, K. L., Zhang, R., Huang, Y., Patzer, R. E., & Kutner, N. G. (2012). Association of
    race and insurance type with delayed assessment for kidney transplantation among
    patients initiating dialysis in the U.S. *Clinical Journal of the American Society of
    Nephrology, 7*(9), 1490–1497.
Johnson, J. G., Firth, J., Bird, S. M., & Mander, A. (2001). The effect of altering eligibility
    criteria for entry onto a kidney transplant waiting list. *Nephrology Dialysis Trans-
    plantation, 16*, 816–823.
Kasiske, B. L., London, W., & Ellison, M. D. (1998). Race and socioeconomic factors
    influencing early placement on the kidney transplant waiting list. *Journal of the American
    Society of Nephrology, 9*, 2142–2147.
Keith, D., Ashby, V. B., Port, F. K., & Leichtman, A. B. (2008). Insurance type and minority
    status associated with large disparities in prelisting dialysis among candidates for kidney
    transplantation. *Clinical Journal of the American Society of Nephrology, 3*, 463–470.
Kucirka, L. M., Grams, M. E., Balhara, K. S., Jaar, B. G., & Segev, D. L. (2012). Disparities in
    provision of transplant information affect access to kidney transplantation. *American
    Journal of Transplantation, 12*, 351–357.

Kutner, N. G., & Brogan, D. (1990). Sex stereotypes and health care: The case of treatment for kidney failure. *Sex Roles: A Journal of Research, 24*(5–6), 279–290.

Kutner, N. G., Johansen, K. L., Kaysen, G. A., Pederson, S., Chen, S-C., Agodoa, L. Y., ... Chertow, G. M. (2009). The comprehensive dialysis study (CDS): A USRDS special study. *Clinical Journal of the American Society of Nephrology, 4*, 645–650.

Mathur, A. K., Ashby, V. B., Sands, R. L., & Wolfe, R. A. (2010). Geographic variation in end-stage renal disease incidence and access to deceased donor kidney transplantation. *American Journal of Transplantation, 10*(Part 2), 1069–1080.

McClellan, W. M., Wasse, H., McClellan, A. C., Kipp, A., Waller, L. A., & Rocco, R. V. (2009). Treatment center and geographic variability in pre-ESRD care associate with increased mortality. *Journal of the American Society of Nephrology, 20*, 1078–1085.

McClenaghan, P. (2000). Social capital: Exploring the theoretical foundations of community development education. *British Educational Research Journal, 26*(5), 565–582.

Mehrotra, R., Marsh, D., Vonesh, E., Peters, V., & Nissenson, A. (2005). Patient education and access of ESRD patients to renal replacement therapies beyond in-center hemodialysis. *Kidney International, 68*, 378–390.

O'Hare, A. M. (2012). Age and access to kidney transplantation. *Journal of the American Geriatrics Society, 60*, 151–153.

O'Hare, A. M., Johansen, K. L., & Rodriguez, R. A. (2006). Dialysis and kidney transplantation among patients living in rural areas of the United States. *Kidney International, 69*(2), 343–349.

Patzer, R. E., Amaral, S., Wasse, H., Volkova, N., Kleinbaum, D., & McClellan, W. M. (2009). Neighborhood poverty and racial disparities in kidney transplant waitlisting. *Journal of the American Society of Nephrology, 20*(6), 1333–1340.

Patzer, R. E., Sayed, B. A., Kutner, N., McClellan, W. M., & Amaral, S. (2013). Racial and ethnic differences in pediatric access to preemptive kidney transplantation in the United States. *American Journal of Transplantation, 13*(7), 1769–1781.

Patzer, R. E., Perryman, J. P., Schrager, J. D., Pastan, S. S., Amaral, S., Gazmararian, J. A., ... McClellan, W. M. (2012). The role of race and poverty on steps to kidney transplantation in the Southeastern United States. *American Journal of Transplantation, 12*(2), 358–368.

Peters, T. G. (2012). Good news regarding race and kidney transplant access in America. *American Journal of Transplantation, 12*(4), 910–911.

Petrou, C. (2011). Making the list: How to get on the kidney transplant waiting list. *Renalife, 28*(2), 6–8.

Powe, N. R. (2003). Early referral in chronic kidney disease: An enormous opportunity for prevention. *American Journal of Kidney Diseases, 41*, 505–507.

Powe, N. R., & Boulware, L. E. (2002). The uneven distribution of kidney transplants: Getting at the root causes and improving care. *American Journal of Kidney Diseases, 40*(4), 86–863.

Powe, N. R., & Melamed, M. L. (2005). Racial disparities in the optimal delivery of chronic kidney disease care. *Medical Clinics of North America, 89*, 475–488.

Ross, C. E., & Wu, C.-L. (1995). The links between education and health. *American Sociological Review, 60*(5), 719–745.

Sanfilippo, F. P., Vaughn, W. K., Peters, T. G., Shield, C. F., III., Adams, P. L., Lorber, M. I., & Williams, G. M. (1992). Factors affecting the waiting time of cadaveric kidney transplant candidates in the United States. *JAMA, 267*(2), 247–252.

Schaeffner, E. S., Mehta, J., & Winkelmayer, W. C. (2008). Educational level as a determinant of access to and outcomes after kidney transplantation in the United States. *American Journal of Kidney Diseases*, *51*, 811–818.

Stack, A. G., & Martin, D. R. (2005). Association of patient autonomy with increased transplantation and survival among new dialysis patients in the United States. *American Journal of Kidney Diseases*, *45*, 730–742.

Thomas, M. A. B., Luxton, G., Moody, H. R., Woodroffe, A. J., Kulkarni, H., Lim, W., … Opelz, G. (2003). Subjective and quantitative assessment of patient fitness for cadaveric kidney transplantation: The "equity penalty." *Transplantation*, *75*, 1026–1029.

Tonelli, M., Klarenbach, S., Rose, C., Wiebe, N., & Gill, J. (2009). Access to kidney transplantation among remote- and rural-dwelling patients with kidney failure. *JAMA*, *301*(16), 1681–1690.

United States Renal Data System (USRDS). (2012). *USRDS 2012 annual data report.* Bethesda, MD: National Institute of Diabetes and Digestive and Kidney Diseases, National Institutes of Health.

Vamos, E. P., Novak, M., & Mucsi, I. (2009). Non-medical factors influencing access to renal transplantation. *International Urology and Nephrology*, *41*, 607–616.

van Ryn, M. (2002). Research on the provider contribution to race/ethnicity disparities in medical care. *Medical Care*, *40*(suppl 1), 140–151.

van Ryn, M., & Burke, J. (2000). The effect of patient race and socio-economic status on physicians' perceptions of patients. *Social Science and Medicine*, *50*, 813–828.

Wan, T. T. H., & Lin, B. Y. J. (2003). Social capital, health status, and health services use among older women in Almaty, Kazakhstan. In J. J. Kronenfeld (Ed.), *Reorganizing health care delivery systems: Problems of managed care and other models of health care delivery: Research in the sociology of health care* (Vol. 21, pp. 163–180). New York, NY: Elsevier.

Ware, J. E., Jr., Kosinski, M., & Keller, S. D. (1994). *SF-36 physical & mental health summary scales: A user's manual.* Boston, MA: New England Medical Center.

Williams, D. R. (2012). Miles to go before we sleep: Racial inequities in health. *Journal of Health and Social Behavior*, *53*(3), 279–295.

Winkelmayer, W. C., Mehta, J., Chandraker, A., Owen, W. F., Jr., & Avorn, J. (2007). Predialysis nephrologist care and access to kidney transplantation in the United States. *American Journal of Transplantation*, *7*, 872–879.

Young, C. J., & Gaston, R. S. (2011). Renal transplantation in black Americans. *New England Journal of Medicine*, *343*(21), 1545–1552.

Zeier, M., Dohler, B., Opelz, G., & Ritz, E. (2002). The effect of donor gender on graft survival. *Journal of the American Society of Nephrology*, *13*, 2570–2576.

Zuber, K., Davis, J., & Rizk, D. V. (2012). Kidney disease education one year after the medicare improvement of patients and providers act: A survey of U.S. nephrology practices. *American Journal of Kidney Diseases*, *59*(6), 891–894.

PART 5
COMPARATIVE AND POLITICAL ISSUES

CONTEXTUALIZING DISPARITIES: THE CASE FOR COMPARATIVE RESEARCH ON SOCIAL INEQUALITIES IN HEALTH

Sigrun Olafsdottir, Jason Beckfield and Elyas Bakhtiari

ABSTRACT

Purpose – *Research on health care disparities is making important descriptive and analytical strides, and the issue of disparities has gained the attention of policymakers in the United States, other nation-states, and international organizations. Still, disparities research scholarship remains US-centric and too rarely takes a cross-national comparative approach to answering its questions. The US-centricity of disparities research has fostered a fixation on race and ethnicity that, although essential to understanding health disparities in the United States, has truncated the range of questions that researchers investigate. In this chapter, we make a case for comparative research that highlights its ability to identify the institutional factors that may affect disparities.*

Methodology/approach – *We discuss the central methodological challenges to comparative research. After describing current solutions*

Social Determinants, Health Disparities and Linkages to Health and Health Care
Research in the Sociology of Health Care, Volume 31, 299–317
ISSN: 0275-4959/doi:10.1108/S0275-4959(2013)0000031015

to such problems, we use data from the World Values Survey to show the impact of key social fault lines on self-assessed health in Europe and the United States.

Findings – *The negative impact of socioeconomic status (SES) on health is more generalizable across context, than the impact of race/ethnicity or gender.*

Research limitations/implications – *Our analysis includes a limited number of countries and relies on one measure of health.*

Originality/value of chapter – *The chapter represents a first step in a research agenda to understand health inequalities within and across societies.*

Keywords: Health; stratification; race/ethnicity; cross-national research

Disparities in health care and health outcomes are key concerns to researchers, providers, and policymakers alike. The Institute of Medicine defines health care disparities as differences in treatment or access between population groups that cannot be explained by different preferences for services or differences in health (McGuire, Alegria, Cook, Wells, & Zaslavsky, 2006). While much of the focus on health care disparities in the United States has focused on differences in access and quality across racial and ethnic groups, there are multiple other social characteristics that potentially matter, including education, income, geographical location, gender, and sexuality. Ultimately, we care about health care disparities as they likely result in health disparities, defined as differences in health outcomes across population groups (Schnittker & McLeod, 2005). Understanding health disparities in a cross-national perspective is important because they can, among other things, reflect (a) differences in treatment; (b) differences in health care system performance; and (c) differential need for health care.

Theoretical frameworks for understanding health care and health disparities often include "upstream" factors such as national social policy arrangements and health care systems as societal determinants of disparities, but too rarely are such factors incorporated into empirical research on disparities (Beckfield & Krieger, 2009, Olafsdottir, 2007; Olafsdottir & Beckfield, 2011). While some research has begun to do this within a single country (e.g., McGuire et al., 2006) and to a lesser extent across selected countries (e.g., Olafsdottir, 2007), a cross-national perspective can offer unique insights into the relationships among broader societal arrangements, individual social location, health care disparities, and health disparities. It is clear that health care disparities identified by empirical research are likely to be understated or misunderstood if they are limited to a single institutional setting. Further, the history of racial inequality in the United States has led to a specific bias when considering inequalities in health care: in the United States, "disparities" tends to mean "racial disparities." While race is a key axis of stratification in the United States, other social contexts may have produced different fault lines that generate different disparities in different social contexts. Only comparative research can reveal the particularities and universals of health and health care disparities.

In this chapter, we (1) specify the advantages of cross-national comparative research; (2) provide an overview of common challenges faced by cross-national comparative research and discuss some working solutions toward these challenges; and (3) provide empirical evidence from 25 European countries and the United States, illustrating how health disparities are shaped across contexts.

WHY COMPARE?

Comparison is essential to describing and interpreting disparities. For example, knowing that an individual utilized a specific type of health services and improved afterward (or not) does not tell us what would have happened if he or she had not used the services. Similarly, an experience of a black woman within the health care system becomes more meaningful when we know how her experience compares to the experiences of black men, white women, and white men. More specifically, comparison allows us to evaluate health disparities as "large" or "small" in relative context. To take a classic, contemporary example of health care disparities research, it has been shown that a 70-year-old black female actor was referred for cardiac catheterization by 73% of the physicians tested, compared to 89% for a 70-year-old white female actor, and 90% for the 70-year-old white male actor (Schulman et al., 1999). The headline-grabbing absolute disparity in this case is 27 percentage points.

We suggest that considering context can aid in the evaluation and interpretation of health disparities. The stratification of people into population groups is society-specific. As an example, a difference between racial and ethnic groups may be the key dividing line in one society, whereas citizenship status or immigration status may play a key role in another, and of course other fault lines such as gender, class, and labor market status also matter for health and health care. A cross-national perspective allows us to evaluate what groups are most likely to be disadvantaged in terms of health, whether there are generalizable patterns in what groups are vulnerable, and how institutional arrangements, history, and culture come together to explain who is most (dis-)advantaged within specific health care systems. Such evaluations can, for instance, draw on measures such as the concentration index and the fairness gap, which are expenditure-based measures developed by health economists and used in international comparisons (Fleurbaey & Schokkaert, 2009; van Doorslaer et al., 1992; Wagstaff, 2009; Wagstaff & van Doorslaer, 2000).

As McKinlay (1996) powerfully demonstrated, medical providers play a critical role in the social construction of heart disease rates. The way in which medical providers interact with patients and the social organization and norms guiding medical practices are likely to impact health disparities. Health and health care disparities can be created in at least two ways by different norms and organization of the medical profession. On the one hand, providers can systematically provide different care to different patients based on their characteristics (McKinlay, 1996; Schulman et al., 1999). On the other hand, differences in the social organization of medical care can result in health disparities, by excluding certain groups from various rights in society (e.g., health care, family benefits, unemployment benefits). Furthermore, the state and the professions adopt different roles in different societies regarding the logic of appropriateness applied to the social practice of medicine. Finally, population health varies greatly across societies, and disease distribution may influence the social practice of medicine in systematically varying ways. Recent research has shown that a diagnosis of an identical situation varies across contexts. A comparison of medical doctors in the United States, Germany, and the United Kingdom revealed that American doctors were most certain in diagnosing a coronary heart disease when presented with a scenario on a videotape, and German doctors were the least certain. In addition, to the cross-national differences, it was found that physicians were more insecure about their diagnosis when the patient was younger or female (Lutfey et al., 2009). What all this means is that, while the finding that older white women are more likely than older black women to be referred for cardiac catheterization despite presenting identical symptoms in an experimental context is extremely important and deserves the attention it received, we should not forget that this disparity may well be larger or smaller in other institutional settings, and may translate differently into health disparities across contexts. This variation goes directly both to our theoretical understanding of what causes health and health care disparities, and to the policy lessons that can be drawn from disparities research.

The promise of comparative research on health disparities can further be illustrated by considering the "fundamental cause" theory of health disparities. Link and Phelan (1995) argue that socioeconomic position is a fundamental cause of health disparities in that removing one mechanism linking socioeconomic position to health will merely result in the generation of new linking mechanisms. For instance, while in some contexts poor sanitation may be a risk factor for poor health among the poor, in other contexts smoking may be a risk factor for poor health among the poor (Link & Phelan, 1995, p. 86). We think a useful next step in the development of the fundamental cause approach would be a better specification of the kinds of contexts that moderate the effects of position in stratified societies – and the contexts that create systems of stratification themselves.

An advantage of the fundamental cause approach is that it redirects attention to the quality and quantity of social inequality itself; that is, processes of ranking and goods allocation that characterize stratification systems become the focus. We argue that stratification systems are generated and reproduced by institutional mechanisms, such that a comparative perspective is necessary to understand how and why socioeconomic position can have different effects on health (and how health can have different impacts on socioeconomic position) in different settings. That is, to understand the societal causes of health disparities, it is essential to incorporate variation in societal structure (Olafsdottir & Beckfield, 2011). Olafsdottir (2007) offers one model of how cross-national variation (here, between the United States and Iceland) can be used to examine the role that national institutions such as the welfare state play in generating health disparities. With such disparities gaining the attention of US policymakers and international organizations such at the World Health Organization and the European Union, cross-national research has a role to play in exploring what policies are more and less effective in reducing disparities (see Crane, Davis, Reinhardt, & Saltman, 2010) for comparative lessons for health care reform in the United States).

Methodological Problems and Current Solutions

While methodological challenges are common to all research, they provide a special kind of challenge in cross-national research. Consequently, we review a few of the major challenges associated with such research and discuss some common approaches. Comparative research faces a number of methodological challenges, some of which are shared with individual-level research (which of course is itself "comparative" in the sense that we always compare cases), and some of which are specific to macro-level research.

Comparability
In order to evaluate health and health care disparities in different settings, comparability of data is essential. This means that variables should be measured consistently across cases, a substantial challenge when measuring health and health care disparities across societies with different legal systems, languages, cultures, and social structures. Even something as seemingly simple as access to care can be difficult to measure in a way that affords cross-national comparison. Fortunately, cross-nationally comparable data on health care arrangements and national institutions are available to researchers. These data can be crudely divided into two types: data on the scope and the nature of the health care system itself and survey data on the publics' evaluations of health care system.

Both the Organisation for Economic Co-operation and Development (OECD) and the World Health Organization offer data on health care systems, with the former limited to the 30 OECD countries (mostly advanced, industrialized nations) and the latter offering a larger sample of nations. Data include spending on health care, the proportion of the population with access to health care, the number of certain medical procedures performed annually, and the number of medical doctors. Some research has used this kind of data to evaluate differences in health care systems and develop typologies (Wendt, Frisina, & Rothgang, 2009; Wendt, Grimmeisen, & Rothgang, 2005).

Several cross-national studies offer insights into how the public evaluates the health care system. For example, the International Social Survey Program (ISSP) offers questions on the role of the government in health care and the European Social Survey (ESS) has included rotating modules in health care. Research using this kind of data has shown that health care trajectories are important in explaining what role the public views as appropriate for the government in the health care system (Kikuzawa, Olafsdottir, & Pescosolido, 2008). Further, it is possible to use this data to evaluate group differences in attitudes toward the health care system. An analysis of public attitudes in 33 countries showed that those in the labor force consistently evaluate the effectiveness of the health care system more negatively. Age and education also correlate with evaluations of health care systems (Olafsdottir & Pescosolido, 2010). Still, even though the given data is collected with the goal of comparability, the problem does not disappear. Other ways to address comparability include comparing relative and absolute differences. Further, multiple measures of key concepts can be used in an effort to triangulate associations: a good example is education, where the analyst often has data on years of schooling and degree attained, which can be harmonized using an International Standard Classification of Education (ISCED) educational classification scheme.

Black Boxes andnd Lag Structures
While the strengths of comparative research include its ability to identify the institutional correlates of health care disparities and place health care disparities into a broader context, such research also faces the challenge of analyzing causal mechanisms in divergent settings. The inability to examine processes inside the black boxes theorized to connect cause and effect is related to the problem of complex lag structures, where an institutional change at time t may not affect the outcome until $t+1$, $t+2$, $t+3$, etc. Theoretical development and the measurement of mechanisms are both required to address these problems. Theoretical work that traces the possible connections from social institutions to disparities in health and health care is ongoing, and stress and material resources are two commonly proposed sets of mechanisms. Research at the intersection of genetics and sociology is currently opening the "black box of the body" in spelling out how social structure (of which the health care system can be conceptualized as one element) causes health and illness (Bearman, 2008; Pescosolido et al., 2008). The challenge of identifying causal mechanisms is probably the most difficult one that stands in the way of comparative research on health care disparities. Two very general approaches to identifying causal social mechanisms in ways that link theory tightly to data are discussed by Gross (2009), who draws on pragmatist theory, and Lieberson and Horwich (2008), who develop implication analysis.

Galton's Problem
Many statistical techniques rely on the assumption that the cases analyzed are independent, but this is not a reasonable assumption where the cases are nation-states (to say nothing of its reasonability where the cases are individuals). Galton's problem is perhaps more problematic than ever in the so-called "era of globalization," which finds national societies deeply embedded in transnational networks. Europe is arguably the clearest example of how health care systems can influence each other, given the efforts of the European Union toward the harmonization of social systems.

One of the aims of that effort is labor mobility, and so there is pressure for the "portability" of health care benefits, and pressure on healthcare institutions to provide similar qualities of service across increasingly permeable national boundaries. A variety of regression-based techniques have been developed to address the nonindependence of cases, including spatial regression. Moran's I is a common test for spatial autocorrelation in data. Beck and Katz (2009) have developed the technique of Ordinary Least Squares (OLS) regression with panel-corrected standard errors, based on a covariance matrix estimator that adjusts for the nonindependence of cases; this approach has been applied in comparative research on welfare states by political scientists and sociologists.

Case Selection and Unmeasured Heterogeneity
The importance of carefully defining the population of interest (Krieger, 2011) applies as well to comparisons of nation-states as it does to research on individuals. For example, discrepant findings on the role of income inequality at the national level in explaining international variation in population health sometimes result from the use of narrower versus broader selection of cases. While an association between income inequality and population health may exist among a sample of nine countries (Wilkinson, 1992), such an association does not generalize to a broader sample of countries (Beckfield, 2004). The importance of case selection in this literature has been noted by Kondo et al. (2009) in a meta-analysis. A deeper problem related to case selection is "methodological nationalism" (Wimmer & Glick-Schiller, 2002), or the tendency for comparative researchers to take the nation-state as the "natural" unit of analysis. Lynch (2009) illustrates an alternative approach, where subnational regions are taken as the units of analysis. This is currently a forefront area with more questions than answers, so our recommendation for those interested in conducting comparative healthcare disparities is to allow for variation in the geographical scale of the institutional factors that might relate to disparities (Krieger, 2011).

Comparative researchers use a range of guidelines in selecting cases for comparison (Bollen, Entwisle, & Alderson, 1993). Mill's method of agreement, for instance, leads to the selection of cases with similar outcomes or effects. The logic is that if some candidate causes are absent from cases where effects are present, those candidate causes can be ruled out, in favor of causes that are present in all cases. In contrast, Mill's method of difference leads to the selection of cases with different outcomes of effects, and candidate causes that hold true for all cases can be ruled out, in favor of causes that are only present where effects are observed. Mill's methods are most often used in conjunction with comparative research on a small number of cases; Ragin's work on Qualitative Comparative Analysis generalizes Mill's approach to larger-N comparisons and comparisons that involve larger sets of causes and effects.

Practical considerations often drive case selection in comparative research, irrespective of whether these considerations are reported or not by researchers (Bollen et al., 1993). Comparable data on health care institutions and health care disparities, although they exist to a greater degree than is recognized by many researchers, are still very limited. Such research will make little progress until harmonized, individual-level data are made available to the research community as the Luxembourg Income Study has done with income data. Currently, comparative researchers select cases based on familiarity, convenience, data availability, or heterogeneity on the variables of interest. As Beckfield and Krieger (2009) note, most comparative research on health inequities is conducted with data on advanced capitalist democracies, which obviously limits our knowledge of the generalizability of findings. Even more importantly, the range of research questions has been drastically truncated by data considerations. Lieberson and Horwich (2008) offer an extremely useful guide to elaborating the empirical implications of theory, in the context of the realities of social research.

Two methodological approaches – Bayesian inference for apparent populations, and panel estimation techniques – are particularly helpful in strengthening causal inferences from comparative data. Often, comparative research relies on a sample that can be characterized as an "apparent population" in that the sample cannot be replicated (Berk, Western, & Weiss, 1995). Examples include research using OECD nation-states, where clearly one could replicate a random sampling of individuals within OECD nation-states, but one has complete or near-complete macro-data on all the member countries of the OECD. Bayesian techniques for the analysis of cross-national survey data are discussed by Garip and Western (2009). Where the researcher has repeated observations on the same units over time, such as are available on health care systems from the OECD Health Data, fixed-effects and random-effects approaches can be used to address the problem of unmeasured heterogeneity (Halaby, 2004). As usual, though, there is no free lunch, as random-effects estimation requires the assumption that the errors are uncorrelated with the regressors (this assumption can be tested using the Hausman framework), and fixed-effects estimation requires the assumption that the unit effects do not vary over time (we are unaware of any available statistical assessment of this strong assumption).

Operationalizing Race and Ethnicity outside of the US Context

Health services researchers in the United States often focus on racial and ethnic disparities when discussing disparities. This is natural given the critical relevance of "the problem of the color line" (DuBois, 1903) to understanding social inequality in the United States, but such a focus masks the uniqueness of the US case as a social context with a specific history of troubled race relations, and a specific structure of racial/ethnic stratification. Consequently, it is important to understand whether similar relationships are found in other contexts, as well as critically evaluate the appropriateness of focusing on race and ethnicity as a key fault line in other societies.

To understand how the European context is different, Table 1 shows the number of respondents in the 2002 ESS self-identifying as a minority, and

Table 1. Percentage of Respondents Belonging to Various Minority Categories in Each European Country.

	Minority	Either Parent Not Born	Majority %	Largest Minority (%)
Belgium	3.16	17.51	Flemish (58)	Walloon (31)
Switzerland	6.61	29.53	German (65)	French (18)
Czech Republic	2.89	8.72	Czech (90)	Moravian (3.7)
Germany	4.02	14.11	German (92)	Turkish (2)
Denmark	2.16	9.54	NA	NA
Estonia	20.67	35.39	Estonian (69)	Russian (26)
Spain	3.21	8.37	NA	NA
Finland	.54	3.47	Finn (93)	Swede (6)
France	3.58	17.45	NA	NA
United Kingdom	6.68	16.06	White (92)	Black (2)
Greece	3.54	15.29	Greek (93)	Foreign citizens (7)
Hungary	3.69	6.15	Hungarian (92)	Roma (2)
Ireland	1.94	7.08	Irish (87)	Other white (8)
Netherlands	4.73	14.70	Dutch (81)	EU (5)
Norway	3.58	11.36	Norwegian (94)	Other European (4)
Portugal	1.83	4.44	NA	NA
Sweden	2.16	16.62	NA	NA
Slovenia	1.96	17.38	Slovak (86)	Hungarian (10)
Slovakia	5.95	8.74	Slovene (83)	Serb (2)
Ukraine	5.07	24.69	Ukrainian (78)	Russian (17)

Notes: Data for minority status and foreign-born parent come from the 2002 ESS; Data for % majority and % minority are from the *World Factbook* (https://www.cia.gov/library/publications/the-world-factbook/).

the number of respondents who report having a parent born outside the country the respondent resides in. With the exception of Estonia, fewer than 10% self-report minority status, and Switzerland, the United Kingdom, Slovakia, and Ukraine are the only countries with between 5% and 10% of respondents identifying as a minority. All other countries have fewer than 5% identifying in such a way. The percentage goes up in most cases when we consider whether the respondents have at least one foreign-born parent. Here, the proportions are highest in Estonia (35%), Switzerland (30%), and Ukraine (25%).

Comparing these percentages to those obtained from the World Fact Book highlights the problem associated with constructing race and ethnicity in a meaningful way within the European context. While in some cases, it can be argued that there is a "true" ethnic minority, for example Turks in Germany, it is more common that the largest minority group is culturally similar to the majority population. For example, both Estonia and Ukraine have a large minority population, yet the largest minority consists of Russians. The issue is further complicated by deciding which information to use to capture race and ethnicity. For example, 95% of those residing in Estonia and Ukraine are either Estonian/Ukrainian or Russian, yet over 20% identify as a minority in Estonia and only about 5% in Ukraine. This reality highlights the importance of a careful understanding of each national context as well as the likelihood that race or ethnicity may not be the central axis of disparities in the European context. Consequently, we provide an illustration of the impact of different social fault lines on health across these same European countries and the United States.

Data

To examine dimensions of health disparities in Europe, we pool five rounds of the ESS (2002, 2004, 2006, 2008, 2010) for comparisons across 20 European countries. As already discussed, a cross-national analysis of race/ethnicity faces the problems of low numbers of minorities/immigrants in some countries and as a solution, we pool the data across years. Other researchers have used similar strategies when working with the ESS. The ESS is a cross-national study that was initiated and seed-funded by the European Science Foundation, with the aim of comparing attitudes across European countries. Countries were dropped if missing data for two or more ESS rounds or if the foreign-born population was too small for comparison. The 20 countries that met the criteria for inclusion in the final dataset were: Belgium, Switzerland,

Czech Republic, Germany, Denmark, Denmark, Estonia, Spain, Finland, France, United Kingdom, Greece, Hungary, Ireland, Netherlands, Norway, Portugal, Sweden, Slovenia, Slovakia, and Ukraine.

For the United States, we pooled corresponding years from the General Social Survey (GSS), which is conducted by National Opinion Research Center (NORC) and uses a full probability sampling design of noninstitutionalized adults 18 years of age or older in the United States. It is possible to add the US case to our analysis, as there are identical questions in the GSS and the ESS for our survey years. For both datasets, missing values were imputed using a multiple imputations by chained equations (ICE) approach in the Stata statistical package (Marchenko, 2011). ICE is an iterative multivariate regression technique that allows imputed datasets based on a set of imputation models for each specified variable with missing values (Royston, 2004). All variables listed below were included in the model, and 5 imputation cycles were performed.

Measures

Our dependent variable is self-assessment of health. Self-assessed measures of health can be powerful predictors of mortality and morbidity (Idler & Benyamini, 1997) and have been recommended as suitable for comparative research by the World Health Organization (de Bruin, Picavet, & Nossikov, 1996). Respondents to the GSS were asked, "Would you say your own health, in general, is excellent, good, fair, or poor?" with excellent coded 1 and poor coded 4. The ESS measures health on a five-point scale ranging from very good (coded 1) to very bad (coded 5) in response to the question, "How is your health in general?" Responses were dichotomized with "fair," "bad," and "very bad" indicating poor health in the ESS and "fair" and "poor" indicating poor health in the GSS. Although the question wording and coding differs between the two surveys, dichotomizing the variables as poor or less-than-good health allows for comparison across the datasets.

For independent variables, immigration status is measured as a binary variable indicating if the respondent is foreign-born (1 = immigrant). Age is measured in years. Sex is measured with a binary variable (0 = male, 1 = female). For unemployment status, GSS respondents were coded as 1 if they reported being laid off or temporarily not working, and ESS respondents were coded 1 if they reported being unemployed and either looking or not working for work in the previous seven days. In order to more easily compare across contexts, education and income were coded based on relative in-country comparisons. Respondents in the ESS were coded as having relatively low education if they had less than tertiary education (based on UNESCO's ISCED), levels 1–3); GSS respondents were coded similarly if they reported less than 12 years of education. In both surveys, low relative income was coded as the bottom quartile within each country based on a continuous measure of household income.

Both surveys rely on self-reported assessments of minority status, however they differ in the level of details provided. The ESS asks respondents to identify whether they belong to an ethnic minority group in their country, but it does not ask respondents to specify the particular minority group. The GSS follows the procedures used in the US decennial Census and asks respondents for a racial self-identification, recording up to three mentions. Respondents were coded as belonging to a minority group if they reported any race or ethnicity other than white. Descriptive statistics for all variables are listed in Table 2.

Table 2. Descriptive Statistics for 21 Countries.

	Immigrant (%)	Minority (%)	Female (%)	Low Edu. (%)	Rel. Poverty (%)	Unemployed (%)
Belgium	9.4	3.2	51.0	33.0	26.0	6.0
Switzerland	20.0	6.8	52.0	25.0	25.0	2.3
Czech Republic	2.8	2.7	51.0	15.0	19.0	4.7
Germany	9.6	4.6	50.0	16.0	25.0	5.7
Denmark	5.8	2.6	50.0	24.0	26.0	3.4
Estonia	19.0	21.0	58.0	25.0	26.0	4.6
Spain	7.8	3.2	51.0	57.0	27.0	7.1
Finland	2.8	1.2	52.0	34.0	28.0	4.6
France	8.9	3.9	53.0	32.0	24.0	6.0
United Kingdom	11.0	7.3	52.0	50.0	21.0	4.7
Greece	9.0	4.6	55.0	46.0	30.0	8.7
Hungary	2.3	4.8	55.0	41.0	23.0	5.6
Ireland	12.0	3.5	54.0	39.0	22.0	7.6
Netherlands	8.0	5.8	54.0	43.0	20.0	2.6
Norway	8.0	3.6	48.0	19.0	31.0	2.6
Portugal	6.0	2.4	58.0	75.0	21.0	7.0
Sweden	11.0	2.7	50.0	41.0	33.0	3.7
Slovenia	8.2	2.6	54.0	28.0	40.0	5.7
Slovakia	2.9	6.3	55.0	17.0	20.0	7.0
Ukraine	10.0	5.8	61.0	17.0	39.0	7.0
United States	13.0	24.0	54.0	16.0	22.0	6.5

Illustrating Health Disparities

For each country we ran a baseline weighted binary logistic regression model to test the effects of the combined independent variables on self-assessed poor health status. For post-estimation analysis, we calculated the change in predicted probability of poor health as each independent variable moves from 0 to 1.

Fig. 1 graphs the change in predicted probabilities for immigration status, minority status, and gender, revealing both between-country and within-country variation in the magnitudes of health differences between groups. For instance, while minorities appear to have a higher probability of poor health in France, the United States, and parts of Eastern Europe, in many countries there is no significant association between minority identification and self-rated health. Similarly, the coefficients for immigration status range from negative (indicating better self-reported health status for immigrants, relative to natives) to positive (indicating poor health for migrants). For gender, as well, predicted changes in probabilities of poor health varied substantially, from a small probability that women are less likely to report

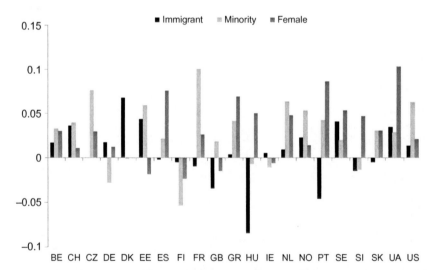

Fig. 1. Marginal Change in Predicted Probability for Poor Health by Minority Status, Immigration, and Gender. Values represent change in predicted probability when variables change from 0 to 1. Based on logistic regression of poor health with age, low education, gender (1 = female), relative poverty, minority status (1 = minority), immigration status, and unemployment status as independent variables. Data from the ESS and GSS (2002, 2004, 2006, 2008, 2010)

poor health in Finland to a substantial probability of poorer health for women in Ukraine.

Fig. 2 similarly graphs changes in predicted probability of poor health for each of the indicators of socioeconomic status (SES). Low education, relative poverty, and unemployment are more consistently associated with poor self-reported health than the demographic variables in Fig. 1, and nearly all coefficients are positive. However, there are also significant differences in the magnitude of each effect across countries.

Table 3 shows the Spearman rank correlations for the marginal change coefficients in Figs. 1 and 2. There does not appear to be a significant correlation between any two of the independent variables. Both the figures and the correlation coefficients suggest that the relevant indicators of health disparities may differ across context. Race/ethnicity, gender, migration status, and socioeconomic position all appear to be potential cleavages for health disparities, but cross-national comparisons may better reveal how and why each matters in a particular social, economic, and political conditions.

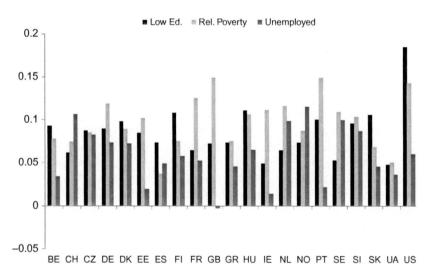

Fig. 2. Marginal Change in Predicted Probability for Poor Health by SES. Values represent change in predicted probability when variables change from 0 to 1. Based on logistic regression of poor health with age, low education, gender (1 = female), relative poverty, minority status (1 = minority), immigration status, and unemployment status as independent variables. Data from the ESS and GSS (2002, 2004, 2006, 2008, 2010)

Table 3. Spearman Rank Correlations for Marginal Effects of
Immigration, Gender, Education, Unemployment, Minority Status,
and Citizenship.

	Immigrant	Minority	Female	Low Ed.	Poverty	Unemployed
Immigrant	1					
Minority	0.1156	1				
	(0.6178)					
Female	−0.2169	0.1766	1			
	(0.3450)	(0.4437)				
Low Ed.	−0.3481	−0.1455	−0.1052	1		
	(0.1221)	(0.5293)	(0.6500)			
Poverty	−0.2519	0.1078	−0.1610	0.0844	1	
	(0.2706)	(0.6419)	(0.4856)	(0.7160)		
Unemployed	0.2740	0.0636	0.0519	0.0156	−0.0909	1
	(0.2294)	(0.7841)	(0.8230)	(0.9465)	(0.6951)	

p-values in parentheses.

DISCUSSION

We have argued that comparative analysis of health disparities is essential, because without comparison we do not know how large or small disparities are in a given context, or how and why disparities are related to social institutions – the "rules of the game" that generate, entrench, and reproduce the social inequalities that are at the root of health care disparities. We have acknowledged that comparative research of the sort we advocate faces a number of specific challenges, and we have identified the solutions to these problems that are currently being implemented by comparative researchers in the fields of sociology, political science, and economics. We have also illustrated a comparative approach to health disparities using data from the ESS and the GSS.

Substantively, we have shown that there is more variation in the association between health and social characteristics such as being an immigrant, a minority or female, than to characteristics that reflect economic advancement (or lack therefore) within a country. This indicates that residing on the lower end of the social hierarchy within the market translates fairly generally into worse health across advanced, industrialized nations. However, understanding health disparities based on gender or race/ethnicity is more complex in a cross-national perspective, as the impact of such group membership appears to be more country-specific and embedded within specific national arrangements. Here, we have provided a starting point for exploring this variation and pointed out both the promise and challenges of cross-national work on health disparities. We argue that engaging in such work has the potential to help us solve some of the major questions of health disparities research, most importantly by linking together the macro-levels of social policy, cultural traditions, and institutional arrangements and the lived health experiences of individuals residing in different nations.

ACKNOWLEDGMENTS

This work was supported by grants from the National Institutes of Health (1R03HD066013-01), the Robert Wood Johnson Foundation, and a National Science Foundation Graduate Research Fellowship under Grant No. DGE-1247312. Views expressed are those of the authors, not the funding agencies. The authors are grateful to Bernice A. Pescosolido for comments on a previous version.

REFERENCES

Bearman, P. S. (2008). Introduction: Exporing genetics and social structure. *American Journal of Sociology, 114*, 5–10.

Beck, N., & Katz, J. N. (2009). *Modeling dynamics in time-series cross-section political economy data.* Social Science Working Paper 1304, California Institute of Technology.

Beckfield, J. (2004). Does income inequality harm health? New cross-national evidence. *Journal of Health and Social Behavior, 45*, 231–248.

Beckfield, J., & Krieger, N. (2009). Epi + demos + cracy: A critical review of empirical research linking political systems and priorities to the magnitude of health inequities. *Epidemiologic Reviews, 31*(1), 152–177.

Berk, R. A., Western, B., & Weiss, R. E. (1995). Statistical inference for apparent populations. *Sociological Methodology, 25*, 421–458.

Bollen, K., Entwisle, B., & Alderson, A. S. (1993). Macrocomparative research methods. *Annual Review of Sociology, 19*, 321–351.

Crane, R., Davis, K., Reinhardt, U., & Saltman, R. (2010). Health care reform: What the United States can learn form the experience of other developed nations. *Health Services Research, 45*, 588–601.

de Bruin, A., Picavet, H. S. J., & Nossikov, A. (1996). *Health interview surveys: Towards international harmonization of methods and instruments.* Copenhagen, Denmark: World Health Organization Regional Office for Europe.

DuBois, W. E. B. (1903). *The souls of black folk.* Chicago, IL: McClurg and Co.

316   SIGRUN OLAFSDOTTIR ET AL.

Fleurbaey, M., & Schokkaert, E. (2009). Unfair inequalities in health and health care. *Journal of Health Economics, 28*, 73–90.

Garip, F., & Western, B. (2009). *Model comparison and simulation for hierarchical models: Analyzing rural–urban migration in Thailand.* Working Paper, No. 2008-0056 Harvard University, Cambridge, Mass.

Gross, N. (2009). A pragmatist theory of social mechanisms. *American Sociological Review, 74,* 358–379.

Halaby, C. (2004). Panel models in sociological research: Theory into practice. *Annual Review of Sociology, 30*, 507–544.

Idler, E. L., & Benyamini, Y. (1997). Self-rated health and mortality: A review of twenty-seven community studies. *Journal of Health and Social Behavior, 38*, 21–37.

Kikuzawa, S., Olafsdottir, S., & Pescosolido, B. A. (2008). Similar pressures, different context: Public attitudes to government intervention for health care in 21 nations. *Journal of Health and Social Behavior, 49*, 385–399.

Kondo, N., Sembajwe, G., Kawachi, I., van Dam, R. M., Subramanian, S. V., & Yamagata, Z. (2009). *British Medical Journal, 339*: b4471.

Krieger, N. (2011). *Epidemiology and the people's health: Theory and context.* New York, NY: Oxford University Press.

Lieberson, S., & Horwich, J. (2008). Implication analysis: A pragmatic proposal for linking theory and data in the social science. *Sociological Methodology, 38*, 1–49.

Link, B. G., & Phelan, J. (1995). Social conditions as fundamental causes of disease. *Journal of Health and Social Behavior, 35*, 80–94.

Lutfey, K. E., Link, C. L., Marceau, L. D., Grant, R. W., Adams, A., Arber, S., ... McKinlay, J. B. (2009). Diagnostic certainty as a source of medical practice variation in coronary heart disease: results from a cross-national experiment of clinical decision making. *Medical Decision Making, 29*, 606–618.

Lynch, J. (2009). The political geography of mortality in Europe. *Perspectives on Europe, 1*, 13–17. Retrieved from http://tinyurl.com/5k2xbc.

Marchenko, Y. (2011). *Chained equations and more in multiple imputation in Stata 12.* 2011 United Kingdom Stata Users' Group Meetings, Stata Users Group.

McGuire, T., Alegria, M., Cook, B. L., Wells, K. B., & Zaslavsky, A. M. (2006). Implementing the institute of medicine definition of disparities: An application to mental health care. *Health Services Research, 41*, 1979–2005.

McKinlay, J. B. (1996). Some contributions from the social system to gender inequalities in heart disease. *Journal of Health and Social Behavior, 37*, 1–26.

Olafsdottir, S. (2007). Fundamental causes of health disparities: Stratification, the welfare state, and health in the United States and Iceland. *Journal of Health and Social Behavior, 48*(3), 239–253.

Olafsdottir, S., & Beckfield, J. (2011). Health and the social rights of citizenship: Integrating welfare state theory and medical sociology. In B. A. Pescosolido, J. K. Martin, J. D. McLeod & A. Rogers (Eds.), *Handbook of sociology of health, illness, and healing: A blueprint for the 21st century* (pp. 101–115). New York, NY: Springer.

Olafsdottir, S., & Pescosolido, B. A. (2010). *Successful health care systems: Variations in and determinants of public attitudes in 33 nations.* Presented at the *Duke Center for European Studies*, Durham, N.C.

Pescosolido, B. A., Perry, B. L., Long, J. S., Martin, J. K., Nurnberger, J. I., & Hesselbrock, V. (2008). Under the influence of genetics: How transdisciplinarity leads us to rethink social pathways to illness. *American Journal of Sociology, 114*, S171–S201.

Royston, P. (2004). Multiple imputation of missing values. *Stata Journal, 4*(3), 227–241.

Schnittker, J., & McLeod, J. D. (2005). The social psychology of health disparities. *Annual Review of Sociology, 31,* 75–103.

Schulman, K. A., et al. (1999). The effect of race and sex on physicians' recommendations for cardiac catheterization. *New England Journal of Medicine, 340*(8), 618–626.

van Doorslaer, E., et al. (1992). Equity in the delivery of health care: Some international comparisons. *Journal of Health Economics, 11,* 389–411.

Wagstaff, A. (2009). Correcting the concentration index: A comment. *Journal of Health Economics, 28,* 516–520.

Wagstaff, A., & van Doorslaer, E. (2000). Measuring and testing for inequity in the delivery of health care. *Journal of Human Resources, 35,* 716–733.

Wendt, C., Frisina, L., & Rothgang, H. (2009). Healthcare system types: A conceptual framework for comparison. *Social Policy and Administration, 43,* 70–90.

Wendt, C., Grimmeisen, S., & Rothgang, H. (2005). Convergence or divergence of OECD health care systems. In B. Cantillon & I. Marx (Eds.), *International cooperation in social security: How to cope with globalization* (pp. 15–46). Antwerp: Intersentia.

Wilkinson, R. (1992). Income distribution and life expectancy. *British Medical Journal, 304,* 165–168.

Wimmer, A., & Glick-Schiller, N. (2002). Methodological nationalism and beyond: Nation-state building, migration and the social sciences. *Global Networks, 2*(4), 301–334.

POLITICAL IDEOLOGY, PARTY IDENTIFICATION, AND PERCEPTIONS OF HEALTH DISPARITIES: AN EXPLORATORY STUDY OF COGNITIVE AND MORAL PREJUDICE

Harry Perlstadt

ABSTRACT

Purpose – *This chapter explores public perceptions of health disparities by taking political ideology and political party identification into account and applies theories of cognitive dissonance, cognitive prejudice, and moral prejudice to understand the impact of political ideology on perceptions of health disparities.*

Methodology/approach – *A statewide telephone survey asked 1,036 people about health disparities. Eight independent variables – political ideology, political party identification, gender, race, age, community type, income, and education achieved – were entered in an additive stepwise regression containing one of four dependent variables – unfair treatment*

Social Determinants, Health Disparities and Linkages to Health and Health Care
Research in the Sociology of Health Care, Volume 31, 319–337
ISSN: 0275-4959/doi:10.1108/S0275-4959(2013)0000031016

based on health insurance, unfair treatment based on ability to speak English, minorities unable to get care when needed, and quality of care for minorities.

Findings – *Political ideology entered all four equations while political party identity entered only two. Liberals were most likely to believe that minorities were unable to get routine care when needed and democrats that ability to speak English meant differential treatment. Respondents with low education were most likely to believe people were treated unfairly based on insurance, while those with lower incomes were more likely to believe that minorities received higher quality of care than whites.*

Research limitations/implications – *A public opinion survey in one state cannot be generalized for the whole country. The survey was conducted in the spring of 2009 just as the debate over the proposed health care reform legislation was reaching a crescendo, which may explain the importance of political ideology on perceptions of health disparities.*

Originality/value of chapter – *This chapter explicitly examines the effect of political ideology and party identification on perceptions of health disparities by utilizing theories of cognitive and moral prejudice. Political ideology reflecting cognitive and moral prejudice may combine with support for a social movement or political faction that supports or opposes reducing health disparities.*

Keywords: Health disparities; political ideology; party identity; public opinion survey; cognitive dissonance

INTRODUCTION

While public health professionals and researchers know about the social determinants of health and their relationship to health disparities, the perceptions of the general public have not been fully explored. The former often define health disparities as any differences among populations that are statistically significant and differ from a reference group by at least 10% (AHRQ, 2006). However, political activists may hold a more subjective definition: health disparities are differences in health that are not only unnecessary and avoidable but, in addition, are considered unfair and unjust (Whitehead, 1991, p. 220).

Of greatest concern are differences in health status or quality of care experienced by racial or ethnic groups, people with lower socioeconomic status (SES), and people living in rural or inner city areas. Studies have documented the existence of a variety of health disparities in the United States, Europe, Latin America, and the Caribbean, and have proposed strategies to minimize them based on a social justice paradigm (Aday, 2000; European Commission, 2009; PAHO, 2001). In 2008, the National Institutes of Health (NIH) sponsored a summit focusing on health disparities research and generated recommendations bridging science, practice, and policy that called for action on social determinants of health, community engagement, broad partnerships, capacity-building, and media outreach (Dankwa-Mullan et al., 2010). The Institute of Medicine, the World Health Organization, and the Robert Wood Johnson Foundation have made raising public awareness of health inequalities a major policy goal (Lynch & Gollust, 2010).

In addition, Lynch and Gollust (2010) found that in a nationally representative, Internet-based survey Americans believed inequalities in access to and quality of health care are more unfair than unequal health outcomes. The focus is on the means or opportunities rather than the outcome of health status. One strategy, built into the Affordable Care Act of 2010, is to reduce disparities in health insurance coverage and access to care. This will be accomplished through health insurance exchanges which are encouraged to overcome language barriers in the delivery of health care (USDHHS, 2011).

Lewis, Saulnier, and Renaud (2000) assert that universal access has done little to change the way health status is distributed across population groups and that health promotion efforts have failed to alter the distribution of health status among groups or classes. They suggest that reducing health disparities may depend on political will which in turn is driven by political ideology and perceptions of health inequality.

Navarro et al. (2006) examined the complex interactions between political traditions, policies, and public health outcomes over a 50-year period in a set of wealthy countries belonging to the Organization for Economic Cooperation and Development (OECD). They found that political parties with egalitarian ideologies tend to implement redistributive policies aimed at reducing social inequalities. Using data from several European social surveys covering 29 European countries, Subramanian, Huijts, and Perkins (2009) found that political conservatives are less likely to self-report poor health controlling for age, gender, and SES.

This study extends our understanding of public perceptions of health disparities by taking political ideology and political party identification into account. It utilizes theories of cognitive dissonance, cognitive prejudice, and moral prejudice to understand the impact of political ideology on perceptions of health disparities.

THEORETICAL CONSIDERATIONS

Until now most research on health disparities has focused on their causes with the aim of providing appropriate treatment and improving health status. Very little research has looked at the nature of public opinion on health disparities (Prevention Institute, 2007). Blaxter (1997) combined the results from a large British survey with qualitative studies on lay attitudes toward health in Western industrialized societies. She tentatively concluded that survey respondents tended to overlook the structural causes of health and illness. Lay people participating in her qualitative studies rarely talked about inequalities in health. She thought that if they acknowledged structural socioeconomic-based inequalities, they would assign an inferior moral status to themselves and their peers.

A similar conclusion was reached by Popay et al. (2003) in a study of four localities in two cities in the north west of England. An analysis of open-ended questions on why health differences can be observed between residential areas revealed that those living in disadvantaged areas were reluctant to accept the notion of inequalities in health between areas and social groups. In follow-up interviews they found that respondents who lived in the relatively affluent areas did not dispute the existence of health inequalities between areas while respondents living in the relatively dis-advantaged study areas questioned the findings.

Although respondents in disadvantaged areas denied the existence of inequalities, they did talk about their own negative health conditions and that of others. Popay et al. suggest that people resolve this contradiction by reconstructing a moral and social identity in which strength of character and personal control are emphasized. These individualistic values and explana-tions are compatible with politically conservative ideologies.

According to Lewis et al. (2000), when calls for health for all confront the inegalitarian realities of societies, the cognitive dissonance for some individuals becomes almost overwhelming. Lord, Ross, and Lepper (1979) found that people holding strong opinions on complex social issues are likely to accept confirming evidence while viewing disconfirming evidence skeptically and search for alternative explanations. This may lead to a polarization of attitudes and two types of prejudice – cognitive and moral (Farley, 2000, pp. 18–19; Sun, 1993). Cognitive prejudice refers to what a person believes to be true. It is a distorted perception of the standard of social reality ("what is") which may involve the formation of social attitudes despite or in ignorance of objective evidence. Moral prejudice is an incongruity between perceptions or attitudes which deviates from group or societal principles of fairness, justice, equality, or need ("what ought to be").

Political ideologies and parties address the problem of balancing the "what is" with the "what ought to be" in many sectors including health care. In American society this involves balancing market justice and social justice. Market justice holds that people are entitled to what they have acquired through their own efforts, actions, or abilities by following agreed upon fair rules, while social justice seeks to ensure that all people are entitled equally to key ends such as health protection (Beauchamp, 1976). While economic resources, social privileges, and political power are not divided and distributed in identical shares, Gil (2006) argued that such distributions should be thoughtfully allocated given individual differences, and everyone's different needs are acknowledged equally.

Rawls (1971) posited that the circumstances of justice include a moderate scarcity of material goods within a society holding a plurality of world views regarding the concepts of moral, religious, and secular good. This means that social and economic inequalities should function to the greatest benefit of the least advantaged members of society (Rawls, 2001). But unlike Rawl's hypothetical veil of ignorance behind which people are unaware of their relative economic, social, and political strength, in the real world, people's perceptions are determined by a wide variety of factors including gender, race, class, status, and party (Kivisto & Hartung, 2007; Weber, 1946). Self-interest leads many not to acknowledge evidence revealing differences in access to care, provision of treatments, and health outcomes between racial and ethnic groups.

Health care may become a zero sum game in which gains for one group, the medically indigent, come at the costs to those who already have health insurance and a regular source of care. The public may choose not to address health inequality if they believe it may reduce the quality or accessibility of their own health care services (Gamble & Stone, 2006; Lewis et al., 2000). The end result is often a lack of consensus so that legislators may be disinclined to commit themselves to health goals to reduce disparities (Lewis et al., 2000).

The political ideology of the party in power may also play a role in recognizing and dealing with health disparities. Social problems may not become public issues, much less public policy, even if research has documented that they exist (Gamble & Stone, 2006; Mauss, 1975). In

2004 the George W. Bush Administration belittled the conclusions of the
National Healthcare Disparities Report 2004 that linked race and SES to
health inequalities (Bloche, 2004; Kaiser, 2004). Krieger (2005) observed
that conservatives continually promote a political climate that favors
individualistic explanations of population health and discounts concerns
about social determinants of health disparities.

It follows that if health and health disparities are debated as a political
rather than a moral philosophical right then "doing the right thing" to
improve population health may not necessarily be the same as "doing the
right thing" politically (Lewis et al., 2000). In August 2009, former vice
presidential candidate Sarah Palin contended that the health reform bill
included 'death panels' that would decide if a person was worthy of health
care based on their level of productivity in society. At the time the House
bill contained no such provision, nor did the 2010 Affordable Care Act
(ACA). Nyhan, Reifler and Ubel (2013) conducted an experiment in 2011 to
determine if fact-checking could correct this false belief. When respondents
who knew the length of congressional terms were told that nonpartisan
health care experts concluded that Palin was wrong, disapproval of the ACA
decreased among those with cold feelings towards Palin but increased
among those with warm feelings towards her. This could be applied to
perceptions about health disparities.

RESEARCH ON PERCEPTIONS OF HEALTH
DISPARITIES

Most of the health disparities research has documented disease-specific
differences between racial, ethnic, gender, and income groups in terms of
access, treatment, and outcome. In 1999, the Kaiser Family Foundation
sponsored the first national survey of public perceptions and experiences
concerning health care. The survey found that the majority of Americans
were unaware of the gap in infant mortality and life expectancy between
blacks and whites and that Latinos were less likely than whites to have
health insurance (Lille-Blanton, Brodie, Rowland, Altman, & McIntosh,
2000). The survey asked how often the health care system treats people
unfairly based on whether or not they have health insurance and how well
they speak English. Approximately 70% of the respondents thought people
were treated unfairly very or somewhat often based on health insurance,
and 58% thought that people were treated unfairly very or somewhat often

based on how well they spoke English. About 49% believed that a person's race or ethnic background very or somewhat often affects whether they can get routine medical care when they need it. Only one % thought that African Americans receive higher quality health care than most whites and 60% thought it was about the same (Kaiser Foundation, 1999).

A community study asking many of the same questions was conducted a few years later in Durham County, NC which includes Duke University and its medical school (Friedman et al., 2005). It found that white, African American, and Latino residents were more aware of health disparities than their counterparts in the national Kaiser study. Benz, Espinosa, Welsh, and Fontes (2011) compared a 2010 National Opinion Research Center (NORC) national telephone survey of 3,159 respondents with the earlier 1999 Kaiser Study. They found an increase in public awareness of disparities between Hispanics and whites between 1999 and 2010, while the perceived disparities between blacks and whites changed moderately over time. In addition, respondents with at least a high school education were more aware of health disparities than those with less than a high school diploma.

Although most national surveys ask questions about political views/ ideology and party identification, the previously mentioned survey research studies (Benz et al., 2011; Friedman et al., 2005; Lille-Blanton et al., 2000) using the Kaiser Foundation questions failed to take political beliefs and identifications into account. However, a 2006–2007 survey of Wisconsin residents asked if they favored government intervention to address health disparities, and if they still supported this policy if it meant raising taxes or shifting resources from the healthier to less healthy groups (Rigby, Soss, Booske, Rohan, and Robert (2009). Overall respondents were more likely to favor closing the health gap between economic groups than between racial groups. Respondents who held egalitarian values, democrats, and those opposed to limited government were more likely to support government intervention. Gender, education, income, and age did not significantly load on supporting government intervention. Respondents also identified lack of health insurance, along with the physical environment and genetics but not individual health habits, as possible causes of health disparities. Attitudes about health disparities varied significantly when controlling for race, economic status, or education, and were greater than the more conventional predictors of support for health policy such as party identification, gender, or age.

From a sociological perspective, social contexts influence people's attitudes and perceptions of social justice, in this case, health disparities. Abend (2008) identified two types of beliefs: a factual or scientific belief, such as the earth is about 4.5 billion years old, and a religious, philosophical, or moral belief such as slavery is wrong. Social groups can differ on the truth or falsehood of both factual and moral beliefs. He proposed that the sociological research question should be: What social factors caused the group to believe that something is factually or morally true or false?

The present study takes the next logical step by adding political ideology and party identification as well as community of residence as possible explanatory variables for the four Kaiser Foundation indicators of health disparities. In essence we have four models, one for each of the dependent variables: (1) lack of health insurance, (2) how well a person speaks English, (3) minorities unable to access routine health care when needed, and (4) quality of care received by members of minority groups. We want to discover how political ideology and party identification affect the four dependent variables controlling for the standard demographic variables (race, gender, community of residence, age, income, and education). An exploratory approach using stepwise additive regression analysis will be used to determine the relative importance of each independent variable on the key measures of health disparities and how they change in the presence of the other variables.

DATA AND METHODS

Data and Sampling

Four questions from the 1999 Kaiser Foundation Survey on health disparities were placed on the 52nd round of the State of the State Survey (SOSS) conducted by the Michigan State University Institute for Public Policy and Social Research (IPPSR). The quarterly survey was administered via telephone between May 26 and June 30, 2009, just as several committees in the US House of Representatives were voting on initial drafts of what would become the Affordable Care Act of 2010. The sample was stratified into six regions of contiguous counties plus the city of Detroit. Each case was weighted so that the proportion of cases in the total sample matched the proportion of adults in the state's 2000 census from the sampling regions on key variables (sex, race, age, and multiple phone lines). The random digit dialing survey reached 1,036 residents in households with landline telephones. The margin of sampling error was $\pm 3\%$ and the completion rate was 46% (see IPPSR, 2009).

Dependent Variables

The four questions from the Kaiser Survey became the dependent variables. Respondents were first asked how often do you think the health care system treats people unfairly based on whether or not they have health insurance with 81.1% indicating very or somewhat often. This is higher than the 70% found in the 1999 Kaiser Foundation survey. Next they were asked how often you think the health care system treats people unfairly based on how well they speak English, with 67.2% indicating very or somewhat often. This is also higher than the 58% in the 1999 Kaiser survey.

The third question was how often do you think that a person's race or ethnic background affects whether they can get routine medical care when they need it, with 52.9% indicating very or somewhat often. This is very close to the 49% in the 1999 Kaiser survey. The last question was when going to a doctor or health clinic for health care services, do you think people from minority groups receive higher quality, about the same quality, or lower quality of health care as whites, with 24.7% believing that minorities received low-quality care and 70.8 believing about the same quality of care. The Kaiser survey ask specifically about African Americans and found that 29% thought African Americans received lower quality than whites and 60% thought they received about the same quality of care as whites.

Independent Variables

The survey included a set of demographic variables and eight were included as independent variables. The respondent characteristics are show in Table 1. Political ideology was measured on a seven-point scale ranging from very conservative to very liberal with four being the middle of the road category. Approximately 51.5% of respondents indicated that they were conservatives, 6.7% middle of the road, and 37.6% liberals. Similarly political party identification was on a seven-point scale ranging from strong republican to strong democrat with four being independent or neither. About one-third (31.4%) of respondents identified themselves as republicans, 14.8% as independents or neither, and 53.9% as democrats.

Self-reported race was grouped into white (82.6%), African American (15.0%), and other (2.3%). Slightly more than half the respondents were women (52.1%). Community of residence was categorized as rural and small

Table 1.   Characteristics of Respondents.

Political ideology	Conservative	Moderate	Liberal
	51.5%	6.7%	37.6%
Party identity	Republican	Independent	Democrat
	31.4%	14.8%	53.9%
Race	White	African American	Other
	82.6%	15.0%	2.3%
Gender	Men	Women	
	47.9%	52.1%	
Community	Rural small town	Suburban	Large city
	53.5%	32.7%	13.7%
Age	Under 40	40–60	60 +
	40.2%	37.2%	22.6%
Income	LT $40,000	$40–$89,999K	$90,000 +
	29.0%	43.5%	27.5%
Education	High school or less	Some college	College degree
	28.9%	30.2%	40.8%

town (53.5%), suburban (32.7%), and urban/large city (13.7%). Age was a continuous variable ranging from 18 to 96 years old with a mean age of 46.

Total household income from all sources was reported in eleven categories from less than $10,000 a year to over $150,000 a year, with 29.0% having incomes less than $40,000, 43.5% with incomes between $40,000 and $90,000, and 27.5% with incomes over $90,000. Finally number of years of education completed was continuous and ranged from 8th grade to 16 or more years, with 28.9% completing high school or less, 30.2% completing some college, and 40.8% earning at least a college degree.

Statistical Procedure

Additive stepwise regression supports a pragmatic exploratory approach to discover how people perceive causes of health disparities. The eight independent variables – political ideology, political party identification, sex, race, age, community type, income, and education achieved – were entered in an additive stepwise regression, one for each of the dependent variables: unfair treatment based on health insurance, unfair treatment based on ability to speak English, minorities unable to get care when needed, and quality of care for minorities.

One limitation of stepwise regression is that it does not rest on an established theory or previous research findings. As discussed above, political ideology and party identification have not been extensively studied with respect to perceptions of health disparities. Two more limitations are (a) some variables may not be added into the model and their contribution ignored, and (b) for those variables that are added, they remain in the model although their significance may decline due to multicollinearity as further variables are included. In this study, only eight independent variables are listed for inclusion which means that so-called nuisance variables are not considered. We will compare the final rank order (β) of the independent variables across the four models to better understand how they affect perceptions of health disparities.

Table 2 shows the zero order correlations for each model or source of perceived health disparities. In the first model, that lack of insurance leads to unfair treatment, political ideology ($r = .307$) has the highest correlation followed by party identification ($r = .255$). This suggests the importance of

Table 2. Zero Order Correlations.

	Model 1 Insurance: Never to often	Model 2 Speak English: Never to often	Model 3 Access care: Never to often	Model 4 Quality: Low to high
Ideology Conservative to liberal	.307*	.015	.184*	−.264*
Party identity GOP to Dem	.255*	.283*	.258*	.127*
Race White, AfroAmer, other	.005	.192*	.238*	−.011
Gender Men and women	.086*	−.110*	−.084	.038
Community Rural to urban	.009	.221*	.152*	.055
Age Young to old	.078	.107	.024	.025
Income Low to high	−.018	−.055	−.039	−.269*
Education Years completed	−.183*	−.009	−.094*	−.172*

*Correlation is significant at the 0.01 level (2-tailed).

political ideology and party on perceptions that link health insurance with health disparities. In the second model, party identity has the highest correlation with believing that ability to speak English leads to unfair treatment ($r = .283$) followed by community ($r = .221$), with urban residents and democrats more likely to perceive unfair treatment.

The highest correlations in the third model, that minorities lack access to health care when needed, are party identity ($r = .258$) and race ($r = .283$). This suggests that democrats and minorities are more likely to perceive ethnicity as a barrier to health care and subsequent unfair treatment. Finally, in the fourth model, income has the highest (negative) correlation with level of quality of care received by minorities ($r = -.269$) followed by ideology, which is also negative ($r = -.264$). In essence, respondents with high incomes and liberal ideologies were more likely to claim that minorities received lower quality health care.

The intercorrelations between the independent variables must be examined since multicollinearity can have a significant impact on the quality and stability of the fitted regression models. The additive stepwise regression will systematically readjust them so that only the unique contribution of each independent variable on the dependent variable remains when all the listed variables are accounted for. Table 3 shows these intercorrelations. Not surprisingly the highest intercorrelations are between income and education ($r = .480$) and between political ideology and political party identity ($r = .447$). Race is moderately intercorrelated with party identity ($r = .279$), community ($r = .275$), and income ($r = -.274$). Essentially, minorities are more likely to be democrats, live in urban areas, but have lower incomes. The intercorrelations of these pairs will influence their final contributions in each model.

Table 3. Inter-Correlations of Independent Variables.

	Ideology	Party	Race	Gender	Income	Age	Community
Party	.447*						
Race	.035	.279*					
Gender	.099*	.119*	.036				
Income	.120	−.192*	−.274*	−.081			
Age	−.202*	−.104*	−.151*	.025	−.133*		
Community	.063	.210*	.275*	−.013	−.025	−.191	
Education	−.034	−.119*	−.193*	.052	.480*	−.031	.042

*Correlation is significant at the 0.01 level (2-tailed).

RESULTS

Four separate additive stepwise regressions were performed, one for each model (Table 4). The final regression for Model 1 examined perceptions that the health care system often treats people unfairly based on health insurance. Table 4 shows that in the final additive regression, education had the greatest effect on perceiving that lack of insurance led to unfair treatment ($\beta = -.448$), followed by race, gender, ideology, and income. This suggests that respondents with lower educations, whites, women, liberals, and high incomes were more likely to state that lack of insurance led to unfair treatment in health care. Interestingly party identity, which had the second highest correlation ($r = .255$) with lack of health insurance after ideology ($r = .307$), was not entered into the equation, most likely due to its intercorrelation with ideology.

The second model in Table 4 concerns perceptions that the health care system often treats people unfairly based on how well they speak English. In this model, political party identity, which had the highest zero order correlation with ability to speak English ($r = .283$) has the strongest effect of all variables entered ($\beta = .356$). Community, which had the second highest zero-order correlation ($r = .221$), ended up third ($\beta = .246$). Overall, democrats, men, urban residents, conservatives, older respondents, and

Table 4. Additive Regressions Final β Ranking for Each Dependent Variable.

Basis of Disparity							
Model 1 Have health insurance		Model 2 Ability to speak English		Model 3 Minorities unable to access care routine when needed		Model 4 Perceived quality of care	
Final order	β	Final order	β	Final order	β	Final order	β
Education	$-.448^{***}$	Party	$.356^{***}$	Ideology	$.305^{***}$	Income	$-.426^{***}$
Race	$-.262^{***}$	Gender	$-.249^{***}$	Gender	$-.244^{***}$	Community	$.302^{***}$
Gender	$.257^{***}$	Community	$.246^{***}$	Race	$.222^{***}$	Ideology	$-.166^{***}$
Ideology	$.253^{***}$	Ideology	$-.223^{***}$	Income	$-.173^{***}$	Party	$-.142^{***}$
Income	$.153^{**}$	Age	$.206^{***}$	Community	$.163^{***}$	Age	$-.072^{*}$
Party	Ns	Race	$.162^{***}$	Age	$.127^{***}$	Race	ns
Community	Ns	Income	ns	Party	ns	Education	ns
Age	Ns	Education	ns	Education	ns	Gender	ns

*Significant at the <0.05 level (2 tailed).
**Significant at the <0.01 level (2 tailed).
***Significant at the <0.001 level (2 tailed).

minorities were more likely to state that ability to speak English affected fair health care treatment.

The third model in Table 4 shows that ideology had the strongest impact ($\beta = .305$) on perceived ability of minorities to get routine medical care when needed followed by gender, race, income, community of residence, and age. The final equation suggests that conservatives, men, minorities, urban residents, respondents with low income, and older respondents claimed that a person's race or ethnic background affects whether or not they can get routine medical care when they need it. It should be noted that party identity, which had the highest zero order correlation with lack of ability to get care ($r = .285$) was never entered into the equation, most likely due to its intercorrelation with ideology.

In the fourth model in Table 4, income, which had the highest zero order correlation ($r = .269$) with quality of care, had the highest effect ($\beta = -.426$) in the final equation. Ideology, with the second-highest zero order correlation ($r = -.264$) ended up third ($\beta = -.166$). Essentially, respondents with low incomes, urban residents, conservatives, republicans, and younger respondents believed minorities received high quality care. Interestingly race was not entered along with education and gender.

As can be seen in Table 4 in each model a different independent variable had the greatest impact (β). Education had the most impact on perceptions of unfair treatment due to lack of insurance, with low-educated respondents more likely to perceive people who lack health insurance often receive unfair treatment ($\beta = -.448$). Party identity had the most impact on perceptions of unfair treatment due to ability to speak English, with democrats more likely to perceive unfair treatment when people had difficulty speaking English ($\beta = .356$). Ideology was most important regarding perceptions of race or ethnic background affecting access to routine care when needed, with liberals more likely to perceive race or ethnicity as a barrier to health care ($\beta = .305$). Finally income had the highest impact on perceptions of quality of care ($\beta = -.426$), with low income respondents believing that minorities received high-quality care.

DISCUSSION

The main research question was what social factors influence a person's perception of health disparities, with specific attention to the impact of political ideology and party identity controlling for race, gender, community of residence, age, income, and education. The Agency for Healthcare

Quality and Research (AHRQ, 2010) analysis reported many significant differences for various indicators of health disparities based on education and income. In this sample of Michigan residents, education and income were significantly correlated ($r = .480$). Education, which only appears in the regression equation for disparities based on lack of health insurance, had the highest impact ($\beta = -.448$). Respondents with higher education were less likely to perceive having insurance as a source of health disparities. Income ranked first on quality of care for minorities ($\beta = -.426$), with low income respondents believing that minorities received high-quality care.

As expected political ideology and party identity were significantly correlated ($r = .447$). Political ideology entered all four regressions, and was ranked first for unable to get routine care when needed ($\beta = .305$). Political party identification entered only two regression, language and quality of care, and was ranked first for disparities based on ability to speak English ($\beta = .356$). The failure of party to enter two of the regressions suggests that for this sample at this time period, political ideology outweighed party identity. Assuming that liberals are likely to be democrats and conservatives to be republicans, then ideology and party identification were congruent for perceived quality of care with democrats and liberals maintaining that minorities received lower quality of care, but noncongruent with democrats and conservatives more likely to perceive disparities based on problems speaking English.

The survey was administered from late May through the end of June, 2009, when the US House of Representatives committees were voting on initial drafts of what would become the Affordable Care Act. A month later, town hall meetings called to explain and discuss the proposed health care reform became raucous, unruly, and in a few instances violent as passions exploded over the issue.

The finding that political ideology is generally stronger than party identification on perceptions of health disparities in this study may reflect the rise of the Tea Party movement and the emerging salience of ideology in American politics. Individuals who hold a set of beliefs based on their particular ideology are true believers who can dismiss findings on health disparities from the congressionally mandated national health care disparities reports (i.e., AHRQ, 2006, 2010) that documented inequalities in health care delivery for minority and low income groups. This supports the Lord et al. (1979) argument that opinions on some public issues may polarize when certain groups are likely to deny or ignore scientific facts.

One explanation is that as people holding strong conservative ideological views realized that with the election of President Obama and 60 democratic

Senators who could end a filibuster, health care reform was a real possibility. They faced the prospect that they might have to change their attitudes and behavior with respect to health insurance and access to care. They experienced cognitive dissonance which could be ameliorated by adopting attitudes and beliefs that distort the social reality of what would be in "Obamacare" as they labeled health care reform. This is transformed into cognitive and moral prejudice about health disparities.

Applying Festinger's (1957) theory of cognitive dissonance, one can argue that strong conservatives reached out through the internet and other media to find others like them who reinforced their beliefs about what would be included in health care reform. The result was the formation of a social movement or political faction (the Tea Party) that upholds a set of moral standards on what ought to be considered fairness, justice and equality in the health care system. The debate shifts from normative action that can be negotiated to one over values which polarizes and solidifies the political ideologies. This makes it very hard for the public health and scientific community to persuade the opponents of health care reform with the facts on health disparities and what health reform would mean.

The challenge facing those seeking to reduce health disparities is that it will require increasing political will and public support in order to overcome opposition in the form of political ideology and party identity to achieve success in the policy arena. Rational appeals to social justice will not persuade them to support legislation to reduce health disparities.

Limitations

This study has limits with respect to both external and internal validity. External validity is the degree to which the results are generalizable to individuals other than those in the current survey sample. A public opinion survey in one state at one point in time cannot be generalized to the whole country. The survey was conducted just as the debate over the proposed health care reform legislation was reaching a crescendo. This may account for the somewhat higher perceptions in the current study that people are treated unfairly whether or not they have health insurance compared to the 1999 Kaiser study (81.1% vs. 70.0%). It may also explain the importance of political ideology on perceptions of health disparities.

Internal validity is the degree to which the results are attributable to the independent variable and not some other rival explanation. This study attempted to explore the contribution of political ideology and party identity to perceptions of health disparities. While the results indicate that political ideology entered all four health disparity models and political party two of the four, this does not overcome other threats to internal validity. These threats might include the historical context in which the survey was administered as well as concerns about using an additive stepwise regression procedure to enter variables. But as pointed out in the methods section, the number of independent variables was restricted to standard demographics, thereby avoiding the introduction of nuisance variables into the regression equations.

Future Research

This study indicates that future research on public perceptions of health disparities should include political ideology and party identification along with income, education, race, and community of residence. It also proposes a theoretical explanation linking micro concepts of cognitive and moral prejudice with macro concepts of political ideology. Future research should include a national sample with oversampling for minority groups and as well as questions to assess cognitive and moral prejudice.

REFERENCES

Abend, G. (2008). Two main problems in the sociology of morality. *Theory and Society, 37,* 87–125.

Aday, L. A. (2000). An expanded conceptual framework for equity: Implications for assessing health policy. In G. L. Albrecht, R. Fitzpatrick & S. Scrimshaw (Eds.), *Handbook of social studies in health and medicine* (pp. 481–492). Thousand Oaks, CA: Sage.

Agency for Healthcare Research and Quality (AHRQ). (2006). *National healthcare disparities report,* Rockville, MD.

Agency for Healthcare Research and Quality (AHRQ). (2010). *National healthcare disparities report 2009,* Rockville, MD.

Beauchamp, D. E. (1976). Public health as social justice. *Inquiry, 13,* 3–14.

Benz, J. K., Espinosa, O., Welsh, V., & Fontes, A. (2011). Awareness of racial and ethnic health disparities has improved only modestly over a decade. *Health Affairs, 30,* 1860–1867.

Blaxter, M. (1997). Whose fault is it? People's own conceptions of the reasons for health inequalities. *Social Science and Medicine, 44,* 747–756.

Bloche, M. G. (2004). Health care disparities – Science, politics, and race. *New England Journal of Medicine, 350,* 1568–1570.

Dankwa-Mullan, I., Rhee, K. B., Williams, K., Sanchez, I., Sy, F. S., Stinson, N., Jr., & Ruffin, J. (2010). The science of eliminating health disparities: Summary and analysis of the NIH summit recommendations. *American Journal of Public Health, 100*(S1), S12–S18.

European Commission. (2009). *Solidarity in health: Reducing health inequalities in the EU.* Brussels: COM(2009) 567/4. Retrieved from http://ec.europa.eu/health/ph_determinants/socio_economics/documents/com2009_en.pdf

Farley, J. E. (2000). *Majority-minority relations* (4th ed.). Upper Saddle River, NJ: Prentice Hall.

Festinger, L. (1957). *A theory of cognitive dissonance.* Stanford, CA: Stanford University Press.

Friedman, J. Y., Anstrom, K. J., Weinfurt, K. P., McIntosh, M., Bosworth, H. B., Oddone, E. Z., ... Schulman, K. (2005). Perceived racial/ethnic bias in healthcare in Durham county, North Carolina: A comparison of community and national samples. *North Carolina Medical Journal, 66,* 267–275.

Gamble, V. N., & Stone, D. (2006). U.S. policy on health inequities: The interplay of politics and research. *Journal of Health Politics, Policy and Law, 31,* 93–126.

Gil, D. G. (2006). Reflections on health and social justice. *Contemporary Justice Review: Issues in Criminal, Social, and Restorative Justice, 9,* 39–46.

Institute for Public Policy and Social Research. (2009). *State of the State Survey-52 (spring).* Michigan State University, East Lansing, MI. Retrieved from http://www.ippsr.msu.edu/SOSS

Kaiser, J. (2004). Democrats blast a sunny-side look at U.S. health disparities. *Science, 303,* 451.

Kaiser Foundation. (1999). *Race, ethnicity & medical care: A survey of public perceptions and experience.* The Henry J. Kaiser Family Foundation. Report #1529. Retrieved from http://www.kff.org/minorityhealth/loader.cfm?url = /commonspot/security/getfile.cfm&PageID = 13294

Kivisto, P., & Hartung, E. (2007). *Intersecting inequalities: Class, race, sex and sexualities.* Upper Saddle River, NJ: Prentice Hall.

Krieger, N. (2005). Stormy weather: "Race," gene expression, and the science of health disparities. *American Journal of Public Health, 95,* 2155–2160.

Lewis, S., Saulnier, M., & Renaud, M. (2000). Reconfiguring health policy: Simple truths, complex solutions. In G. L. Albrecht, R. Fitzpatrick & S. Scrimshaw (Eds.), *Handbook of social studies in health and medicine* (pp. 509–524). Thousand Oaks, CA: Sage.

Lille-Blanton, M., Brodie, M., Rowland, D., Altman, D., & McIntosh, M. (2000). Race, ethnicity, and the health care system: Public perceptions and experiences. *Medical Care Research and Review, 57*(Suppl. 1), 218–235.

Lord, C. G., Ross, L., & Lepper, M. R. (1979). Biased assimilation and attitude polarization: The effects of prior theories on subsequently considered evidence. *Journal of Personality and Social Psychology, 37,* 2098–2109.

Lynch, J., & Gollust, S. E. (2010). Playing fair: Fairness beliefs and health policy preferences in the United States. *Journal of Health Politics, Policy and Law, 35,* 849–887.

Mauss, A. (1975). *Social problems as social movements.* Philadelphia, PA: J. B. Lippincott.

Navarro, V., Muntaner, C., Borrell, C., Benach, J., Quiroga, A., Rodríguez-Sanz, M., ... Pasarín, M. I. (2006). Politics and health outcomes. *The Lancet, 368,* 1033–1037.

Nyhan, B., Reifler, J., & Ubel, P. A. (2013). The hazards of correcting myths about health care reform. *Medical Care, 51,* 127–132.

Pan American Health Organization (PAHO). (2001). *Equity and health: Views from the Pan American Sanitary Bureau.* Washington, DC: PAHO (Occasional Publication No. 8). Retrieved from http://whqlibdoc.who.int/hq/2001/9275122881.pdf#page = 31

Popay, J., Bennett, S., Thomas, C., Williams, G., Gatrell, A. C., & Bostock, L. (2003). Beyond "beer, fags, egg and chips"? Exploring lay understandings of social inequalities in health. *Sociology of Health & Illness, 25*, 1–23.

Prevention Institute. (2007). *Laying the groundwork for a movement to reduce health disparities.* REPORT 07-01. Retrieved from http://www.preventconnect.org/downloads/2009/DRA_II_Laying_the_GroundWork_FINAL.pdf

Rawls, J. (1971). *A theory of justice.* Cambridge, MA: Belknap Press.

Rawls, J. (2001). In E. Kelly (Ed.), *Justice as fairness: A restatement.* Cambridge, MA: Belknap Press.

Rigby, E., Soss, J., Booske, B. C., Rohan, A. M. K., & Robert, S. A. (2009). Public responses to health disparities: How group cues influence support for government intervention. *Social Science Quarterly, 90*, 1321–1340.

Subramanian, S. V., Huijts, T., & Perkins, J. M. (2009). Association between political ideology and health in Europe. *The European Journal of Public Health, 19*, 455–457.

Sun, K. (1993). Two types of prejudice and their causes. *American Psychologist, 48*, 1152–1153.

U.S. Department of Health and Human Services (USDHHS). (2011). *HHS action plan to reduce racial and ethnic disparities: A nation free of disparities in health and health care.* Washington, DC. Retrieved from http://minorityhealth.hhs.gov/npa/files/Plans/HHS/HHS_Plan_complete.pdf

Weber, M. (1946). Class, status, party. In H. H. Gerth & C. W. Mills (Trans. and Ed.), *From Max Weber: Essays in sociology* (pp. 180–195). New York, NY: Oxford University Press.

Whitehead, M. (1991). The concepts and principles of equity and health. *Health Promotion International, 6*, 217–228.